Aromatherapy: The Science of Essential Oils

Edited by

Pradeep Kumar Shukla
Department of Biological Sciences
Faculty of Science, Sam Higginbottom
University of Agriculture
Technology and Sciences, Prayagraj
Uttar Pradesh, India

Ajeet Kumar Srivastav
Redcliffe Hygiene Private Limited
Gurugram-122016
Haryana, India

Department of Biochemistry
Babu Banrasi Das University
Lucknow, India

Deepti Chopra
Photobiology Laboratory, Systems Toxicology and Health Risk Assessment Group
CSIR-Indian Institute of Toxicology Research
Vishvigyan Bhavan 31, P.O. Box No. 80, M.G. Marg
Lucknow-226001, India

Shikha Agnihotry
Department of Computational Biology and Bioinformatics
Jacob Institute of Biotechnology and Bio-Engineering
Sam Higginbottom University of Agriculture Technology and Sciences
Prayagraj (Allahabad)
Uttar Pradesh, India

Pragati Misra
Centre for Tissue Culture Technology, Jacob Institute of Biotechnology and Bioengineering
Sam Higginbottom University of Agriculture Technology and Sciences, Prayagraj
Uttar Pradesh, India

&

Jyoti Singh
Photobiology Laboratory, Systems Toxicology and Health Risk Assessment Group
CSIR-Indian Institute of Toxicology Research
Vishvigyan Bhavan 31, P.O. Box No. 80, M.G. Marg
Lucknow-226001, India

Aromatherapy: The Science of Essential Oils

Editors: Pradeep Kumar Shukla, Ajeet Kumar Srivastav, Deepti Chopra,
Shikha Agnihotry, Pragati Misra & Jyoti Singh

ISBN (Online): 978-981-5136-20-3

ISBN (Print): 978-981-5136-21-0

ISBN (Paperback): 978-981-5136-22-7

First published in 2024.

Bentham Science Publishers Pte. Ltd.
80 Robinson Road #02-00
Singapore 068898
Singapore
Email: subscriptions@benthamscience.net

BENTHAM SCIENCE

CONTENTS

FOREWORD

One of humanity's greatest legacies is the extensive knowledge about plants, which forms the basis of culture itself. The fascination of ambient pancha-mahabhutas in plant bodies is the first step in the biological process of producing essential oils. Owing to their distillation of "essential" components from "nonessential", essential oils are the most significant plant wealth. They are frequently referred to as the "plant's soul" or the "quintessence for healing". Aromatherapy is a form of traditional, alternative, or harmonizing therapy that uses volatile plant metabolites, known as essential oils, and other aromatic plant compounds to change a person's mind, body, and spirit. Essential oils are so-called "essential," not for their indispensable role in life, but because "essential" is the attribute of "essence", and these oils comprise the essence of a plant's fragrance. Aromatherapy encompasses not only the artistic application of essential oils to induce virtuous changes on aesthetic and mystical levels but also the scientific application of essential oils to effect salutary changes in the physical realm. Essential oils have a tremendous impact on the body's and mind's deepest levels.

Nowadays, there is rising attention to the use of alternate and complementary therapies along with core medicine. This empirical discovery suggests that human immune responses may be stimulated, augmented, or somehow refined by persistent exposure to aromatic compounds. Aromatherapy is the practice of using essential oils as the major therapeutic agent to treat several diseases. Essential oils have been used for millennia by humans for their paramount importance in traditional and alternative medicinal approaches. Furthermore, their applications are also documented in Ayurveda, Chinese medicine, and homeopathy. There is a curiosity to unveil/rediscover the possible paradoxes of synthesis, mechanisms, and applications of essential oils and provide validated information on a common platform.

The book **"Aromatherapy: The Science of Essential Oils"** shows a broad picture of essential oils-based aromatherapy in several sub-sections, including historical perspective, aromatherapy evolution, essential oils biochemistry and biosynthesis, therapeutic applications, and pharmacological aspects of essential oils, essential oil toxicities, and regulatory aspects. The major highlights of the book pertain to correlation studies on essential oils mediated skin remediation; the use of a combination of different essential oils for aromatherapy; understanding of the molecular mechanism behind aromas and the role of aromatherapy; essential oils characteristics and properties against particular condition; current status and future prospective of aromatherapy. The book effectively presents many perceptions, and replicas, and a treasure of brilliant articles, both detailed overviews and studies, which can broaden our understanding of all aspects of essential oils as limitless molecules meant for numerous applications. The material in this book was gathered from reliable, reputable sources. It provides a great comparison to help grasp the principles of aromatherapy based on essential oils.

The chapters, written by professionals and experts in their corresponding fields, cover a profuse spectacle of topics and provide a groundwork in the natural chemistry of essential oils and their major applications. This comprehensiveness of the book brands it as a 'one-stop platform' and devising it as equally valuable for physiochemists, medical professionals, plant scientists, pharma-industrialists, microbiologists, ayurveda experts, biotechnologists, herbal-drug scientists, and physicians. Beyond multidisciplinary, interdisciplinary, and transdisciplinary research that incorporates the viewpoints of several disciplines, integrated, theory- and issue-driven aromatherapy procedures/protocols have vast scope. The intricacy of essential oils is being revealed with continual investigation, and it is becoming more and more clear how important they are to many businesses and how they may be used in healthcare.

Future discoveries and creative uses might result from the continued investigation and comprehension of their intricate biological makeup. Furthermore, research and documentation on aromatherapy must eventually be placed within the larger frameworks of protecting biodiversity, managing resources sustainably, and protecting intellectual and biological property rights. This book will additionally accommodate as a wide-ranging outline of traditional and current information on the health effects of aromatherapy, that will be pertinent to the advancing back to nature crusade of today's world.

This book is intended to satiate the requirements of EO manufacturers, purveyors, and consumers as well as the scientific fraternity, academicians, and legislators who will find the most recent knowledge given by exclusive experts under one cover. I am certain that readers in the field of life sciences would find this book very useful. The authors, editorial team, and publisher deserve congratulations and best compliments for publishing this useful book.

Ir. Jonathan A. Lal
Sam Higginbottom University of Agriculture
Technology and Sciences
Prayagraj, Uttar Pradesh-211007
India

PREFACE

Writing the first edition of a book on the fascinating topic of aromatherapy, The Science of Essential Oils, is a privilege and an honour for us.

Since about 6,000 years ago, essential oils have been utilised to boost one's health or disposition. Aromatherapy is "the therapeutic application or the medical use of aromatic compounds (essential oils) for holistic healing," according to the National Association for Holistic Aromatherapy (NAHA). Numerous essential oils are thought to contain antiviral, nematocidal, antifungal, insecticidal, and antioxidant characteristics in addition to varying degrees of antibacterial action. Applications for aromatherapy include inhalation, topical use, and massage. Users should be mindful that "natural" goods are actually chemicals and might be dangerous if used improperly.

When using essential oils, it is critical to follow the advice of a trained professional. This book also discusses how commonly used therapeutic drugs, personal care products, and other chemicals, when consumed or applied to the body, can be toxic if not thoroughly researched. Although there is a growing awareness of the benefits of Aromatherapy, it is still underutilised, and people need to be educated about how Aromatherapy is safe for users through therapeutic application and what precautions can be taken before use. All of the authors in this book are highly skilled researchers who have extensive and up-to-date knowledge of the subject matter and are actively conducting research in the relevant fields.

We made every attempt to give information compiled from research articles already published on the topic for each chapter, and we organised it into subsections to make it easier to read. We did our best to utilise plain language that readers of all reading levels might understand. We anticipate that after reading the book, the reader will be better informed about the advantages of routine use of essential oils, aromatherapy in general, and about how other plants and natural elements interact with aromatherapy on the skin and inside the body.

Pradeep Kumar Shukla
Department of Biological Sciences
Faculty of Science, Sam Higginbottom University of Agriculture
Technology and Sciences, Prayagraj
Uttar Pradesh, India

Ajeet Kumar Srivastav
Redcliffe Hygiene Private Limited
Gurugram-122016
Haryana, India

Department of Biochemistry
Babu Banrasi Das University
Lucknow, India

Deepti Chopra
Photobiology Laboratory, Systems Toxicology and Health Risk Assessment Group
CSIR-Indian Institute of Toxicology Research
Vishvigyan Bhavan 31, P.O. Box No. 80, M.G. Marg
Lucknow-226001, India

Shikha Agnihotry
Department of Computational Biology and Bioinformatics
Jacob Institute of Biotechnology and Bio-Engineering
Sam Higginbottom University of Agriculture
Technology and Sciences
Prayagraj (Allahabad)
Uttar Pradesh, India

Pragati Misra
Centre for Tissue Culture Technology, Jacob Institute of Biotechnology and Bioengineering
Sam Higginbottom University of Agriculture
Technology and Sciences, Prayagraj
Uttar Pradesh, India

&

Jyoti Singh
Photobiology Laboratory, Systems Toxicology and Health Risk Assessment Group
CSIR-Indian Institute of Toxicology Research
Vishvigyan Bhavan 31, P.O. Box No. 80, M.G. Marg
Lucknow-226001, India

DEDICATION

In grateful remembrance of **Professor Ramesh Chandra Pant**, whose love for learning continues to inspire us through the pages of life.

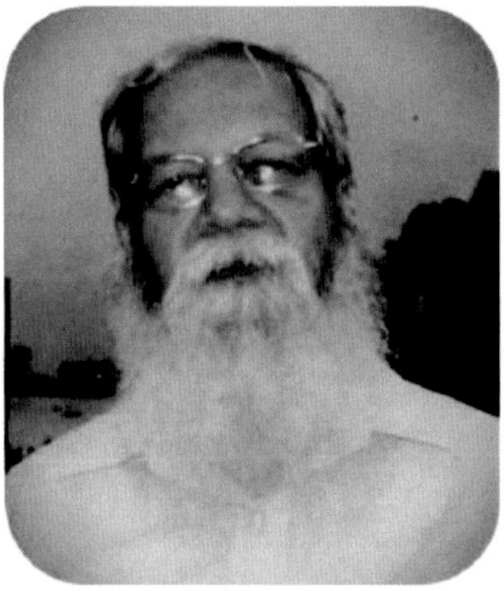

In the tapestry of our lives, there are threads woven by exceptional individuals who leave an indelible mark on our hearts and minds. You were one such luminary, a beacon of wisdom, compassion, and inspiration. You havc ignited our curiosity, fuelled our dreams, and left an indelible mark on our hearts. Your legacy lives on, in the hearts of those who were fortunate enough to be your students. As we continue to learn and grow, we carry the torch of your teachings, forever grateful for the privilege of having known and learned from you. Your teachings continue to resonate in our hearts, guiding us throughout life.

List of Contributors

Alka Sagar	Department of Microbiology and Biotechnology, Meerut Institute of Engineering and Technology, Meerut, UP, India
Ashwani Kumar	Department of Entomology, Naini Agricultural Institute, Sam Higginbottom University of Agriculture, Technology and Sciences, Prayagraj, Uttar Pradesh, India
Archana Shukla	Department of Biological Sciences, Faculty of Science, Sam Higginbottom University of Agriculture, Technology and Sciences, Prayagraj, Uttar Pradesh, India
Angel Kushwaha	Department of Molecular and Cellular Engineering, Jacob Institute of Biotechnology and Bioengineering, Sam Higginbottom University of Agriculture, Technology and Sciences, Prayagraj, Uttar Pradesh, India
Ajeet Kumar Srivastav	Redcliffe Hygiene Private Limited, Gurugram-122016, Haryana, India Department of Biochemistry, Babu Banrasi Das University, Lucknow, India
Arun K. Chaurasia	Department of Genetics and Plant Breeding, Naini Agricultural Institute, Sam Higginbottom University of Agriculture, Technology and Sciences, Prayagraj, Uttar Pradesh, India
Chirag Maheshwari	ICAR-Central Institute of Agricultural Engineering, Navi Bagh, Bhopal, Madhya Pradesh-462038, India ICAR-Indian Agricultural Research Institute, Pusa, New Delhi-110012, India
Deepti Chopra	Photobiology Laboratory, Systems Toxicology and Health Risk Assessment Group CSIR-Indian Institute of Toxicology Research Vishvigyan Bhavan 31, P.O. Box No. 80, M.G. Marg Lucknow-226001, India
Divya Dubey	Photobiology Laboratory, Systems Toxicology and Health Risk Assessment Group, CSIR-Indian Institute of Toxicology Research, Vishvigyan Bhavan 31, P.O. Box No. 80, M.G. Marg, Lucknow-226001, India
Eugenia P. Lal	Department of Biological Sciences, Faculty of Science, Sam Higginbottom University of Agriculture, Technology and Sciences, Prayagraj, Uttar Pradesh, India
Gagan Sharma	Redcliffe Hygiene Private Limited, Gurugram-122016, Haryana, India
Ghanshyam Pandey	Department of Plant Protection and Plant Pathology, Naini Agricultural Institute, Sam Higginbottom University of Agriculture, Technology and Sciences, Prayagraj, Uttar Pradesh, India
Jyoti Singh	Photobiology Laboratory, Systems Toxicology and Health Risk Assessment Group, CSIR-Indian Institute of Toxicology Research, Vishvigyan Bhavan 31, P.O. Box No. 80, M.G. Marg, Lucknow-226001, India
Jaya Upadhyay	Department of Gastroenterology, Sanjay Gandhi Post graduate Institute of Medical Sciences, Lucknow, Uttar Pradesh, India
Lakshmi Bala	Department of Biochemistry, Babu Banrasi Das University, Lucknow, India
Muzaffar Hasan	ICAR-Central Institute of Agricultural Engineering, Navi Bagh, Bhopal, Madhya Pradesh, India

Mohd. Danish Kamar	Photobiology Laboratory, Systems Toxicology and Health Risk Assessment Group, CSIR-Indian Institute of Toxicology Research, Vishvigyan Bhavan 31, P.O. Box No. 80, M.G. Marg, Lucknow-226001, India Academy of Scientific and Innovative Research, AcSIR Headquarters, CSIR-HRDC Campus, Sector 19, Kamla Nehru Nagar, Ghaziabad-201002, Uttar Pradesh, India
Manoj Kumar Tripathi	ICAR-Central Institute of Agricultural Engineering, Navi Bagh, Bhopal, Madhya Pradesh-462038, India
Pragati Misra	Centre for Tissue Culture Technology, Jacob Institute of Biotechnology and Bioengineering, Sam Higginbottom University of Agriculture, Technology and Sciences, Prayagraj, Uttar Pradesh, India
Pradeep Kumar Shukla	Department of Biological Sciences, Faculty of Science, Sam Higginbottom University of Agriculture, Technology and Sciences, Prayagraj, Uttar Pradesh, India
Priyanka Spring	Department of Botany, Abhilashi PG Institute of Science, Mandi, Himanchal Pradesh University, Himanchal Pradesh, India
Rahul M. Srivastava	Maulana Azad National Institute of Agricultural Engineering, Bhopal, Madhya Pradesh, India
Rajpal S. Jadam	ICAR-Central Institute of Agricultural Engineering, Navi Bagh, Bhopal, Madhya Pradesh-462038, India
Shikha Agnihotry	Department of Computational Biology and Bioinformatics, Jacob Institute of Biotechnology and Bio-Engineering, Sam Higginbottom University of Agriculture, Technology and Sciences, Prayagraj (Allahabad), Uttar Pradesh, India
Sandeep Negi	Photobiology Laboratory, Systems Toxicology and Health Risk Assessment Group CSIR-Indian Institute of Toxicology Research Vishvigyan Bhavan 31, P.O. Box No. 80, M.G. Marg Lucknow-226001, India
Shambhavi Pandey	Department of Forensic Sciences , Faculty of Science, Sam Higginbottom University of Agriculture, Technology and Sciences, Prayagraj, Uttar Pradesh, India
Suman Sanju	Department of Botany, Abhilashi PG Institute of Science, Mandi, Himanchal Pradesh University, Himanchal Pradesh, India
Suchit Ashish John	Department of Biological Sciences, Faculty of Science, Sam Higginbottom University of Agriculture, Technology and Sciences, Prayagraj, Uttar Pradesh, India
Shailesh Marker	Department of Genetics and Plant Breeding, Naini Agricultural Institute, Sam Higginbottom University of Agriculture, Technology and Sciences, Prayagraj, Uttar Pradesh, India
Saumya Shukla	Photobiology Laboratory, Systems Toxicology and Health Risk Assessment Group, CSIR-Indian Institute of Toxicology Research, Vishvigyan Bhavan 31, P.O. Box No. 80, M.G. Marg, Lucknow-226001, India Department of Biochemistry, School of Dental Sciences, Babu Banarasi Das University, BBD City, Faizabad Road, Lucknow-226028, Uttar Pradesh, India

Sakshi Yadav Photobiology Laboratory, Systems Toxicology and Health Risk Assessment Group, CSIR-Indian Institute of Toxicology Research, Vishvigyan Bhavan 31, P.O. Box No. 80, M.G. Marg, Lucknow-226001, India
Department of Botany, University of Lucknow, Lucknow-226007, India

CHAPTER 1

Aromatherapy Evolution and Blending Basics of Essential Oils

Shikha Agnihotry[1,*], Deepti Chopra[3], Jyoti Singh[3], Sandeep Negi[3], Ajeet Kumar Srivastav[2,5], Jaya Upadhyay[4] and **Gagan Sharma[2]**

[1] *Department of Computational Biology and Bioinformatics, Jacob Institute of Biotechnology and Bio-Engineering, Sam Higginbottom University of Agriculture, Technology and Sciences, Prayagraj (Allahabad), Uttar Pradesh, India*

[2] *Redcliffe Hygiene Private Limited, Gurugram-122016, Haryana, India*

[3] *Photobiology Laboratory, Systems Toxicology and Health Risk Assessment Group CSIR-Indian Institute of Toxicology Research Vishvigyan Bhavan 31, P.O. Box No. 80, M.G. Marg Lucknow-226001, India*

[4] *Department of Gastroenterology, Sanjay Gandhi Post graduate Institute of Medical Sciences, Lucknow, Uttar Pradesh, India*

[5] *Department of Biochemistry, Babu Banrasi Das University, Lucknow, India*

Abstract: The history of aromatherapy begins over 3500 years BC. Aromatics were at the time for religious purposes, perfume, and medicine. Then, in 1910, René-Maurice Gattefossé, a chemical engineer from Lyon, discovered the therapeutic properties of pure lavender after an explosion in his laboratory, which left him with major burns. He treated them with lavender essential oil. Won over by that "miracle", he founded the French Society of Aromatic Products and published around twenty works that are still considered references today. These works would give aromatherapy its reputation and its very name, as it was Gattefossé who coined the term "aromatherapy", in 1935. He conducted many rewarding personal and scientific experiments on essential oils. Other scientists, such as Charles Chamberland, a biologist and assistant to Louis Pasteur, had already examined their spectacular antimicrobial action. In the 5th century BCE, Hippocrates was already treating patients with aromatic vapours. Aromatherapy is a branch of phytotherapy that uses the volatile active ingredients of aromatic plants. These are plants that have the ability to synthesize an essence. This science focusses on the use of essential oils for therapeutic, curative, or preventive purposes. For the most part, the essential oils are extracted by steam distillation of parts of the plant (such as leaves, flowers, or bark). Only the essences of citrus pericarp (such as orange or mandarin zest) tend to be obtained *via* mechanical cold pressing. In 1929, Sévelinge, a pharmacist from Lyon, demonstrated the antibacterial efficacy of certain essential oils.

* **Corresponding author Shikha Agnihotry:** Department of Computational Biology and Bioinformatics, Jacob Institute of Biotechnology and Bio-Engineering, Sam Higginbottom University of Agriculture, Technology and Sciences, Prayagraj (Allahabad), Uttar Pradesh, India;
E-mail: shikha25agnihotry@gmail.com

Pradeep Kumar Shukla, Ajeet Kumar Srivastav, Deepti Chopra, Shikha Agnihotry, Pragati Misra and Jyoti Singh (Eds.)

Then, in the 1950s, a military physician used them to treat injured soldiers in Indochina. In 1975, Pierre Franchomme, a pharmacologist and aromatologist, brought about decisive progress by proposing that the concept of "chemotype", the "plant's true chemical ID card", should be taken into account, listing the key aromatic compounds characterizing each plant and how they affect its properties. Today, aromatherapy is more frequently the focus of scientific studies. It is recognized as a fully-fledged branch of medicine. Over 17,000 articles on aromatherapy have appeared in an international high-level scientific publications.

Keywords: Aromatherapy, Essential Oil, Therapeutic, Phytotherapy and Chemotherapy.

1. INTRODUCTION

A subset of phytotherapy denoted as aromatherapy makes utilization of the volatile active components of fragrant plants. The application of essential oils (EOs) for medicinal, curative, or preventative reasons is the main accentuation of this science. The term "aromatherapy" was first utilized in 1935 by Lyon-born chemist René-Maurice Gattefossé, who used EOs in several fruitful scientific and personal studies. Notwithstanding their olfactory resemblance, EOs are compounds with distinct chemical characteristics because of their composition, which gives them a uniqueness that cannot be superseded by other synthetic molecules. Since they have a categorical chemical makeup, synthetic products—referred to as "essences"—function in a constrained way inside the body, whereas EO acts more broadly [1, 2]. Because of their numerous biological benefits and therapeutic applications, EOs are among the most consequential natural products made from plants [3, 4]. For millennia, essential oils have played a consequential role in many diverse civilizations all over the world. Even the most archaic races understood that scent essences had a particular influence. Essential oils were employed for ceremonial and medicinal purposes by the Chinese, Indians, and Egyptians. Archaic Egyptians were well vigilant of the physiological effects of scents and the first types of aromatherapy. Sanskrit is the pristine language of the old Indian book recognized as Ayurveda. Derived from the terms Veda, which betokens "erudition," and ayur, which denotes "life." The most revered book in India, the Vedas, lists approximately 700 distinct herbs and aromatics, codifying the utilization of these substances for both religious and medicinal purposes. Herbs have been utilized by humans for medicinal purposes since the dawn of time. One of the first inscribed records of humans is the Rig Veda, which was composed about 5,000 years ago in India. It verbalizes how herbs can be remedied. The textbooks for the age-old medicinal science of Ayurveda, which is still in utilization today, are included in a number of texts. Herbal recipes abound in these publications. Virtually all therapeutic plants are fragrant plants, just as they were in the past. Like virtually all other medicinal traditions that have persisted through the ages, Ayurveda was drawn to the fragrances of plants and engendered methods to extract their scents. One of the sacred plants in India is basil, which is verbalized to arouse the mind and heart and give love and devotional spirit. However, it took considerably longer for the methodical extraction of essences for medicinal or cosmetic uses to emerge. Essential oil use is growing these days, and aromatherapy is becoming more widely accepted.

Interest in utilizing coalesced essential oils in aromatherapy as therapeutically efficacious agents has significantly increased recently. There is a dearth of research on the aromatherapy benefits of coalesced essential oils on humans, even though these oils are being utilized more and more to enhance patients' quality of life and palliate a variety of illnesses. Applying an amalgamation of essential oils might have a synergistic impact and be efficacious in treating solicitousness and melancholy [5]. Essential oils are fascinating natural compounds derived from aromatic plants that play a paramount role in conventional pharmacopeia. There has been an abundance of attention lately on utilizing sundry EOs as substitute medicinal and antibacterial agents. Furthermore, more focused and logical research is still required to address how to apply those efficacious EOs and their individual constituents in the pabulum and agriculture sectors in order to engender novel natural pharmaceutical drugs and incipient health-oriented products [6].

2. AROMATHERAPY EVOLUTION

The therapeutic use of aromatic plants seems to be as old as human civilization itself. Plants such as fennel, coriander seeds, cumin, and many others have been found at the sites of ancient burial grounds. Many texts from Asia to Ancient Egypt, and much of the Mediterranean area, describe the various procedures and rituals involved in the making of healing ointments, medicated oils, poultices, and healing perfumes [7, 8].

Aromatic oils have been a part of human history for more than 3,500 years BC and appear with regularity throughout all major civilisations down the ages, with uses ranging from religious ritual, food flavouring, medicine, perfumery and masking of bad odours [9]. It is impossible to date exactly when the plants were first used medicinally, since such a development would have occurred over thousands of years [10]. In ancient times, our ancestors relied on a combination of experimentation and observation to explore the diverse uses of plants. They engaged in trial and error, testing various parts of plants, such as leaves, roots, or berries, to discern their potential applications as food, medicine, or in other aspects of daily life. This hands-on approach allowed them to discover the valuable properties and benefits offered by different plants, gradually building a repository of knowledge that has been passed down through generations. Such knowledge would have been passed on to succeeding generations as part of a verbal tradition, eventually becoming the herbal medicine that we recognise today, and out of which aromatherapy developed [11].

Furthermore, during the Neolithic period (7000 B.C. to 1000 B.C.) in the Eastern world, there is evidence that humanity discovered certain plants containing fatty oil – plants such as olive, castor, flax and sesame – which could be extracted by pressing and then used to cook with, anoint with, and for their own medicinal preparations [12]. The practice of using aromatic fumigations to uplift the spirit and help cure diseases has also been used by the world's greatest civilizations throughout history [13]. The use of aromatic plants was originally part of herbal medicine. Herbal medicine dates back thousands of years and is not confined to any one geographical area. Residual patterns of use and trade in contemporary society suggest that nearly every part of the world has some history of the use of aromatic plants in its healthcare system [14]. The use of technology in the distillation of essential oils from aromatic plants that forms the basis for contemporary "aromatherapy," as we know it, is much more recent [15]. However, among the many countries that have a documented history of using aromatic plants in their healing traditions are India, China, Egypt, France, Greece, Iraq, Syria (part of Mesopotamia), Switzerland, Tibet, UK, and the United States (Native Americans) [16]. Early aromatics were used in the form of steams, smokes, inhalants, fumigants, snuffs, salves, lotions, compresses, poultices, waters, colognes, perfumes, and baths. Egypt, One of the most famous manuscripts concerning aromatic medicine is the Papyrus Ebers manuscript written around 2800 BC. Another document, written about 800 years later, mentions "fine oils and choice perfumes." These manuscripts, written while the Great Pyramid was being built, show that frankincense, myrtle, galbanum, and eaglewood were used as medicine during the time of Moses (from the Old Testament) and myrrh was used to treat hay fever. When Tutankhamun's tomb was opened in 1922, thirty-five alabaster jars of perfume were found in his burial chamber and they were still faintly aromatic. All of them were broken or empty and the contents—frankincense and myrrh (highly valued commodities)—stolen [17].

Aromatherapy is a highly popular form of complementary medicine, usually entailing the application of essential plant oils to the skin by gentle massage. It has relaxing effects but other claims have not been substantiated by reliable trial evidence. Allergic airborne contact dermatitis occurred in a patient who had previously used several essential oils for aromatherapy. The toxicity of essential oils has already been reviewed [18].

Nearly six thousand years ago, aromatics were first used by the Egyptians for religious ceremonies like burials as a means of 'cleansing the spirit', and to enhance their existing practice of prayer. During that period, one of the common methods to unlock the medicinal properties of certain herbs and spices was through the practice of burning them as incense. Their initial belief was that the smoke created when burning those plants would act as a passage for their prayers to be carried to the heavens, directly to the deities they worshipped [19]. In addition, during healing ceremonies, different combinations of herbs and spices were burned to drive the 'evil spirits' from the bodies of the sick. Evidence of these events is depicted in many discovered ceramic jars and pots, as well as hieroglyphic messages in the tombs of the buried. Both births and burial were accompanied by herbs like frankincense and Myrrh, which are both referenced in the Bible as well as other historic religious texts for their value and ties to deities [20].

At around the same time, the Chinese were also practicing medicine using plants, and "Yellow Emperor's Classic of Internal Medicine" was written to depict their knowledge of plant medicine. This text is believed to be the oldest surviving medical book in the history of China and contains briefings on over 300 different plants and their medicinal value [21]. Some historians argue that because this text was written to highlight the actual medicinal properties of plants, it is a proof that the Chinese recognized aromatics as a form of medicine prior to the Egyptians. Regardless of the timeline, "Yellow Emperor's Classic of Internal Medicine" is still used by many of the writers and authorities in the realm of Aromatherapy when referencing the medicinal properties of many different plants, thousands of years after it was written [22].

Long after the origin of aromatics, the Egyptians, through further refined practice, began using plants and herbs in oils for topical use on their skin as perfumes. Often, they were used after bathing to protect their skin and hair from drying out in the sun, but they were also used in festivals and celebrations simply as a fragrance. This evolutionary step for essential oils was incredibly important to their continued use, as perfumes became tremendously popular around the world. So much so, in fact, it's said that when Julius Caesar returned to Rome from Egypt with Cleopatra, he threw perfume bottles into the crowds of people welcoming him home [23].

Across the Mediterranean in Greece, a physician by the name of Asclepius made a name for himself through his use of herbs and oils while performing surgeries. It wasn't until the fall of the Egyptian empire, nearly 900 years later, that Europeans began to gain notoriety for their use and knowledge of aromatherapy, in part because of the legendary status of the Egyptian methods of aromatics. However, in the absence of the Empire, Greek physicians began developing more widely recognized methodologies by which to extract many medicinal properties of essential oils [24].

After that historical period, a significant figure emerged in the medical field, Ibn Sina, who lived from 980 to 1037 A.D. He is widely acknowledged as one of the most influential Islamic physicians, both during his time and in subsequent eras. He is responsible for writing 'Al-Qanun fi al-Tibb' which translates to 'The Canon of Medicine', and is a 14-volume dissertation of all existing medical knowledge. He included the stories and findings of influential physicians before him, as well as his own findings, and became a medical textbook for hundreds of years following its release. Ibn Sina is responsible for discovering over 100 methods of treatment using plants, and many of his methods are still in use today [25].

Fast forward to the late 16th century, when the physician John Gerard published 'Herball or General Historie of Plantes' which became a reference text and book of learning for apothecaries living in Britain at that time [26]. Such apothecaries had previously been only mixing medicines that were being prescribed by doctors, but now were experimenting with plants and herbs on their own and began treating patients. It was at this time that the Black Death made it's second appearance in Europe, and it was nearly as deadly as the first time it hit. This time around, however, it was apparent that there were effective medicinal properties in plants, as the only people who were reported to not succumb to the disease were apothecaries and people who were in constant contact with herbs and medicinal plants. Although there is not substantial enough evidence to prove this was the case, it's an interesting piece of lore regarding aromatherapy and the medicinal value of plants [9].

Aromatherapy preferences and complications in 3000 otolaryngology patients have been studied. Among these patients, 1.67% had some form of complication induced by essential oils used in aromatherapy, including skin eruptions, respiratory distress, and other symptoms. Some patients (0.93%) refused aromatherapy because of individual preference and unpleasant smell. People were advised to follow instructions at all times and to never use these oils for an extended period or overuse them [27].

It was not until 1830, in Grasse, France, a city of perfume makers and a venerated centre of distillation, that the study of essential oils came into being. Very quickly, some of the leading scientists of the time, such as Louis Pasteur, took an interest in it. From as early as 1887, Charles Chamberland, a disciple and assistant to Pasteur, began scientifically measuring the antiseptic effects of oregano, clove, and cinnamon essential oils on anthrax [28].

Then, in 1910, René-Maurice Gattefossé, a chemical engineer from Lyon, discovered the therapeutic properties of pure lavender after an explosion in his laboratory, which left him with major burns. He treated them with lavender essential oil. Won over by that "miracle", he founded the French Society of Aromatic Products and published around twenty works that are still considered references today. These works would give aromatherapy its reputation and its very name, as it was Gattefossé who coined the term "aromatherapy", in 1935 He's most known for that reason, but he is also a legend for the book he wrote on aromatherapy titled, "Aromatherapie: Les Huilesessentielles hormones vegetales" [28, 29].

In 1929, Sévelinge, a pharmacist from Lyon, demonstrated the antibacterial efficacy of certain essential oils. Then, in the 1950s, a military physician used them to treat injured soldiers in Indochina war. Aromatherapy was on its way and nothing could stop it. In 1975, Pierre Franchomme, a pharmacologist and aromatologist, brought about decisive progress by proposing that the concept of "chemotype", the "plant's true chemical ID card", should be taken into account, listing the key aromatic compounds characterising each plant and how they affect its properties [30].

Enter Hippocrates, widely regarded as the father of medicine, who founded a line of thinking regarding the use of essential oils and plants that would become the basis by which aromatherapy centralizes its focus: Holistic medicine. Hippocrates argued that the body as a whole should be treated as although it is a single organism, and the methods by which to treat any illness should be applied to the body in its entirety [31, 32].

It was a contribution of all these researchers, and many many others, that built the foundation for the practice of aromatherapy and aromatics that we still take part in today. Now, we enter the Modern Era of aromatherapy, where essential oils are abundant and those who use them for their healing and therapeutic properties have endless resources available. In today's world, one can customize the methods by which they practice their aromatherapy to fit their needs, and the options are continuing to expand [33].

2.1. India

Ancient India, was one of the first civilizations that aimed at treating people holistically. Traditional Indian medicine, known as Ayurvedic (means 'life knowledge'), is the oldest form of medical practice in the world, with plants and plant extracts being in continuous use from at least 5000 years ago up to the present day [34, 35].

One of the earliest books on plants is called "Vedas," and it was written in India around 2000 BC. It describes the many applications of over 700 plants and substances, including sandalwood, ginger, myrrh, cinnamon, and coriander, for both sacred and therapeutic purposes [36].

2.2. China

The ancient Chinese were extremely knowledgeable about the medicinal properties of plants. The Chinese healing system, which included medical treatments such as acupuncture, shiatsu, and herbal remedies, can be traced back to 2500 BC and served as the foundation for what is now known as "Traditional Chinese Medicine" (TCM) [37]. The balance of Qi (energy), Yin, and Yang (passive, negative, and positive active forces), and the five elements (Fire, Earth, Metal, Water, and Wood) the primary focus for health. Around 2800 BC, the Yellow Emperor, Huang Ti wrote a book called "Internal Medicine" about disease causes and treatment, which included information on many plants and herbal remedies [38]. It is one of the world's oldest books, and still available in print today. However, China's main contribution to the aromatherapy story lies within the citrus family, since it is believed that nearly all citrus species originated in this country, eventually reaching the Mediterranean world in the 10th century *via* the Arabs [39, 40].

2.3. Egyptians

The ancient Egyptians are widely regarded as the forefathers in the use of aromatic plants. They used fragrant oils not only in incense, medicine, massage, skincare, and cosmetics but also in their highly refined embalming process [41].

During this period, the ancient Egyptians did not have records of distillation, which means they likely employed alternative methods like 'enfleurage' and 'maceration' to create aromatic oils. In the absence of distillation, they had to rely on these techniques to extract fragrances from plants. In the 'enfleurage' process, they would immerse the plant material in oil and then squeeze the mixture through a cloth to capture the aromatic essence. On the other hand, 'maceration' involved heating the aromatic substances in oil to achieve a similar outcome. These resourceful methods allowed the ancient Egyptians to harness the captivating scents of plants for various purposes. During this time, a wide variety of medicinal herbs from around the world were grown in the pharaohs' gardens. However, the therapeutic preparations made from aromatic oils and the creation of perfumes for the Pharaohs were used to anoint them in times of prayer, war, and love were under the supervision of temple priests and physicians of the day [42].

Egyptians valued personal hygiene, and the Ebers Papyrus from 1500 BC offers one of the first known recipes for body deodorant. This proves that Egyptian doctors were well-versed in the medicinal benefits of a wide variety of herbs [43].

The Egyptians placed a high value on perfume, which was closely associated with religion. It was so important that each Egyptian God was assigned a specific fragrance, which was frequently used to anoint their statues. Some prescriptions and formulae for improving sanitation have also survived, having been recorded on stone tablets. One of the most popular methods of applying perfume was to place a cone of solid unguent on the head, which would slowly melt in the heat covering the head and body with the aromatic mixture [44].

The ancient Egyptians were the experts at embalming and perfuming temples with plant resins and essences. Indeed, when Howard Carter and his team opened Tutankhamen's tomb in 1922, they discovered several pots and jars that still contained scented unguents of frankincense, Indian Spikenard, and kyphi - they had been sealed for over 3000 years [45]. The strong antiseptic and antibacterial properties of the oils were used to embalm the dead, preventing the flesh from rotting, with the goal of preserving mummies for 3000 years, as it was believed that this was how long it took for the soul to pass through all animals of the earth and then back into a human being [46]. However, one of the most popular perfumes among the Egyptians was known as "kyphi," which was used for much more than just perfume because it could also be used as an antiseptic, incense, poison antidote, a balsamic, and, according to Plutarch, a tranquilizer that "lulled one to sleep, allayed anxieties, and brightened dreams." A potent narcotic called calamus, cassia, cinnamon, peppermint, citronella, pistacia, juniper, acacia, henna, cyperus, "resin," cedarwood, frankincense, myrrh, and raisins were among the 23 elements that made up the concoction known as kyphi.

Kyphi was so deeply ingrained in Egyptian culture that the sun God, Ra, was worshipped in Heliopolis (the City of the Sun) by burning incense three times a day - a "resin" at sunrise, myrrh at noon, and kyphi at sunset. Kyphi was also used by both the Greeks and the Romans [45]. Aromatic woods, herbs, and spices were also burned to honour their Gods; Egyptians believed that as the smoke rose, their prayers would be carried with it [47]. When this magnificent civilization eventually collapsed, Europe became the new center of medicine [44].

2.4. Greeks

The Nile Valley in Egypt, known as the "Cradle of Medicine," is where the Greeks learned a great deal about fragrant herbs. Herodutos and Democrates visited this area in about 500BC. Assyrian women would "bruise with stone, wood of cypress, cedar, and frankincense, and upon it poured water until it became of a specific consistency," according to Herodotus. To impart a really pleasant odour, they coated the body and face with this. A medical school was later founded on the Greek island of Cos, and it gradually gained notoriety thanks to Hippocrates' support [48]. Greek-born Hippocrates (460–377 BC), regarded as the "Father of Medicine," wrote about the medicinal qualities of plants and herbs, thereby preserving all knowledge gleaned from the Egyptians. His therapy would involve herbal infusion, massage, internal herb use, baths, and physical therapy. He believed in the idea of holism, which is the idea that surgery should only be done as a last option [49].

Hippocrates understood the benefits of burning certain aromatic plants as a Preventive measure against infectious diseases as early as the fourth century BC. His understanding of fragrant essence was once even employed to fumigate Athens and purge it of the plague. Hippocrates preached about the "healing power of nature" together with Galen (2 AD). He is recorded as saying that "the road to health is to take an aromatic bath and scented massage every day" and that "the physician must be experienced in many things, but surely in rubbing... Nothing can tighten a joint that is too loose and nothing can relax a joint that is too rigid [48 - 50].

Greek medicine was built on the principles of mental, emotional, and physical equilibrium. The return to healthy condition was considered as re-establishing the balance, which was disturbed by the disease; this approach was known as holism [49]. Hippocrates is perhaps better recognized today for the Hippocratic Oath, which all newly licensed doctors are required to take [50].

The first dissertation on smell, titled "Concerning Odours," was written by Theophrastus (370–285 BC), a Greek philosopher who studied under both Plato and Aristotle and eventually served as the head of the Peripatetic School. He compiled a list of all Greek and foreign aromatics and discussed possible applications for each. Theophrastus was the one who made one of the greatest that using aromatic oils topically can still have an impact on how the body functions. His work "Enquiry into Plants" shows the earliest attempts to carefully record plant observations and list them based on commonalities, such as whether they were annual, biennial, or perennial [51]. The Greeks thought that divine origins might be traced to sweet, aromatic scents. In their earliest mythologies, Gods arrived on scented clouds while dressed in fragrant essence-drenched robes. The Greeks also held that the dead travelled to a place called Elysium after passing away, where the air was perpetually perfumed with delectable scents from perfumed rivers [52].

The perfume "Megaleion," which was made by a Greek named Magallus using a combination of myrrh, cinnamon, and cassia, became well-known throughout the nation, due to its ability to heal wounds and reduce inflammation. The Greek troops would also carried an ointment containing myrrh into combat due to its great antibacterial and wound-healing capabilities, this was no surprise [53]. Marestheus, a great physician and another well-known Greek realized that certain aromatic plants frequently had stimulant qualities and that the scents of roses, fruit, and spices could enliven drained minds [54].

2.5. Romans

Numerous Greek physicians worked in Rome as well, sharing their expertise with yet another highly developed civilization. However, the Romans increased the use of aromatic plants in hygiene and beauty products in addition to using them as medicines. In addition to being utilized in water and in massage mixtures, aromatic oils and essences were frequently employed in public baths [55].

As the Roman Empire grew, it gained access to a wide range of plants and herbs. As a result, they used fragrances and aromatic oils excessively. They utilized three different types of perfume: "diapasmata," which is a powdered perfume, "ladysmata," which were solid unguents, "stymmata," which were scented oils. These were used as after-shower massage oils and to scent hair body, clothes, and bedding. According to legend, Cleopatra expertly used fragrant fragrances to seduce Mark Antony. Additionally, according to the legend, Nero allegedly consumed more incense at his wife's burial than Arabia could produce in a year. Interestingly, the phrase "perfume" refers to the lighting of incense and is derived from the Latin phrase "per fumum," which means "through the smoke" [56].

Greek military doctor Pedanius Dioscorides (40–90 AD) served in Nero's Roman emperor's army. He wrote a book titled "De Materia Medica" and was able to travel far (to Germany, Italy, and Spain) (the oldest surviving Greek herbal). This vast five-volume work includes information on the habitat of over 500 plants, how to prepare them, as well as more than 1,000 herbal remedies [57]. For at least the following 1200 years, this book served as the primary medical reference for the Western world, earning Dioscorides, the moniker "The Father of Pharmacology." The most authoritative historical source on the medications used by the Greeks, Romans, and other ancient cultures is De Materia Medica, with much of the herbal knowledge included in Dioscorides' book still having an impact on herbal medicine today [58]. Claudius Galen, a well-known Roman surgeon, physician, and philosopher, was of Greek ancestry. He studied medicine and began his medical profession by using medicinal plants to treat the wounds of Roman gladiators, providing him the chance to learn about wounds. Galen is credited with saving every gladiator who came under his care, and as a result of his achievements, he swiftly advanced to the position of personal physician with numerous Roman emperors. Galen was the person who asserted that the brain, not the nose, interprets smells [59].

The Roman Empire expanded throughout time to encompass a sizable portion of thc globe, and with it, their understanding of the therapeutic properties of plants. The Romans are credited with introducing perfumery to the British Isles. Plants like fennel, parsley, sage, rosemary, and thyme were among the seeds and plants that were gathered from all over the world and eventually made it to Britain's coastline where they gradually naturalized [60]. But as this vast empire crumbled and Christianity spread, many Roman doctors fled to Constantinople, bringing with them priceless medical writings that were later translated into a wide range of other languages [61].

2.6. Hebrews and Early Christians

The Origins of Christianity Around 1240 BC, the Jewish people began their 40-year journey from Egypt to Israel, bringing with them a variety of precious gums and oils, as well as the knowledge of how to use them. In the Old Testament book of Exodus, God told Moses to make a 'holy anointing oil' out of myrrh, sweet cinnamon, calamus, cassia, and olive oil. Such a combination had extremely potent antiviral and antibacterial properties, protecting anyone who came into contact with it. Not only that, but myrrh's wound-healing properties were well-known even before this time [62]. Purification of Hebrew women occurred during a year in the Hebrew civilisation and was accomplished during the first six months by regular anointing with 'oil of myrrh,' with other aromatics being used for the latter six months. During the Exodus and other times when bathing was impractical for Jewish women, a small linen bag containing myrrh and other aromatics was hung on a cord between the breasts to act as a deodorant [63].

Whereas ancient Indian temples were made of sandalwood, King Solomon's temple in Jerusalem was made of aromatic cedarwood ("cedars of Lebanon"). Perhaps they recognized the need for a soothing atmosphere when attending religious ceremonies [64, 65].

According to the records, Phoenician merchants brought precious cinnamon, frankincense, ginger, and myrrh from the Orient, under the fact that there is a competition in the world. They symbolized his deity status (frankincense for a

God) and his death (myrrh was used to embalm the dead). Gold, incidentally, was symbolic of his royal status (gold for a king) [66] Spikenard was said to have been imported from India and was used by Mary to anoint Jesus before his crucifixion, and the sponge that was held up to him while he hung on the cross was a mixture of vinegar and myrrh, possibly to ease the pain of crucifixion victims [62].

2.7. Middle Ages (500-1500AD)

Age (500–1500 AD) aromatic essences and waters were brought back to Europe by the Knights of the Crusades. The popularity of these aromatic oils grew to such an extent that it sparked the creation of perfumes. However, it was not until the bubonic plague made its way to Europe in the fourteenth century that the true worth of these plants and herbs was realized [67]. On-street corners, fires were to be lit at night and to burn frankincense, benzoin, and pine, among other things. Using incense, perfumed candles, and aromatic "strewing" herbs that were thrown on the floors to be walked on, producing their own fragrances to stop infection and cover up what must have been terribly unpleasant, the smell of death and the fight against infection were waged indoors. and unhealthy bodily odours [68]. In order to combat the Black Death at the time, aromatic plants were widely used. People frequently carried or wore pomanders—oranges that had been packed with cloves—or herbal bouquets. The finest antiseptic defence against the plague at the time was provided by these fragrant plants, and people were aware of this. It is important to note that because they frequently handle aromatic plant materials, apothecaries and perfumers were believed to be resistant to the Plague [14]. To filter their breathing and create an environment that was believed to be antiseptic and resistant to the bubonic plague, doctors of the time frequently wore nasal bags filled with fragrant herbs like cinnamon and cloves.

To further purify the air, they inhaled; they waved in front of them while walking a long stick on an open work top that was also filled with fragrant herbs. Throughout the Middle Ages and until the 17th century, physicians continued to apply these techniques [69]. But at this time, monks were the primary growers of fragrant herbs, like thyme and melissa, which had come to these shores from Italy. When botany was added to the study of medicine, these aromatic gardens were carried on by medical universities. Eventually, during the Renaissance, they evolved into botanical gardens, or what came to be known as "physic" gardens.

In Britain, Oxford became home to the first of these physic gardens in 1621 [70]. A German abbess by the name of St. Hildegard of Bingen (1098–17, September 1179) planted lavender in the 12th century and used its essential oil for medicinal purposes. She was renowned for her healing abilities, which included the effective use of medicines, herbs, and priceless stones [71]. The principal commercial route for Arab civilization during the Middle Ages was through Venice, and it was from this city that the passion for perfumed leather gloves first emerged. It's probable that Catherine D'Medici, an Italian noble woman, introduced this style to the rest of Europe when she wed the future French king, and took her perfumer to France in 1533.

The major product of Grasse, France, at the time was leather, but when this trend caught on, the town's shrewd, businessmen started scenting their leather with the aromatic plants that grew nearby, eventually turning to flowers like tuberose, acacia, violets, lavender, and roses. Grasse's leather sector was gradually supplanted by perfume production as the need for leather declined, and this is still the case today [72]. In the 16th century, a man by the name of Paracelsus rose to fame as a surgeon, astrologer, physician, and alchemist, revolutionized medicine and laid the groundwork for both modern and alternative forms of treatment.

He was the first to be successful in isolating active chemical agents in plants, a procedure that is now common place in the pharmaceutical industry. This involved separating the more obvious parts of plants from their more subtle parts. In a book titled "The Great Surgery Book," which he wrote in 1536, he made it abundantly clear that the primary purpose of alchemy—the original term for modern chemistry; was not to turn common metals into gold but rather to make curative medicines from specific plants extracts, which he referred to as "quintessential" or "essential" oils. Certain oils, such as cedarwood, cinnamon, frankincense, myrrh, rose, rosemary, and sage, were popular because of his focus on the necessity of distillation for the release of the most significant component of plants known to pharmacists by 1600 [73].

2.8. Medieval Islam

Islam Avicenna (Ibn Sina), an Arab philosopher and physician, was born in Bukhara, Persia, in the years AD 980–1037 [74]. At the age of 16, he started studying medicine, and by the time he was 20, he had been named a court physician and had been awarded the title "Prince of Physicians." He published numerous publications outlining how various herbs affect the human body. His "Al-Qanun fi al-Tibb" or "The Canon of Medicine," was a massive medical encyclopaedia that contained the Hippocratic and Galenic traditions and was written in 14 volumes. Over a period of 700 years, it was the only accepted medical textbook and instruction manual in Western Europe and the Islamic world. He is also credited with creating the chilled coil, a technique that included lengthening the cooling pipe and coiling it to enable the steam to cool more rapidly and effectively. This innovation furthered the then very straight forward method of distillation. The creation of Rosa centifolia essential oil was his first significant achievement using this improved distillation technique. Finally, it was Damascus in Syria, which gave the Damask Rose its name, that developed into a significant rose-producing region in the 13th century. Perfuming the mortar used to build their mosques was another particularly unusual use on which the Arabs put their essence. This curious practice had been passed down to them by the ancient Babylonians [75, 76].

2.9. Tudor Times (1485-1603)

Elizabeth I was the first British monarch during whom the art of fragrance really took off. Sadly, the lack of cleanliness in the West persisted from the Middle Ages all way until the Tudor era. It was necessary to use a variety of techniques to cover up the offensive odours and perhaps neutralise potentially harmful "miasmas" as a result. One such instance is Carmelite Water, or Eau des Carmes, which was developed by French Carmelite nuns in 1611 and would be used extensively for generations because it included Melissa [77].

Another innovation at this time (1665) was Aqua Mirabilis, or "beautiful water," which was brought by an Italian former Franciscan priest who had moved to Cologne. Finally, his recipe became known as "Eau to Cologne" because of the efforts of his nephew, J M Farina. It is an ethyl alcohol-based lotion that is diluted with bergamot, orange, lemon, rosemary, lavender, thyme, and neroli essential oils. Another innovation from the 16th century was Royal Hungarian Water (also known as Hungary Water), which included fresh rosemary blooms, sage, rose, and lavender that had been distilled over alcohol [78].

2.10. 17th Century

Due to the widespread usage of medicinal herbs at the time, unfortunately, charlatans and quacks were able to make quick money. Unfortunately, as a result, herbal medicine started to lose the trust of the time's doctors and medical establishment [36]. The great British herbalists, like Culpeper and Gerarde, were at their peak at this time. Botanist, herbalist, and physician Nicholas Culpeper lived from 18 October 1616 to 10 January 1654. Culpeper wrote books in English to make medical and pharmaceutical knowledge available to healers who could not read Latin, drawing inspiration from the work of medical reformers like Paracelsus who disregarded conventional medical authority.

The Complete Herbal, written by Culpeper and first published in 1653, contains hundreds of therapeutic herbs and has influenced herbal therapy ever since. It has been reprinted 41 times [79]. Many essential oils were now included in the "materia medica" of the herbalists as a result of the advancements made in the distillation process. Additionally, many houses had their own "still rooms" where the ladies would make their own home remedies, vinegars, wines, and distilled spirits. This practice was known as "simpling," and it was a common practice in addition to growing their own culinary herbs.

By the century's conclusion, the apothecary, physician, and alchemist professions had diverged from one another. As a result, all interest in the interrelationship of matter and spirit was extinguished, thus severing the link between medicine and psychology. Alchemy gave rise to the chemistry and pharmacy professions that we know today [36].

2.11. 18th Century and Industrial Revolution

Economic Revolution, The use of essential oils, entered the mainstream of medicine around 1700, and it persisted until the study of chemistry advanced to the point that synthetic materials could be produced in a laboratory. For instance, salicylic acid, the active component of willow, was created synthetically in 1852. During this time, the laboratory started to overtake the herb garden as the primary source of medicine [80].

The use of herbs and samples was not an exception. Unfortunately, as in so many other instances, the industrial revolution in Britain led to the downfall of many traditional practices. People from the countryside migrated into industrial towns and cities to obtain more lucrative employment; they lived in terraced homes with limited or no access to garden land. Sadly, as a result, the skills of cooking with fresh herbs and making basic dishes were lost [81].

2.12. 19th Century Scientific Approach

A laboratory test on the antibacterial properties of essential oils, was conducted for the first time in 1887. This was initially prompted by the widespread spread of tuberculosis and observations that people managing the processing of flowers and herbs were largely free of respiratory illnesses [82]. The first formal scientific investigation of essential oils and their impact on microorganisms started in 1887. Chamberland conducted additional research in France, which was later verified by Cadac and Meunier. The study found that essential oils could destroy the microorganisms that cause glandular fever and yellow fever [83].

The creation of synthetic and less expensive versions of the essential oil components made it easier to extract oils from plants as a result of new chemical procedures. Instead of creating customized natural formulae for each person, this resulted in the commercial mass manufacture of treatments with artificial substances. When compared to proven scientific remedies, herbal therapy quickly gained the reputation of "quackery" [84].

As chemical chemistry continued to advance, a scientific revolution was underway by 1896. The new approach entailed separating an active chemical ingredient from a plant and synthesizing it for mass manufacturing, allowing for the consistent production of large quantities at a low cost. Sadly, as a result of this decision, the synthetic versions only had a very small amount of the original drug's medicinal characteristics [85].

Therefore, essential oils were disassembled molecule by molecule and, for the first time, chemists were able to name many chemical elements of these ancient oils and their enigmatic properties, giving us geraniol, citronellol, and cineol from which affordable, synthetic replicas could be manufactured. Modern medications are based on these synthetic replicas because they were found to be extremely potent. Unfortunately, experimenting in this way with natural materials led to a variety of negative effects when utilizing synthetic medications. These side-effects then frequently necessitate treatment on their own, which causes further side effects and issues to arise. With just a few exceptions for those with carminative and flavouring qualities, natural essences were regrettably mostly excluded from the official pharmacopeias. In addition to the original natural essences, the perfume business also underwent steady development at this time and enthusiastically embraced the usage of these new fragrant synthetics. Around this time, the French town of Grasse officially rose to prominence as the world's primary location for the cultivation and extraction of essence. Unfortunately, as the scientific approach to medicine developed, herbal remedies and aromatic cures lost credibility as effective treatments and were viewed as "quackery" and "old wives' tales [86].

2.13. Development of Aromatherapy in the 20th Century

Based on Schroeder and Messing's study, Maurice Girault created the "aromatogram" in 1969, furthering the therapeutic application of aromatherapy in France. A laboratory method known as an aromatogram identifies the antibacterial properties of particular essential oils in connection with particular microbiological infections. The antibacterial property of essential oils has been the subject of numerous further studies as a result of this breakthrough [87]. Daniel Penoel, a medical and naturopathic student in France, developed an interest in Jean Valnet's work in the meantime. In order to create what is now known as "scientific aromatherapy," he worked with a chemist named Pierre Franchomme.

The emphasis was on treating infections with essential oils, and this approach is now known as 'aromatology' or 'aromatic medicine' [15]. Professional organisations representing the industry were established over time. The International Federation of Aromatherapists was the first of several professional organizations that were created over time to represent the business and provide the newly emerging therapy structure and credibility. As a result, educational standards for aromatherapy have greatly improved, with various bodies formed to address issues such as essential oil quality, industry self-regulation, an umbrella body for aromatherapy associations, EC legislation, and NHS registration. The educational abilities of specific essential oils in relation to specific microbial pathogens were also improved. As a result of this development, many further investigations have been carried out into the antimicrobial potential of essential oils [87, 88].

Aromatherapy is now one of the most popular and effective forms of complementary medicine. Even though the usefulness of these little oils has been empirical knowledge for thousands of years, the positive effects of aromatherapy are finally being proven through clinical research in laboratories all over the world [89].

3. ESSENTIAL OILS

Essential oils are usually classified simply as being top note, middle note, and base note [90].

3.1. Top Notes

Top notes are oils that mainly consist of small energetic molecules and are said to be uplifting, revitalizing, energizing, and stimulating. Top note, oils are often used in the morning or after a nap invigorate *eg*.: Bergamot and Sweet Orange.

3.2. Middle Notes

Middle note oils are slightly less energetic and slightly heavier than the top notes. They are said to balance and normalize the various systems of the body. For *e.g.*, the digestive system and the circulatory system. This group of oil is generally the most popular for general use *eg*.: Lavandin, Geranium.

3.3. Base Notes

Base notes are oils with mainly heavier molecules that take longer to evaporate and are less energetic than middle notes. They are said to be sedative, relaxing, and calming. Base note oils are usually used at bedtime, after activities or play *eg*.: Cedarwood and Sandalwood.

4. SAFETY GUIDELINES

In general, those essential oils which are commonly available are safe to use for aromatherapy or household purposes [91].

Following are the safety measures:

The specific data: Always check the specific safety data before using a new oil.

4.1. Internal Use

Do not use essential oils internally. This rule is in accordance with the guidelines of safety recommended by the International Federation of aromatherapy [92]. Essential oils do not mix with water, and in an undiluted form they may damage the lining of the digestive tract. In addition, some essential oils are toxic if taken internally.

Storage: Store in dark bottles, away from the light and heat and away from the reach of children & pets.

4.2. Hazardous Oils

Some essential oils can be dangerous, especially in inexperienced hands, due to high toxicity levels or the potential for severe dermal irritation. Oils to be avoided in this content are:

- Bitter Almond
- Arnica
- Camphor
- Camphor (brown and yellow)
- Cinnamon (bark)
- Sage (Common) *etc.*

4.3. Toxicity

Essential oils which should be used in moderation (only in dilution and for a maximum of 2 weeks at a time) because of toxicity levels *eg.*:

- Ajowan
- Cedarwood (vigiman)
- Aniseed, Basil (exotic)
- Camphor
- Fennel

- Eucalyptus.

4.4. Patch Test

Always perform a patch test before applying any new oil to the skin, even as a perfume. Apply a few drops to the back of your wrist cover with a plaster, and leave for an hour or more. If irritation or redness occurs, bathe the affected area in cold water. Reduce the concentration level by half for future use or avoid altogether.

4.5. Dermal/Skin Irritation

Oils which may cause irritation to the skin, especially if used in high concentration [93]. These are: Ajowan, Aniseed, Basil, Black Pepper, Borned, Cinnamon, Garlic, Ginger, Lemon, Peppermint, *etc*.

4.5.1. Sensitization

Some oils can cause irritation to only those who have sensitive skin or can cause an allergic reaction to some individuals. Even some widespread oils, such as tea tree or jasmine, have been known to cause sensitization in a few cases. It is important for those with sensitive skin always to do a patch test before using a new oil to check for individual sensitization. Oils which may cause sensitization include Basil, Cedarwood, Chamomile, Citronella, Garlic, Lemon, Lemongrass, Lemon Balm, Vanilla, *etc* [94].

4.5.2. Phototoxicity

Some oils are phototoxic, *i.e.*, they cause skin pigmentation if exposed to direct sunlight. Do not use the following oils either heat or in dilution with the skin, if the area or skin is going to be exposed to the sun.: Angetica roots, bergamot (except bergapten free types), Cumin, Ginger, Lemon, Lime, Lovage, Mendarin, Orange,Verbeve [95, 96].

4.5.3. Pregnancy

Due to the sensitivity of the developing baby, only use half the recommended dose of essential oils during pregnancy [97]. Oils that could be poisonous or include an emmenagogue (a chemical that stimulates uterine muscles) are not recommended. Several oils should never be used:

Use only rose and lavender (after 4 months of Pregnancy)

High blood pressure: Avoid the following oils in case of high hypertension:

- Hyssop
- Resomary
- Sage
- Thyme

4.5.4. Epilepsy

Avoid the following oils in case of epilepsy, due to their strong action on the nervous system:

- Fennel (Sweet)
- Hyssop
- Rosemary

4.5.5. Diabetes

Avoid angelica oil in case of diabetes.

4.5.6. Homeopathy

Homeopathy treatment is not compatible with the following;

- Black Pepper
- Camphor
- Eucalyptus
- Peppermint *etc*

4.5.7. Neat Application

Generally speaking, skin shouldn't be directly applied with essential oils. Always rehydrate them in cream or carrier oil first. Using neat lavender for cuts, spots, burns, and other wounds is an exception to this guideline. Ylang-ylang and sandalwood are two examples of non-irritating essential oils that can be used straight on the skin as a perfume. Do a patch test first of all. Keep a good distance from the eyes.

4.5.8. Babies and Children

Always increase the dilution for babies and infants to at least half the recommended amount. For babies, avoid the possibility of toxic and irritant oils altogether.

A. **Babies 0-12 months**: Use only 1 drop of lavender, rose, or chamomile (German or roman) essential oils, diluted in 1 top carrier oil for massage or bathing.
B. **Infants 1-5 years**: Use only 2-3 drops of safe oils, *i.e.*, those which are nontoxic and non-irritant, diluted in 1 tsp carrier oil for massage and bathing.
C. **Children 6-12 years:** Use as for adults but in half the stated concentrations.
D. **Children over 12 years:** Use as directed for adults.

4.5.9. Assessing Condition

The process begins with a comprehensive gathering of information about the client, encompassing their environment, lifestyle, nutrition, and any existing health concerns. Collaboratively, the practitioner and the client prioritize the issues based on their significance. By closely considering the client's individual needs and concerns, the primary presenting condition is pinpointed. Once this primary condition is determined, a list of all essential oils associated with addressing that condition is compiled below it. This approach ensures a personalized and tailored essential oil selection, promoting a holistic and effective wellness plan for the client's unique situation. It is simple to choose the precise oils required by using the common denominators. In most cases, it is preferable to priority and emotional state. For instance, despair, apathy, and stress anxiety. This is due to the fact that a person's mood influences the healing process, and by restoring the emotional balance, the physical body can be relaxed, encouraging the reduction of tension and improvement of health *e.g.*: Sleeplessness: Surroundings + Mental conditions.

5. SELECTING OILS

Typically, two or three oils are used for mixing, but occasionally more. A mix created by combining many oils is referred to as a "synergistic blend." These two Greek words, from which this is derived, essentially imply to work together. Except under certain circumstances, essential oils shouldn't ever be applied neatly to the skin. They must be diluted in appropriate carriers. Air, water, and vegetable oils are the most often used carriers.

- Vegetable oil for massage
- Water for baths
- Water and air for vaporizers

5.1. For Cold And Flu

- Eucalyptus
- Rosemary

- Tea Tree
- Peppermint

5.2. For Skin Care

- Lemon/Lavender
- Chamomile/ Sandalwood
- Bergamot / Sandalwood

5.3. For Headache

- Lavender/Chamomile
- Lavender/ Peppermint

5.4. For Wounds

- Chamomile/ Lavender
- Tea Tree/ Lavender

5.5. For Mental Fatigue

- Basil/Peppermint
- Rosemary/Bergamot

5.6. For Cystitis

- Sandalwood/Lavender
- Tea Tree/ Sandalwood

5.7. For Eczyema

- Lavender/ Chamomile
- Lavender/ Juniper

5.8. For Refreshing

- Lemon/Basil
- Bergamot/ Rosemary

5.9. For Stress

- Lavender/ Chamomile
- Lavender/ Ylang Ylang
- Sandalwood/ Lavender

5.10. Sore Throat

- Sandalwood/Lemon
- Sandalwood/ Tea Tree

5.11. Detoxifying/Hangovers/Cellulite

- Juniper/ Rosemary

5.12. For Purifying Sick Room

- Eucalyptus/ Peppermint
- Lavender/ Lemon

5.13. Effects of Essential Oils

- Through Smell
- Through Skin

5.14. Through Smell

1. Emotional Harmony (olfaction Technique)
2. Nose
3. Through olfactory built
4. Limbic System
5. Thalamus
6. Pituitary gland
7. Hormones are secreted
8. Hypothalamus
9. Autonomic nervous system comes into action- hence emotional healing
10. Inhaled air through the trachea
11. Bronchial tubes
12. Lungs
13. With air sacs (aveoli)
14. Around which lies minutes, blood vessels
15. Exchange of gases occurs there
16. Essential oil enters the blood stream with oxygen in minute particles and reach the organs Eg:Purifying, regulating & toning of the uterus.., Anti depressant, nerve tonic, aphrodisicac. Hence used to cure people who have problems conceiving.

5.15. Through Skin

- Physical harmony (absorption technique)
- Through the skin (semi-permeable)

- Molecules enter the blood stream
- Circulates throughout the body
- Benefits the organs of the body
- Imperto benefits – leaves system.

CONCLUSION

People have been improving their physical, intellectual, emotional, and spiritual health with essential oil-predicated aromatherapy for thousands of years. Science has recently commenced to comprehend how the valuable chemical components found in these EOs impact the body and the mind. Presently, EOs hold a relatively trivial position in the Western pharmacy; however, they remain widely utilized in the Ayurvedic medicine of India and other Eastern societies. In addition, EOs are regulated and prescribed in several European nations. Current developments have led to a resurgence of interest in essential oils in the 21st century, as some philomaths are commencing to investigate their potential benefits.

It takes practise to masterfully blend EOs to stimulate uplifting and pleasant aromas. Every EO has a number of constituent components, each of which is in charge of giving the oil its particular characteristics. EOs can be blend to intensify their effects. For instance, combining an antiviral oil with an anti-inflammatory oil mitigates coughs and colds more prosperously. Albeit this is commonly referred to as synergy, concept of synergy is more abysmal to blending. One or many chemical constituents of EOs, are primarily accountable for their medicinal benefits. However, more and more data points to the blending of key and miniscule components as the source of oils' health effects. One of the main ingredients of thyme, thymol, has vigorous antibacterial properties. Studies reveal that the blending of thyme EO has a vigorous antibacterial impact than the separate ingredient. While there is still much to learn about the synergistic effects of EOs, it is conspicuous that blending of EOs offer advantages over isolated chemicals that cannot be duplicated in a laboratory. Albeit there are no set restrictions, aromas conventionally get along well with members of their own family as well as those from nearby families. A diversity of products and treatments may be engendered by coalescing essential oils with other substances.

REFERENCES

[1] Corazza S. Aromacologia: Uma ciência de muitos cheiros. São Paulo: SENAC 2002.

[2] Gnatta JR, Kurebayashi LFS, Turrini RNT, Silva MJP. Aromatherapy and nursing: historical and theoretical conception. Rev Esc Enferm USP 2016; 50(1): 127-33. [http://dx.doi.org/10.1590/S0080-623420160000100017] [PMID: 27007430]

[3] Mancini E, Camele I, Elshafie HS, *et al.* Chemical composition and biological activity of the essential oil of *Origanum vulgare* ssp. hirtum from different areas in the Southern Apennines (Italy). Chem Biodivers 2014; 11(4): 639-51.

[http://dx.doi.org/10.1002/cbdv.201300326] [PMID: 24706631]

[4] Elshafie HS, Mancini E, Camele I, Martino LD, De Feo V. *In vivo* antifungal activity of two essential oils from Mediterranean plants against postharvest brown rot disease of peach fruit. Ind Crops Prod 2015; 66: 11-5.
[http://dx.doi.org/10.1016/j.indcrop.2014.12.031]

[5] Hongratanaworakit T. Aroma-therapeutic effects of massage blended essential oils on humans. Nat Prod Commun 2011; 6(8): 1934578X1100600.
[http://dx.doi.org/10.1177/1934578X1100600838] [PMID: 21922934]

[6] Elshafie HS, Camele I. An overview of the biological effects of some mediterranean essential oils on human health. BioMed Res Int 2017; 2017: 1-14.
[http://dx.doi.org/10.1155/2017/9268468] [PMID: 29230418]

[7] Oumeish OY. The cultural and philosophical concepts of cosmetics in beauty and art through the medical history of mankind. Clin Dermatol 2001; 19(4): 375-86.
[http://dx.doi.org/10.1016/S0738-081X(01)00194-8] [PMID: 11535377]

[8] Calvert RN. The history of massage: An illustrated survey from around the world. Inner Traditions/Bear & Co. 2002.

[9] Damian P, Damian K. Aromatherapy: Scent and psyche: Using essential oils for physical and emotional well-being. Inner Traditions/Bear & Co. 1995.

[10] Abate S, Tsion T, Mohammed O, Mengesha B. A draft training manual on production, processing, utilization and marketing aspects of aromatic plants: Based on experiences of Wondo Genet Agricultural Research Center and other countries. Academia 2009.

[11] Schnaubelt K. The healing intelligence of essential oils: the science of advanced aromatherapy. Simon and Schuster 2011.

[12] Bedigian D, Harlan JR. Evidence for cultivation of sesame in the ancient world. Econ Bot 1986; 40(2): 137-54.
[http://dx.doi.org/10.1007/BF02859136]

[13] Dwivedi A, Rahul M, Chaturvedi M. Aromatherapy a holistic cure: Current approaches and future concerns. Int J Pharmaceut Life Sci 2010; 1(1): 23-9.

[14] Skaria BP, Ed. Aromatic Plants. Volume 1, New India Publishing, India; 2007.

[15] Rhind JP. Essential Oils (Fully Revised and Updated 3rd Edition): A Comprehensive Handbook for Aromatic Therapy. Abe Books 2019.

[16] Máthé Á. Introduction: Utilization/significance of medicinal and aromatic plants. Medicinal and aromatic plants of the world. Dordrecht: Springer 2015; pp. 1-12.

[17] Smith MM. Sacred luxuries: Fragrance, aromatherapy & cosmetics in ancient egypt. Libr J 2000; 125(4): 86-6.

[18] Cooke B, Ernst E. Aromatherapy: A systematic review. Br J Gen Pract 2000; 50(455): 493-6.
[PMID: 10962794]

[19] Ross SM. Aromatic plants, spirituality, and sacred traditions. Holist Nurs Pract 2007; 21(6): 331-2.
[http://dx.doi.org/10.1097/01.HNP.0000298618.34631.49] [PMID: 17978637]

[20] Ozioma E J. Herbal medicines in african traditional medicine. Herbal Medicine. IntechOpen 2019.
[http://dx.doi.org/10.5772/intechopen.80348]

[21] Bao K. Non-scientific classification of Chinese herbal medicine as dietary supplement. Chin J Integr Med 2017; 23(3): 166-9.
[http://dx.doi.org/10.1007/s11655-016-2536-8] [PMID: 28108910]

[22] Ching N. Yellow emperor's classic of internal medicine. Books 1970; 2: 9.

[23] Chaudhri SK, Jain NK. History of cosmetics. Asian J Pharm 2009; 3: 3.

[24] Darriet A. Herbs, spices, and essential oils. In: Hui YH, Ed. Handbook of Food Products Manufacturing. Hoboken, NJ, USA: John Wiley & Sons 2007; pp. 205-20. [http://dx.doi.org/10.1002/9780470113554.ch11]

[25] Edriss H, Rosales BN, Nugent C, Conrad C, Nugent K. Islamic medicine in the middle ages. Am J Med Sci 2017; 354(3): 223-9. [http://dx.doi.org/10.1016/j.amjms.2017.03.021] [PMID: 28918826]

[26] Gerard J, Woodward M. Leaves from Gerard's Herball. AbeBooks 1943.Leaves from Gerard's Herball.

[27] Yoo K. Statistical analysis of aromatherapy preferences and complications for 3000 otolaryngology patients. Int J Aromather 2006; 16(3-4): 181-5. [http://dx.doi.org/10.1016/j.ijat.2006.10.001]

[28] Focà A, Liberto MC. 1 Historical Notes. Aromatherapy. Basic Mechanisms and Evidence Based Clinical Use 2015; 2: 1.

[29] Gattefosse RM. Gattefosse's aromatherapy. Random House 2012.

[30] Baudoux D. Contemporary French Aromatherapy: A Pharmacological and Therapeutic Guide to 100 Essential Oils. Singing Dragon 2019.

[31] Mantri S. Holistic medicine and the Western medical tradition. Virtual Mentor 2008; 10(3): 177-80. [PMID: 23206886]

[32] Fanouriou E, Kalivas D, Daferera D, *et al.* Hippocratic medicinal flora on the Greek Island of Kos: Spatial distribution, assessment of soil conditions, essential oil content and chemotype analysis. J Appl Res Med Aromat Plants 2018; 9: 97-109. [http://dx.doi.org/10.1016/j.jarmap.2018.03.003]

[33] Ali B, Al-Wabel NA, Shams S, Ahamad A, Khan SA, Anwar F. Essential oils used in aromatherapy: A systemic review. Asian Pac J Trop Biomed 2015; 5(8): 601-11. [http://dx.doi.org/10.1016/j.apjtb.2015.05.007]

[34] Tame M. Ayurvedic texts in khotanese literature. Shodoznavstvo 2020; 2020(86): 99-118. [http://dx.doi.org/10.15407/skhodoznavstvo2020.86.099]

[35] Bharadwaj R. Indian knowledge tradition: Ayurveda medicine and contemporary challenges. Institut Hindu Dharma Negeri Denpasar 2018.

[36] Petrovska B. Historical review of medicinal plants' usage. Pharmacogn Rev 2012; 6(11): 1-5. [http://dx.doi.org/10.4103/0973-7847.95849] [PMID: 22654398]

[37] Xiao L J, Tao R. Traditional Chinese medicine (TCM) therapy. Adv Exp Med Biol 2017; 1010: 261-80.

[38] Curran J. The yellow emperor's classic of internal medicine. BMJ 2008; 336(7647): 777. [http://dx.doi.org/10.1136/bmj.39527.472303.4E]

[39] Gmitter FG, Hu X. The possible role of Yunnan, China, in the origin of contemporary citrus species (rutaceae). Econ Bot 1990; 44(2): 267-77. [http://dx.doi.org/10.1007/BF02860491]

[40] Chang N, Luo Z, Li D, Song H. Indigenous uses and pharmacological activity of traditional medicinal plants in Mount Taibai, China. Evid Based Complement Alternat Med 2017; 2017: 1-11. [http://dx.doi.org/10.1155/2017/8329817] [PMID: 28303162]

[41] Inoue M, Hayashi S, Craker L E. Role of medicinal and aromatic plants: Past, present, and future. Pharmacognosy-Medicinal Plants. IntechOpen 2019; pp. 1-13.

[42] Aboelsoud N H. Herbal medicine in ancient Egypt. J Med Plants Res 2010; 4(2): 082-6.

[43] Forshaw R. Before Hippocrates. Healing practices in ancient Egypt. Medicine, Healing and

Performance. Oxbow Books 2014. [http://dx.doi.org/10.2307/j.ctvh1dwj4.6]

[44] Byl SA. 2012.The essence and use of perfume in ancient Egypt

[45] Tatomir R. To cause "to make divine" through smoke: ancient Egyptian incense and perfume An inter-and transdisciplinary re-evaluation of aromatic biotic materials used by the ancient Egyptians Moesica et Christiana—Studies in honor of Professor Alexandru Barnea. Braila: Editura Istros 2016; pp. 665-78.

[46] Koller J, Baumer U, Kaup Y, Weser U. Herodotus'and pliny's embalming materials identified on ancient egyptian mummies. Archaeometry 2005; 47(3): 609-28. [http://dx.doi.org/10.1111/j.1475-4754.2005.00222.x]

[47] Yadav VK, Choudhary N, Heena Khan S, *et al.* Incense and incense sticks: Types, components, origin and their religious beliefs and importance among different religions. J Bio Innov 2020; 9(6): 1420-39. [http://dx.doi.org/10.46344/JBINO.2020.v09i06.28]

[48] Kanellou V. Ancient Greek medicine as the foundation of contemporary medicine. Tech Coloproctol 2004; 8(S1): s3-4. [http://dx.doi.org/10.1007/s10151-004-0095-z] [PMID: 15655635]

[49] Saleem H, Anjum SMM, Awan AB, Ahmed J. A short history of evolution of indigenous plants and medicine system. J Pharm Alt Med 2013; 2: 1-4.

[50] Bhattacharya S, Saha T, Das P, *et al.* Aromatic plants: Role and uses in human prosperity and sustainability. Pharma Innov J 2022; 11(5): 341-8.

[51] Cain WS. History of research on smell. Handbook on Perception: Tasting and Smelling 2012; 6: 197-229.

[52] Classen C, Howes D, Synnott A. Aroma: The cultural history of smell. Routledge 2002. [http://dx.doi.org/10.4324/9780203428887]

[53] Forrest RD. Early history of wound treatment. J R Soc Med 1982; 75(3): 198-205. [http://dx.doi.org/10.1177/014107688207500310] [PMID: 7040656]

[54] Buckle J. Clinical aromatherapy-e-book: essential oils in practice. Elsevier 2014.

[55] Giannenas I, Sidiropoulou E, Bonos E, Christaki E, Florou-Paneri P. The history of herbs, medicinal and aromatic plants, and their extracts: Past, current situation and future perspectives. Feed additives. Academic Press 2020; pp. 1-18. [http://dx.doi.org/10.1016/B978-0-12-814700-9.00001-7]

[56] Djilani A, Dicko A. The therapeutic benefits of essential oils. Nutrition, well-being and health. InTech 2012. [http://dx.doi.org/10.5772/25344]

[57] Staub PO, Casu L, Leonti M. Back to the roots: A quantitative survey of herbal drugs in Dioscorides' De Materia Medica (ex Matthioli, 1568). Phytomedicine 2016; 23(10): 1043-52. [http://dx.doi.org/10.1016/j.phymed.2016.06.016] [PMID: 27444350]

[58] Moscou K, Snipe K. Pharmacology for Pharmacy Technicians-E-Book. Elsevier 2018.

[59] Shoja MM, Tubbs RS, Ghabili K, Griessenauer CJ, Balch MW, Cuceu M. The roman empire legacy of galen (129–200 ad). Childs Nerv Syst 2015; 31(1): 1-5. [http://dx.doi.org/10.1007/s00381-014-2467-7] [PMID: 25034238]

[60] Groom N, Ed. New perfume handbook. Springer 1997.

[61] Grant M. The Antonines: The Roman Empire in Transition. Routledge 2016. [http://dx.doi.org/10.4324/9781315870243]

[62] Wang HM, Yang WL, Wang CA, Tsai YS, Chen CY. Historical and Modern Uses for the Ingredients of the Holy Anointing Compound (Doctoral dissertation, Thesis on Researchgate) 2008.

[63] Koedam A, Margaris MS, Vokou D, editors. Aromatic plants: basic and applied aspects. Vol. 7. Springer; 2012.

[64] Tydlitátová V V. Trees and scents in Tanak. 2007. Available from: https://repositorio.uam.es/bitstream/handle/10486/6567/39096_9.pdf?sequence=1&isAllowed=y

[65] Pullaiah T, Das SC. History of sandalwood. Sandalwood: Silviculture, Conservation and Applications. Singapore: Springer 2021; pp. 9-20. [http://dx.doi.org/10.1007/978-981-16-0780-6_2]

[66] Ben-Yehoshua S, Borowitz C, Ondrej Hanuš L. 1 frankincense, myrrh, and balm of Gilead: Ancient spices of Southern Arabia and Judea. Hortic Rev (Am Soc Hortic Sci) 2012; 39(1): 3-66.

[67] Giblin CH. Mary's Anointing for Jesus' Burial-Resurrection (John 12, 1-8). Biblica 1992; 73(4): 560-4.

[68] Grieve M. A modern herbal. Vol. 2. Courier Corporation; 2013.

[69] Low KEY. Presenting the self, the social body, and the olfactory: managing smells in everyday life experiences. Sociol Perspect 2006; 49(4): 607-31. [http://dx.doi.org/10.1525/sop.2006.49.4.607]

[70] Gould F. Aromatherapy for holistic therapists. Nelson Thornes 2003.

[71] Vender C, Fusani P. Conservation of medicinal and aromatic plants in Italy. Report of a Working Group on Medicinal and Aromatic Plants. 2002.

[72] Sweet V. Hildegard of Bingen and the greening of medieval medicine. Bull Hist Med 1999; 73(3): 381-403. [http://dx.doi.org/10.1353/bhm.1999.0140] [PMID: 10500336]

[73] Martin M. Selling Beauty: Cosmetics, Commerce, and French Society. JHU Press 2009.

[74] Nadeem F, Azeem MW, Jilani MI. Isolation of Bioactive Compounds from Essential Oils–A Comprehensive Review. Int J Chem Biochem Sci 2017; 12: 75-85.

[75] Shamey R, Kirchner E, Amirshahi SH. Ibn Sina (Avicenna) Ca. 980–1037. Pioneers of Color Science. Cham: Springer 2020; pp. 39-43. [http://dx.doi.org/10.1007/978-3-319-30811-1_9]

[76] McGinnis J. Medieval Philosophy of Religion. Routledge 2014.

[77] Widrlechner MP. History and utilization ofRosa damascena. Econ Bot 1981; 35(1): 42-58. [http://dx.doi.org/10.1007/BF02859214]

[78] Johnson RL, Foster S, Kiefer D, Dog TL. National Geographic Guide to Medicinal Herbs: The World's Most Effective Healing Plants. National Geographic Books 2012.

[79] Raghavan S. Handbook of spices, seasonings, and flavorings. CRC press 2006. [http://dx.doi.org/10.1201/b13597]

[80] Culpeper N. Culpeper's complete herbal & English physician. Applewood Books 2007.

[81] Lis-Balchin M. Essential oils and 'aromatherapy': Their modern role in healing. J R Soc Health 1997; 117(5): 324-9. [http://dx.doi.org/10.1177/146642409711700511] [PMID: 9519666]

[82] Guenther E, Althausen D. The essential oils. New York: Van Nostrand 1948; Vol. 1: p. 81.

[83] Maiolini M, Gause S, Taylor J, *et al.* The war against tuberculosis: A review of natural compounds and their derivatives. Molecules 2020; 25(13): 3011. [http://dx.doi.org/10.3390/molecules25133011] [PMID: 32630150]

[84] Navarro M. Larvicidal activity of plant and algae extracts, essential oils and isolated chemical constituents against Aedes aegypti. Nat Prod J 2013; 3(4): 268-91.

[85] AL-Sallami . Alternative medicine, science or quackery. J Trop Nephro-Urol 2007; 5(1): 38-40.

[86] WOLPE PR. The American Medical Ethics Revolution: How the AMA's Code of Ethics Has Transformed Physicians' Relationships to Patients, Professionals, and Society. Baltimore: Johns Hopkins University Press 1999.

[87] Micozzi MS. Fundamentals of complementary and alternative medicine-E-book. Elsevier 2014.

[88] Blackwell R, Smith M. Aromatograms. International Journal of Aromatherapy 1995; 7(1): 22-7. [http://dx.doi.org/10.1016/0962-4562(95)80009-3]

[89] Shah BN. Textbook of pharmacognosy and phytochemistry. Elsevier 2009.

[90] Lee J, Hur MH. The Effects of Aroma Essential Oil Inhalation on Stress, Pain, and Sleep Quality in Laparoscopic Cholecystectomy Patients: A Randomized Controlled Trial. Asian Nurs Res 2022; 16(1): 1-8.
[http://dx.doi.org/10.1016/j.anr.2021.11.002] [PMID: 34954406]

[91] Fischer-Rizzi S. Complete aromatherapy handbook: Essential oils for radiant health. Sterling Publishing Company, Inc. 1990.

[92] Tisserand R, Young R. Essential oil safety: A guide for health care professionals. Elsevier 2013.

[93] Burfield T. Safety of essential oils. Int J Aromather 2000; 10((1-2)): 16-29. [http://dx.doi.org/10.1016/S0962-4562(00)80005-3]

[94] Vostinaru O, Heghes S C, Filip L. Safety profile of essential oils. Essential Oils-Bioactive Compounds, New Perspectives and Applications. IntechOpen 2020. [http://dx.doi.org/10.5772/intechopen.91363]

[95] Schaller M, Korting HC. Allergie airborne contact dermatitis from essential oils used in aromatherapy. Clin Exp Dermatol 1995; 20(2): 143-5.
[http://dx.doi.org/10.1111/j.1365-2230.1995.tb02719.x] [PMID: 8565250]

[96] Kejlová K, Jírová D, Bendová H, Gajdoš P, Kolářová H. Phototoxicity of essential oils intended for cosmetic use. Toxicol In vitro 2010; 24(8): 2084-9.
[http://dx.doi.org/10.1016/j.tiv.2010.07.025] [PMID: 20688147]

[97] Buckle J, Ryan K, Chin KB. Clinical Aromatherapy for Pregnancy, Labor and postpartum. Int J Childbirth Educ 2014; 29: 4.

CHAPTER 2

Plant as Potential Resources for Efficacious Essential Oils: Underpinning Aromatherapy Evolution

Pragati Misra[1,*], **Ghanshyam Pandey**[2], **Shambhavi Pandey**[3], **Atul Singh**[4], **Arun K. Chaurasia**[5], **Eugenia P. Lal**[6], **Shikha Agnihotry**[7], **Ajeet Kumar Srivastav**[8,9] and **Pradeep Kumar Shukla**[6]

[1] *Centre for Tissue Culture Technology, Jacob Institute of Biotechnology and Bioengineering, Sam Higginbottom University of Agriculture, Technology and Sciences, Prayagraj, Uttar Pradesh, India*

[2] *Department of Plant Protection and Plant Pathology, Naini Agricultural Institute, Sam Higginbottom University of Agriculture, Technology and Sciences, Prayagraj, Uttar Pradesh, India*

[3] *Department of Forensic Sciences, Faculty of Science, Sam Higginbottom University of Agriculture, Technology and Sciences, Prayagraj, Uttar Pradesh, India*

[4] *Department of Agriculture, Koneru Lakshmaiah Education Foundation, Vaddeswaram, AP, India*

[5] *Department of Genetics and Plant Breeding, Naini Agricultural Institute, Sam Higginbottom University of Agriculture, Technology and Sciences, Prayagraj, Uttar Pradesh, India*

[6] *Department of Biological Sciences, Faculty of Science, Sam Higginbottom University of Agriculture, Technology and Sciences, Prayagraj, Uttar Pradesh, India*

[7] *Department of Computational Biology and Bioinformatics, Jacob Institute of Biotechnology and Bio-Engineering, Sam Higginbottom University of Agriculture, Technology and Sciences, Prayagraj (Allahabad), Uttar Pradesh, India*

[8] *Redcliffe Hygiene, Private Limited, Gurugram-122016, Haryana, India*

[9] *Department of Biochemistry, Babu Banrasi Das University, Lucknow, India*

Abstract: The basis of healthcare has been medicinal plants from the dawn of humanity. For over 4000 years, people have carefully documented and passed down through generations the various ways in which these have been utilized. The Indian Vedic literature, which dates to roughly 2000 BC, contains a list of around 700 compo-

[*] **Corresponding author Pragati Misra:** Centre for Tissue Culture Technology, Jacob Institute of Biotechnology and Bioengineering, Sam Higginbottom University of Agriculture, Technology and Sciences, Prayagraj, Uttar Pradesh, India; E-mail: pragati.misra@shiats.edu.in

Pradeep Kumar Shukla, Ajeet Kumar Srivastav, Deepti Chopra, Shikha Agnihotry, Pragati Misra and Jyoti Singh (Eds.)

unds. Cinnamon, spikenard, ginger, myrrh, coriander, and sandalwood are a few of these. Since ancient times, aromatic plant parts and oils have been used for their therapeutic and culinary characteristics, as well as to produce incense, perfumes, cosmetics, and for incense sticks. Ritual use was widespread in early cultures, where it served both sacred and therapeutic objectives that were intricately intertwined. Since prehistoric times, plant essential oils have been utilized in foods, aromatherapy, perfumes, cosmetics, spices, and alimentation. They have also been applied in other medical procedures and phytotherapy. In the current era of pharmaceutical science, interest in herbal medicines has grown relative to conventional or synthetic treatments because they are more affordable, more widely accepted, compatible with human physiology, and have fewer adverse effects. The medicinal properties and applications of an expanding number of emerging essential oils have been researched and documented by pharmacists. The interest in analysing their bioactivity has progressed owing to their widespread use, particularly the recently investigated antibacterial, antioxidant, anticancer, and antidiabetic effects. The traditional Indian or Ayurvedic system of medicine, as well as other ecumenical customary systems, would be transformed if plant predicated knowledge were to be incorporated. The uses of numerous plants for therapeutic, medical, aesthetic, psychological, olfactory, massage, aromatherapy, and other associated issues are examined in this chapter.

Keywords: Aromatherapy, Bioactivity, Essential oils, Medicinal plants, Phytotherapy.

1. INTRODUCTION

Essential oils are organic, volatile, and complex chemicals that are produced as secondary metabolites by the corresponding aromatic plants and are distinguished by their aroma [1]. Each part of the plant, either bud, flowers, leaves, stalks, twigs, seeds, fruits, roots, wood, or bark, is capable of producing essential oils (EOs), which are subsequently stored in secretory cells, cavities, canals, epidermic cells, or glandular trichomes [2]. EOs are liquids that are lipid soluble, clear, and rarely coloured. They are insoluble in organic solvents and have a density that is typically lower than that of water. Constituents are secondary plant metabolites that are lipophilic, extremely volatile, and reach masses below 300 molecular weight. They can be physically separated from other parts of the plant or membranous tissue. The most recent applications of EOs include being as antioxidants and preservatives in victuals, fused into foodstuff packing material [3], and significant application as crop protectants [4, 5].

For ages, EOs have been used extensively in the pharmaceutical, agricultural, sanitary, and cosmetic industries. They have also been included in cuisines as herbs or spices [6, 7]. According to [8], a number of variables, including pabulum, temperature, humidity, solar radiation, location, genetics, and harvesting time, can have an impact on EOs. The Thymus plant's thymol and carvacrol have been found to have high antioxidant properties [9]. Thymol also has a number of biological and pharmacological properties, including activities that are antimutagenic, anticancer, antioxidant, and anti-inflammatory [10]. Carvacrol is already being used as a food ingredient to prevent bacterial infection and amplification because of its pleasant scent and antibacterial properties [11]. Numerous essential oils have antioxidant and antibacterial characteristics in addition to serving as food and cosmetic additives [12 - 15].

A phenolic monoterpene called carvacrol (2-methyl-5-isopropylphenol) is found in the EOs produced by several aromatic plants, including *Origanum vulgare L., Nigella sativa L.,* and *Thymus vulgaris* L. [16, 17]. Carvacrol is observed as a safe pabulum adjunct and adds flavour to beverages and chewing gum because it demonstrated low toxicity in rats [18, 19].

The oils of numerous herbs, including *Carthamus tinctorius* L. and *Pandanus odoratissimus* L., contain α-terpineol, an evaporative monoterpene alcohol with a faintly sugary aroma [20, 21]. According to pharmacological research, α-terpineol has antinociceptive, anticonvulsant, and hypotensive properties [22 - 24].

Numerous researchers have hypothesised that (-)-α-bisabolol has a range of biological properties, including antifungal [25], antinociception [26], and anticancer actions [27]. When rats were pretreated with the KATP channel blocker glibenclamide, the gastroprotective effect of (-)-α-bisabolol (100 mg/kg) was overturned, indicating the significance of endogenous prostaglandins in its gastroprotective function [28]. An aromatic chemical called anethole (1-methoxy-4-(1-propenyl)-benzene) is widely consumed in the industry as a flavouring agent for food and beverages. Northeastern Brazil is home to the Euphorbiaceae bush Croton zehntneri Pax et Hoff, also known as "canela de cunh" and "canela de cheiro" [29]. Anethole, a key component of the essential oil of *Croton zehntneri* (EOCZ), is used therapeutically in traditional medicine for a number of adverse conditions, such as too much pain, anxiety and gastrointestinal disturbances. Anetholes can also exhibit anti-inflammatory and anaesthetic activities [30, 31].

2. PLANTS AS SOURCE OF ESSENTIAL OILS

Essential oils are found in many different plants; however, the primary source of essential oils might come from different portions of the plant (Table **1**). These consist of barks, fruits, seeds, peels, roots, leaves, and so on. Typically, complex mixtures of polar and nonpolar natural chemicals make up plant essential oils.

2.1. Salvia

The Lamiaceae family has over 900 species, with the genus Salvia (sage) being remarkably enormous, important medicinal and aromatic genera [32]. It is clear that sage has a history of promoting health and treating illnesses from its Latin name, "Salvia," which means "remedy." Around the world, many species of *Salvia* are used in traditional medicine to cure microbial infections, malaria, cancer and inflammation and to clean sick people's dwellings [33, 34]; tinctures and medications are recognised in a number of pharmacopoeias (*e.g.*, European Pharmacopoeia, 6th ed.; Pharmacopoeia Hungarica, 8th ed.). Herbalists in Lebanon, Syria, and Jordan see Salvia species as a "panacea," or an all-purpose medication that may be used to treat a variety of pulmonary and urinary problems as well as cancer, microbiological infections, asthma, cough, and headaches, stomachaches, and abdominal pain. The most potent active ingredients in sage are the essential oils formed in the foliage (1-2.8%), which contain the monoterpenes α- and β thujone, camphor, borneol and cineole and additionally the sesquiterpenes - humulene and -caryophyllene [35]. Many diseases and their symptoms may be treated naturally, safely, and effectively by *Salvia species*. The above-mentioned herbal medicines with antibacterial, anti-inflammatory, antioxidant, free radical scavenging, and anticancerous activities have been found to be very effective in the development of novel natural drugs to prevent, control, and treat many minor health issues together with more serious and perplexing diseases like diabetes, Parkinson's, and Alzheimer's. In the past few decades, with the increase in pharmacological awareness about the beneficial effects of sage, especially *S. officinalis*, their use in herbal medicines has been enhanced. But until further conclusive trials show the safety, quality, and efficacy of *S. officinalis*, clinicians should exercise caution.

Future research will concentrate on carrying out extensive chemical and pharmacological tests as well as looking into human metabolism because of these worries. Additionally, *S. officinalis* must be used to its full potential in developing therapeutic drugs and serve as a basis for upcoming research on the use of medicinal plants [36]. *Salvia* was popularly used in herbal tea blends before its usage as antibiotics was advised to tuberculosis patients to avoid drowsiness, and was discovered to be an active component in phytotherapy for the treatment of chronic bronchitis [37].

The broad spectrum of biological properties exhibited by *Salvia spp.* such as antibacterial, antimicrobial, antioxidant, antitumour, antidiabetic, anxiolytic, sedative, and anti-inflammatory properties, might provide insight into its remarkable efficacy in treating diverse human disorders [37 - 41].

According to prior studies, *S. bracteata's* aerial parts are distinguished by the presence of antibacterial diterpenoids [42]. The seed extracts have shown effectiveness against *Escherichia coli*, *Staphylococcus aureus*, *Mycobacterium smegmatis*, and *Candida albicans*. The extract was rich in adipose acid, including

9,12-octadecenoic acid, which accounted for 64.3%. [43]. Additionally, the EOs of *S. bracteata* collected from Turkey and Iran [44 - 46] were also investigated [47].

S. lanigera Poir (Lamiaceae) spreading wild in Cyprus was hydrodistilled to isolate the EO, which was then analysed by GC and GC-MS. The principal constituents were revealed to be thymol (12.1%), hexadecanoic acid (6.0%), carvacrol, and a-thujone (5.7%), totaling 67 compounds, or 93.6% of the oil. One of the most researched characteristics of essential oils is their antimicrobial activity, which works in tandem with their antioxidant efficacy to prevent the spread of infectious diseases that affect both humans and animals. Numerous research indicate that a wide variety of essential oils, particularly those from the Lamiaceae family, have potent antibacterial and antiradical properties. It was discovered that *S. lanigera* essential oil exhibits strong antioxidant properties as well as a wide range of antibacterial effects against test strains, particularly Gram-positive bacteria. These findings suggest that *S. lanigera* essential oil may be used to improve the safety and shelf life of food as a natural substitute for conventional food preservatives [48].

S. officinalis L. is widespread, and the food industry frequently uses its leaves as ingredients. Sage essential oil has been demonstrated to have numerous biological properties and is used in the treatment of a number of ailments. The majority of the samples contained a-thujone, camphor, borneol, c-muurolene, and sclareol, however, the percentages of these compounds varied according to the environmental conditions, including height, availability of water, and pedo-climatic variables [49].

2.2. Hyssop

Hyssop is a plant that allures bees, emits delightful fragrance and serves as an ornamental addition [50]. In the pabulum industry, the aerial parts of Hyssop are used as a spice or condiment, having mint-like taste [51 - 53]. The plant has a long record of its use in traditional medicine as a carminative, tonic, expectorant and antiseptic [54] it was also valued for treating rheumatic pain, bruises, wounds, and states of anxiety and hysteria, for regulating blood pressure, and as a muscle relaxant [55]. Hyssop essential oil is used in liqueurs, cosmetics, and phytotherapy. Nevertheless, caution is recommended because it contains epileptogenic pinocamphone and isopinocamphone [56]. Furthermore, oil is also used to flavour alcoholic beverages, meat items, and seasonings. It is also a component of many brands of colognes and fragrances [57, 58, 59, 60]. ISO 9841 has officially classified hyssop oil's chemical composition as ecumenical [61].

2.3. Nepeta

Nepeta, also known as catmints, is a genus that encompasses various species containing a diverse array of secondary metabolites, including terpenoids (monoterpenoids, diterpenoids, triterpenoids, sesquiterpenoids), and phenolics (monoterpenoids, diterpenoids, triterpenoids, sesquiterpenoids). One of the species within this genus is *Nepeta rtanjensis*. Due to its spasmolytic and myorelaxant properties, many *Nepeta species* have historically been used to treat a variety of gastrointestinal and respiratory disorders, including colic, diarrhoea, coughing, and asthma [62, 63]. *Nepeta species* have been revealed to have effects that attract aphids and cats [63, 64] or repel insects, mainly mosquitoes, red poultry mites, and ixodid ticks [65]. During hydro distllation, 30 g of the aerial parts of *N. cataria* at different stages (vegetative, floral budding and full flowering) resulted in EO yields of 0.3, 0.5 and 0.9% (w/w) essential oil, respectively (Table **1**). A total of 13, 12 and 14 compounds accounting for 93.6, 99.6 and 99% of the total composition was found at vegetative, floral budding and full flowering stages, respectively. The major constituents of the oil throughout all growth stages were nepetalactones, specifically 4a-α, 7-α, 7a-β-nepetalactone (55-58%) and 4a-α, 7-β, 7a-α-nepetalactone (30-31.2%) [66].

Table 1. EO Composition (%) of Catnip (*N. cataria*) at three stages of harvest [66].

Component	RI*	Vegetative (%)	Floral Budding (%)	Full Flowering (%)
α-Pinene	936	2.7	3.1	4.6
Sabinene	957	0.0	0.0	0.15
β-Pinene	978	0.8	1.13	1.64
1-Cyclohexen-1-yl-methyl ketone	980	0.5	0.6	0.7
Triplal	1023	0.1	0.4	0.4
Thymol	1294	0.4	0.4	0.57
4a-α,7-α,7a-β-Nepetalactone	1332	55	58	55.03
4a-α,7-β,7a-α-Nepetalactone	1342	30.06	31.1	31.2
trans Caryophyllene	1430	1.1	2.7	2.1
α-Humulene	1446	0.82	0.92	0.87
11-Dodecenol	1500	0.84	0.69	1.1
Spathulenol	1580	0.6	0.4	0.3
Caryophyllene oxide	1569	0.5	0.2	0.12
6,10-dimethyl-2-undecane	1907	0.2	0.0	0.25

Nepeta plants also exhibit antimicrobial activity against a wide range of bacteria and fungi, antioxidant properties, and phytotoxic properties (Table **2**) [63 - 68]. Additionally, according to several studies [63,69-71], these plants manifest antiviral, phytotoxic, and allelopathic properties. Numerous investigations examined the cytotoxic and cytostatic effects of various *Nepeta species* [72 - 75]. The majority of the biological activities listed above for *Nepeta species* are attributed to nepetalactones, which are often the primary components of essential oils [63 - 66, 71, 76, 77]. Nepetalactones (or nepetalactones in iotas) are not produced by some *Nepeta species* [68, 78], hence their biological action may be attributed to other terpenoid or phenolic chemicals [68, 63, 77, 79], Nepetalactones' stereochemistry determines how biologically active they are [68, 80, 81].

Table 2. Antimicrobial activities of different species from the Nepeta genus.

Species	Microorganism	Antimicrobial Activity	References
Nepeta cataria	*Staphylococcus aureus* *Escherichia coli* *Candida albicans*	Strong inhibition Moderate inhibition Mild inhibition	[82]
N. faassenii	*S. aureus*	Strong inhibition	[83]
N. deflersiana	Gram positive bacteria Gram-negative *E. coli* *P. aeruginosa*	Strong inhibition	[84]
N. ispahanica	*S. aureus, S. epidermidis* and *B. subtilis* *E. faecalis* and *E. coli*	Moderate inhibition	[85]
N. nuda	*S. aureus* and *K. pneumoniae*	Strong inhibition	[86]
N. septemcrenata	*B. subtilis, S. aureus* and *E. coli*	Strongest inhibition	[87]
Himalayan *Nepeta* spp., *N. leucophylla*, *N. discolor, N. govaniana, N. clarkei, N.elliptica* and *N. erecta*	P. *aeruginosa, E. coli, P. multocida, P. vulgaris, Serratia marcescens* and *S. aureus*	Moderate to strong inhibition	[88]
N. ucrainica L. spp. *kopetdaghensis*	*S. aureus* *M. luteus* *P. aeruginosa* and *E. coli*	Strong inhibition Moderate inhibition Mild inhibition	[75]
N. transcaucasica	*E. coli*	Moderate inhibition	[89]

Various biological functions of *N. rtanjensis* have been thoroughly documented up to this point, including antibacterial [66, 68], antifungal [66 - 68], and allelopathic (Nest Trans-cis nepetalactone), which is considered the key ingredient primarily responsible for the biological actions [66,68,77], is a prominent component of *N. rtanjensis* essential oil.

The main components widely used in ethnomedical techniques have long been thought to be found in plant species. Different investigations revealed that the medicinal plant species that the locals use for the conventional treatment of ailments are not thoroughly examined for their therapeutic/preventive potential and phytochemical discoveries. The pharmacological effects of *Nepeta spp*. have been documented, and they have antimicrobial, antioxidant, anti-inflammatory, sedative, relaxant, diuretic, cholesterol-lowering, antiasthmatic, carminative, vermifuge, herbicidal, insecticidal, and insect-repellent properties. Some sources also mention them as a topical treatment for snake and scorpion bites [78, 90 - 94].

The categorised chemical makeup, which mostly consists of nepetalactones, an unsaturated lactone, is responsible for all actions stated. *Nepeta species* can be divided into two groups, the first of which has a high percentage of nepetalactone (and its isomers), and the second group has a low percentage of nepetalactones and compounds such as 1,8-cineole, β-caryophyllene, -caryophyllene oxide, β-farnesene, α-citral, and β-citronellol as the main [78].

Because of its antispasmodic, antiseptic, expectorant, diuretic, antitussive, antiasthmatic, carminative, and vermiifuge properties, several species of this genus are frequently used in Iranian traditional medicine [91, 95].

2.4. Thymus

Thymus species are considered medicinal plants due to their pharmaceutical properties [96 - 103]. *Thymus species* revealed a wide range of therapeutic properties in their essential oils, commonly known as thyme oil, which include antirheumatic, antispasmodic, antiseptic, antimicrobial, cardiac, carminative, diuretic, and expectorant effects (Table **3**). *Thymus algeriensis* is an aromatic herbaceous plant and spice that is frequently used as a culinary herb, whether it is fresh or dried [104].

Table 3. Details of bioactive compounds found in the thymus oil after GC–MS analysis, along with the formula, molecular weight and reported activity of each bioactive compound (105).

S. No.	Compound	Molecular Formula	Molecular Weight	Reported Activity	References
1	α-Pinene	$C_{10}H_{16}$	136.24	Antioxidant anti-inflammatory, chondroprotective	[106, 107]
2	Camphene	$C_{10}H_{16}$	136.24	Hypolipidemic, hepatoprotective	[108-109]

(Table 3) cont.....

S. No.	Compound	Molecular Formula	Molecular Weight	Reported Activity	References
3	β-Myrcene	$C_{10}H_{16}$	136.24	Antioxidant, antiulcer, anticancer	[110 - 112]
4	Carene	$C_{10}H_{16}$	136.24	Antioxidant, anti-inflammatory	[113 - 115]
5	*p*-Cymene	$C_{10}H_{14}$	134.21	Antioxidant, antimicrobial	[116, 117]
6	γ-Terpinene	$C_{10}H_{16}$	136.24	Antimicrobial, antioxidant	[118]
7	α-Terpineol	$C_{10}H_{18}O$	154.25	Antimicrobial	[119]
8	Thymol	$C_{10}H_{14}O$	150.22	Antimicrobial, antioxidant	[120]
9	Caryo-phyllene	$C_{15}H_{24}$	204.36	Local anesthesia, antimicrobial	[121]
10	Humulene	$C_{15}H_{24}$	204.36	Larvicidal, anticancer	[122, 123]

The oil has also found its role in strengthening the immune system and can be used to treat flu, chills, and other infectious disorders. It has been demonstrated to play a significant role in urinary antiseptic cystitis and urethritis. The traditional applications of essential oils from *T. serpyllum*, *T. algeriensis*, and *T. vulgaris* were validated scientifically, along with their phytochemical analysis and bioactivity. Thymol has been found as the primary oil component in all three *Thymus* EOs. These three species of *thymus* plants should be used as an antibacterial agent in oral hygiene as well as a therapy for small wounds and oral cavity illnesses, according to research on the antimicrobial activity of EOs. Additionally, Thyme's historic use in the treatment of dyspepsia, gastrointestinal disturbances, bronchitis, laryngitis, tonsillitis, and pertussis is strengthened by its robust antioxidant and anticancer action. The oil from *T. serpyllum* had the highest level of biological activity in all experiments. Thymus oils have a lot of promise for anticancer therapies in addition to being used in food and cosmetics, and they unquestionably need further research [124].

Additionally, this plant is frequently used in traditional medicine and is valued for its antibacterial, antifungal, antispasmodic, and antiseptic effects [125]. In addition to being used in the perfumery, essential oils from aerial components were used as flavouring agents in a range of pabulum, beverages, and confectionary goods [125]. Numerous essential oils can be used as organic herbicides. Additionally, *T. algeriensis* oil with *S. littoralis* has shown extremely strong insecticidal efficacy. As a result, this plant may be a useful source for pest control. *T. algeriensis* oils offer a safe and cost-effective alternative to harmful conventional pesticides for controlling a variety of insect life stages. The value of *T. algereinsis* in Tunisia as an indigenous medicinal plant and a potential source of biologically active chemicals is highlighted by all of these findings. This plant may protect individuals from the harmful effects of free radicals, and it will likely be used to create safe pabulum products and additives [126].

Among the 350 species of the *Thymus* genus particularly known as thyme, *T. vulgaris* L. is primarily originated in the Mediterranean region [97]. *Thymus* species have been widely used as herbal teas, tonics, antitussives, carminatives, and antiseptics, in addition to treatments for constipation, anti-inflammatory, antioxidant, antibacterial and antifungal agents, anthelmintic, and hepato-protective agents, besides as a promiser to treat neuroblastoma. Since thyme essential oils are already used as food preservatives, especially for red meat and poultry. Researchers and the pabulum industry have been very concerned about their phytochemical analysis and medicinal capabilities [127 - 129]. Studies on *Mentha spicata* L. [130], *Rosmarinus officinalis* L. [131], *Ocimum basilicum* L. [165], *Origanum majorana* L. [132], and *T. vulgaris* have all demonstrated that the composition of essential oils can be affected by seasonal variations [133].

2.5. Mentha

Lamiaceae species are regarded as highly significant owing to their widespread usage in essential oil production, traditional medicine, food, cosmetics, and flavouring. *Mentha* constitutes the largest genus in the Lamiaceae family, which includes around 20 species spread all over the world [134]. It consists of common perennial herbaceous plants that are cultivated in temperate regions like those in South Africa, Australia, and the Mediterranean area [135]. Additionally, *Mentha species* have long been valued for their antibacterial quality [136 - 138].

M. suaveolens, *M. rotundifolia*, *M. pulegium*, *M. aquatica*, and *M. longifolia* are only a few of the species where the antimicrobial properties of mint essential oils have been revealed [139, 140]. Today's scientific community shows that plant extracts' antioxidant properties have positive effects on human health [141]. The *Mentha species* are recognised as potent primary antioxidants and free radical scavengers that can interact with one another to prevent ROS attacks on living systems [142]. It is usual to discuss foods or plants and their bioactive components for human consumption in relation to their antioxidant capacity.

Mints are generally used in culinary or medicinal teas to treat digestive problems and intestinal parasites because of their revitalising flavour and scent [143]. Owing to its anti-inflammatory, anti-emetic, antispasmodic, sudorific, analgesic, and stimulant properties, the genus Mentha has reportedly been used in traditional medicine for the treatment of nausea, bronchitis, flatulence, anorexia, ulcerative colitis, and liver problems [144 - 147]. Additionally, it is already reported in the literature that various *Mentha species*, including *M. spicata*, *M. piperita*, *M. arvensis*, *M. rotundifolia*, *M. suaveolens*, and *M. pulegium*, have antibacterial and antioxidant properties in their essential oils or extracts [148 - 150].

The aromatic plant known as the *European pennyroyal*, or *M. pulegium*, is a member of the Lamiaceae family and is native to Southwestern and Central Europe, Asia, Iran, Arab nations, and Ethiopia. Traditional uses for its oil extracts and dry parts include aromatherapy, cosmetics, and medicine (for conditions such as gout, colds, amenorrhea, increased urination, skin ailments, and abortifacients), as well as in cooking (as a culinary herb) [151, 152]. Most research on *M. pulegium* conducted to date has used its essential oil and has occurred in various parts of the world, including Iran [153], Greece [154], Turkey [155], and Portugal [156]. These studies have primarily focused on the chemical makeup of the plant. The *M. pulegium* sultry water extract showed the maximum antioxidant activity and phenol concentration, according to this study's approved conclusions. The essential oil, however, had strong antimicrobial characteristics. As a result, the essential oil and extracts of *M. pulegium* have enormous promise as natural preservative substitutes in the pabulum business. Before thinking about its use in pabulum preservation or therapeutic applications, further research should be done to determine the extracts' safety and toxicity for human consumption [157].

The blooming aerial parts of *M. pulegium* L. have historically played a significant role as an antiseptic for the treatment of bronchitis, TB, pabulum poisoning, algid, and sinusitis, as well as antiflatulent, carminative, expectorant, diuretic, and menstruate [158, 159]. The findings indicated that piperitone and piperitenone made up the majority of the oil from south Iran (71.1%) and that this oil is of the piperitone/piperitenone kind. Depending on the kind of organism, the oil exhibited an inhibitory or germicidal impact that demonstrated antimicrobial activity against Gram-positive bacteria, predominantly *S. aureus*. This study demonstrated the antibacterial properties of *M. pulegium* L.'s oil [160].

2.6. Rosemary

The phenolic and volatile components of the rosemary plant are primarily responsible for the plant's biological actions [161 - 164] such as a-pinene, (_)-bornyl acetate, camphor, eucalyptol, carnosol, carnosic acid, and rosmarinic acid contained in the EO, found in the extract of rosemary respectively [161 - 163]. Owed to the likelihood of a synergistic effect among their components, few components may have a potential impact on biological activity [165].

R. officinalis L. can be utilized as fresh, dried, or as a tea additive. Essential oil and extracts of Rosemary can be purchased and used in food packaging, aromatherapy, and medical treatments [167 - 170]. Rosemary is used in food as a flavouring agent, preservative, in cosmetics [170, 171], or in folk medicine for antimicrobial, antiinflammatory, diuretics, as well as for the prevention and treatment of diabetes, cancer, cardiovascular diseases [161, 163, 165, 172 - 174] and for improvement of nervous system (Fig. **1**). Protein, fibre, vitamins, and minerals found in rosemary are identified to exhibit disease-preventing characteristics (United States Department of Agriculture) [175].

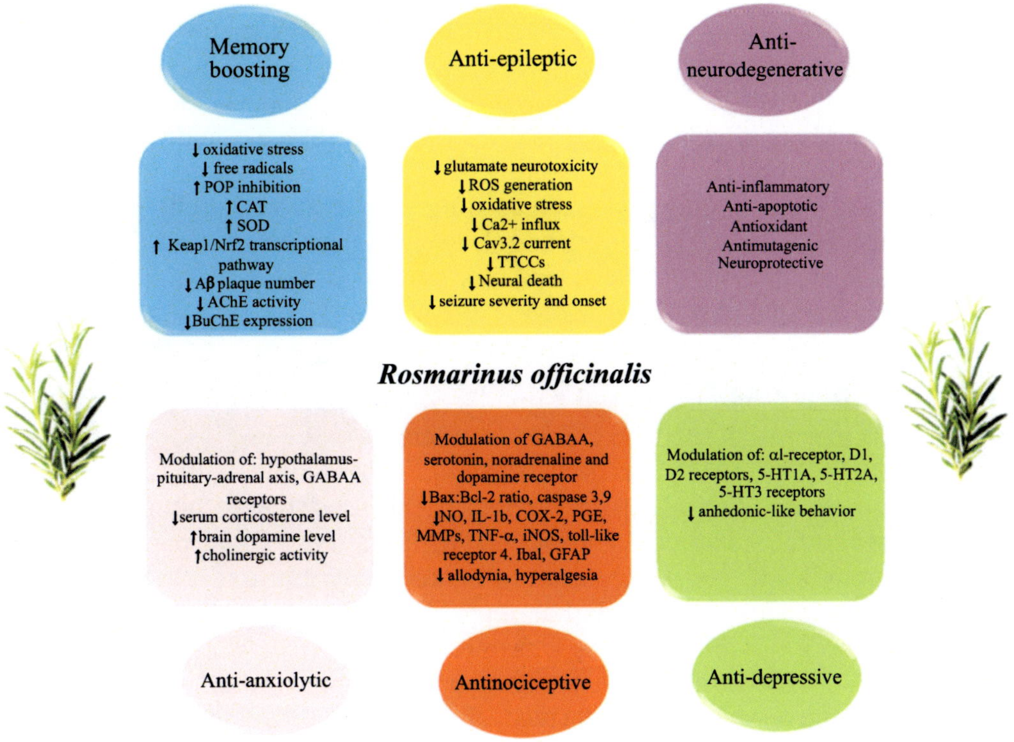

Fig. (1). Neuropharmacological properties of rosemary on the nervous system [166].

2.7. Eucalyptus

The Myrtaceae family includes native Australian eucalyptus trees, which are often known as eucalyptus and include more than 700 distinct species. The EOs from the *Eucalyptus species* are known for their antibacterial properties [176]. The terpene 1,8-cineole, also known as eucalyptol, is the primary component of eucalyptus EOs and variation in its concentration has been observed in different species [176, 177]. This substance's concentration ranges from 44% to 84%, and it is known to have significant antibacterial action [176]. The 18 most popularly traded essential oils in the world are all from *Eucalyptus species* [176]. *E. globulus* and *E. radiata* are two well-known species that produce essential oils (EOs), which are highly sought after by consumers because they can be used as anaesthetics, antiseptics, astringents, deodorants, disinfectants, expectorants, febrifuges, fumigants, inhalants, insect repellants, and as a folk remedy for abscesses, arthritis, asthma, boils [178, 179].

Typically, eucalyptus is produced for its wood, which is used to make cellulose pulp in the first place and then for board and panels [180, 181]. The essential oils produced by steam or hydrodistillation from *Eucalyptus species* are widely known. These are among the most frequently traded oils in the world and have been widely used in the perfume and scent industries [182]. Since ancient times, essential oils from this plant species have been used as an antibacterial, antipyretic, and analgesic [180]. Numerous biological actions, including antibacterial, fungicidal, insect-repelling, fumigant, pesticidal, and acaricidal activities, have been found [182]. According to earlier research, *E. citriodora* essential oil has antibacterial, antifungal, anticandidal, insecticidal, acaricidal, antitrypanosomal, and herbicidal properties [182 - 185].

2.8. Lippia

Northeastern Brazil has long used *Lippia gracilis* Schauer (Verbenaceae), also known as "alecrim-da-chapada" and "candeia-de-queimar," for a variety of therapeutic uses. Different plant parts of *Lippia species* are used as folk medicine for the treatment of skin ailments, wounds, abscesses, burns, cough, influenza, sinusitis, bronchitis, nasal congestion, headache, jaundice, and paralysis. [186 - 188]. Traditionally, its leaves are used to make an alcoholic macerate for topical treatment, infusion or decoction that may be used as a tea [189]. Numerous studies examining the pharmacologic properties of *L. griseus* have demonstrated the antibacterial, larvicidal, molluscicidal, antinociceptive, and anti-inflammatory properties of the essential oil derived from the plant's leaves [190 - 193]. Additionally, the methanolic extract of *L. gracilis* leaves has been shown to exhibit anti-nociceptive and anti-inflammatory properties [194].

2.9. Boswellia

The resin used to make frankincense comes from *Boswellia* tree species. In Chinese and Ayurvedic medicine, frankincense resin, its extract, and essential oil have historically been widely used for a variety of health objectives [195]. Traditional uses of frankincense essential oil (FREO)1 include its ability to reduce inflammation. FREO has recently gained popularity for supporting skin health. First, the research described how FREO affected the levels of 17 important biomarkers related to tissue remodelling, immunological replication, and inflammation in skin cells. Furthermore, using genome-wide analysis of the same cells, the impact of FREO on the expression levels of 21,224 genes was examined. In these cells, FREO had a sizable antiproliferative effect. Collagen III, IP-10, and ICAM-1 were all strongly suppressed by FREO during their development. A genome-wide study of gene expression revealed that FREO influenced the expression of the ecumenical gene. Inflammation and tissue remodeling-related signalling pathways were also severely impacted. An *in vitro* study revealed that FREO caused cell death in J82 bladder cancer cells through oxidative stress that was mediated by NRF-2 [196]. FREO and/or its main component, alpha-pinene, have also been demonstrated to have antiproliferative and proapoptotic effects on a number of different cancer cell types [197, 198]. To understand the biochemical mechanism of action of FREO, more investigation into its actions on cancer cells is required.

2.10. Lavender

A plant known as lavender has sedative, emotional, soothing, antibacterial, analgesic, and antispasmodic rejuvenating qualities. It is also effective in overcoming mild depression [199 - 203]. Linalool, linalyl acetate, 1,8-cineole B-ocimene, terpinen-4-ol, and camphor make up the majority of lavender's chemical composition. This plant's linalyl and linalyl acetate have the ability to activate the parasympathetic nervous system. Linalool works as a sedative, and linalyl acetate produces narcotic effects when combined [202, 204].

2.11. Rose

Rose relieves tension headaches, heart palpitations, dermatitis, sleeplessness, and dejection [205]. Rose has a beautiful, upbeat perfume that helps to reduce anxiety. Citronellal and 2-phenyl ethyl alcohol, which are found in rose, have analgesic and anxiety relieving properties [199, 206].

2.12. Marjoram

Oreganum majorana, often known as marjoram or “khezama” in Tunisia, is extensively used for both culinary and medicinal purposes [207]. Marjoram oil has also been used as an antiseptic, expectorant, and sedative, as well as for the treatment of dyspepsia, insomnia, rheumatism, migraine, dysmenorrhea, and dysentery [208]. This is due to the oil's spicy herbaceous overtones. Infusions of *O. majorana* are also often made and used as stimulants, sudorifics, emmenagogues, and galactagogues to treat a variety of health conditions and disturbances, such as heart and blood disorders, pyrexias, leucoderma, inflammation, asthma, hysteria, and paralysis [209, 210]. Due to the antioxidant, antimicrobial, cytotoxic, and acetycholinesterase properties of O. majorana EO, there is strong evidence to support its potential for being used as a natural agent in a variety of applications, such as cosmetics industry, food preservation, skin disorders, pharmaceutical compositions, and therapeutics. Further *in vivo* studies and clinical trials are required in light of these alluring qualities in order to further validate the potential of this EO and better comprehend the mode of function of its bioactive compounds.

2.13. Pomegranate

Pomegranate juice (POMj) is known to provide a number of health advantages. Pomegranates play a significant role in the treatment of widespread diseases and also play a significant role in the treatment of risk factors, including high blood pressure, hyperlipidemia, oxidative stress, high blood sugar, and inflammatory activity [211 - 213]. When compared to other polyphenols like resveratrol, POMj has a higher bioavailability of its total phenolic content and antioxidant potential [214]. POMj's effectiveness may be linked to the high levels of polyphenols and nitrates in the substance. In fact, earlier studies on polyphenol supplementation have shown an improvement in blood flow, vessel dilation, and endothelial function and a protective role for cardiovascular diseases [215 - 217], oxidative stress, [218 - 220] as polyphenols rich diet may be associated with reduced incidence of cardiovascular disorders. The effect of plasma concentrations of metabolites and other endogenous antioxidants and reducing agents on (i) concentrations of other endogenous antioxidants and reducing agents, and (ii) the absorption of pro-oxidative food components, such as iron, has been used to explain the powerful protective effect of polyphenol-rich foods [221]. Similarly, nitrate supplementation has been shown to improve exercise tolerance and performance while reducing blood pressure [222] and oxygen uptake [223]. It also increases oxygenation (*e.g.*, blood flow) in skeletal muscle [224] and mitochondrial efficiency [225]. Increased endothelial nitric oxide synthase expression and nitric oxide generation might explain this putative ergogenic impact of nitrate-opulent supplements [226, 227]. Among the older population, natural POMj appears to be an effective anti-inflammatory, anti-muscle damage, and anti-thrombocytopenia medication. In light of this, it is encouraged to incorporate such supplements into the behavioural guidelines for the senior population.

2.14. Cinnamon

Known for its antibacterial and anti-inflammation properties, cinnamon has been widely used in traditional medicine to treat diabetes [228, 229], and lipid peroxidation. Cinnamaldehyde (CA) is a key component of cinnamon [230].

Known biological properties of CA include anti-candidal, anti-inflammatory, and free radical scavenging activities [231 - 233]; as well as significant effects on cardiovascular disorders, such as vasorelaxation and reductions in blood pressure associated with diabetes [234].

2.15. Glycyrrhiza

The plant species belonging to *Glycyrrhiza* genus, generally well-known as licorice, is widely used around the globe for food and medicinal purposes. In particular, *G. glabra* L. and the metabolite glycyrrhizin (glycyrrhizic acid) have been studied intensely for their effects on human beings. The genus includes plants having bioactive molecules encompassing triterpene saponins (*e.g.*, glycyrrhizin) and flavonoids (*e.g.*, liquiritigenin, liquiritin) [235]. EOs derived from the aerial parts of *G. triphylla* were assessed for their phytochemicals and biological (antimicrobial, antioxidant, antiseptic, and anticancer) properties. The EOs contained a total of 55 chemicals, mainly present in 99.3% of the oil content, which were composed of β-caryophyllene (25.4%), limonene (16.7%), β-myrcene (16.0%), and ahumulene (4.4%). Sesquiterpene hydrocarbons, which made up 43.6% of the total oil, were the main component of the oil. The oil was resolutely effective against eight bacterial species and one fungus at both its minimum inhibitory concentration (MIC) and minimum bactericidal concentration (MBC). Gram-negative and Gram-positive bacteria were both successfully combatted by the EO's potent antibacterial properties [236]. Due to its significant potential in the treatment of different ailments, research was conducted to examine the possible role of different elicitor concentrations on the biomass enhancement and their effects on different metabolites, particularly phenol, alkaloid, flavonoid and glycyrrhizin [237].

2.16. Dictamnus

Dictamnus species have anticancerous, antinociceptive, antiphlogistic, antiviral, antibacterial, and antioxidant effects, owing to their use in human medicine [238]. The Xinjiang Province of China is home to the *Dictamnus angustifolius* (Rutaceae) plant, a perennial herb with a strong aroma whose roots have been used as an alternative to traditional medicine for various ailments. It is used to cure rheumatism, bleeding, itching, jaundice, chronic hepatitis, and skin infections [239 - 241]. Additionally, it has found its application in febrifugal, detoxicant, and anti-inflammatory medications [242, 243].

CONCLUSION

Essential oils (EOs) are incredibly potent, naturally occurring fragrant liquids produced by the plant. When used carefully, they may be a great asset in aromatherapy, therapies, personal care, and other applications related to health and mind.

Plants generate EOs from various plant components from which they originate. Some plants store their valuable volatile aromatic compounds in their leaves or flowers, whereas others may accumulate them in their bark, roots, peels, seeds, or other plant components.

EOs are extracted by steam or dihydrogen monoxide distillation from the leaves, flowers, wood, buds, bark, roots, and other plant parts of aromatic plants such as citronella, lavender, palmarosa, cedarwood, rose, *etc*. The quality, scent, medicinal advantages, and cost of essential oils vary mostly depending on the plant's rarity, the region of origin, the climate for culture, the engenderment mechanism, and the amount of oil the plants produce. The method which is utilized to get yield oil from different plant components regulates its standard as an essential oil or a carrier oil (vegetable oil). If the oil is engendered through steam distillation, it is a volatile, aromatic essential oil, and if the oil is expeller pressed/cold pressed, it is a lipid-predicated.

With increased pharmacological awareness in recent decades on the safe properties of natural plant-based oils, the use of these oils in herbal remedies has increased. But until further conclusive tribulations show the safety, quality, and efficacy of these EOs, clinicians should exercise caution. The broad spectrum of biological characteristics of plants, including as their species-specific antibacterial, antimicrobial, antioxidant, antitumor, antidiabetic, anxiolytic, sedative, and anti-inflammatory qualities, help to explain why they are so effective in treating a range of illnesses in people.

Despite being extremely effective alternative antimicrobial agents, especially against pabulum-borne microbes, there is a considerable lack of information regarding their toxicity profiles. In the forthcoming days, more studies should be designed with extensive pharmacological and chemical experiments, along with human metabolism.

REFERENCES

[1] Bakkali F, Averbeck S, Averbeck D, Idaomar M. Biological effects of essential oils – A review. Food Chem Toxicol 2008; 46(2): 446-75. [http://dx.doi.org/10.1016/j.fct.2007.09.106] [PMID: 17996351]

[2] Najafian L, Babji AS. Production of bioactive peptides using enzymatic hydrolysis and identification antioxidative peptides from patin (*Pangasius sutchi*) sarcoplasmic protein hydolysate. J Funct Foods 2014; 9: 280-9. [http://dx.doi.org/10.1016/j.jff.2014.05.003]

[3] Kuorwel KK, Cran MJ, Sonneveld K, Miltz J, Bigger SW. Essential oils and their principal constituents as antimicrobial agents for synthetic packaging films. J Food Sci 2011; 76(9): R164-77.

[http://dx.doi.org/10.1111/j.1750-3841.2011.02384.x] [PMID: 22416718]

[4] Adorjan B, Buchbauer G. Biological properties of essential oils: an updated review. Flavour Fragrance J 2010; 25(6): 407-26.
[http://dx.doi.org/10.1002/ffj.2024]

[5] Ali B, Al-Wabel NA, Shams S, Ahamad A, Khan SA, Anwar F. Essential oils used in aromatherapy: A systemic review. Asian Pac. J. Trop. Biomed. 2015; 5(8): 601-11.
[http://dx.doi.org/10.1016/j.apjtb.2015.05.007]

[6] Candan F, Unlu M, Tepe B, *et al.* Antioxidant and antimicrobial activity of the essential oil and methanol extracts of Achillea millefolium subsp. millefolium Afan. (Asteraceae). J Ethnopharmacol 2003; 87(2-3): 215-20.
[http://dx.doi.org/10.1016/S0378-8741(03)00149-1] [PMID: 12860311]

[7] Friedman M. Chemistry and multibeneficial bioactivities of carvacrol (4-isopropyl-2-methylphenol), a component of essential oils produced by aromatic plants and spices. J Agric Food Chem 2014; 62(31): 7652-70.
[http://dx.doi.org/10.1021/jf5023862] [PMID: 25058878]

[8] Tohidi B, Rahimmalek M, Arzani A, Sabzalian MR. Thymol, carvacrol, and antioxidant accumulation in *Thymus species* in response to different light spectra emitted by light-emitting diodes. Food Chem 2020; 307: 125521.
[http://dx.doi.org/10.1016/j.foodchem.2019.125521] [PMID: 31655264]

[9] Sharifi-Rad M, Varoni EM, Iriti M, *et al.* Carvacrol and human health: A comprehensive review. Phytother Res 2018; 32(9): 1675-87.
[http://dx.doi.org/10.1002/ptr.6103] [PMID: 29744941]

[10] Nabavi S, Di Lorenzo A, Izadi M, Sobarzo-Sánchez E, Daglia M, Nabavi S. Antibacterial effects of cinnamon: From farm to food, cosmetic and pharmaceutical industries. Nutrients 2015; 7(9): 7729-48.
[http://dx.doi.org/10.3390/nu7095359] [PMID: 26378575]

[11] Ghasemi Pirbalouti A, Hashemi M, Ghahfarokhi FT. Essential oil and chemical compositions of wild and cultivated Thymus daenensis Celak and Thymus vulgaris L. Ind Crops Prod 2013; 48: 43-8.
[http://dx.doi.org/10.1016/j.indcrop.2013.04.004]

[12] Bozin B, Mimica-Dukic N, Samojlik I, Jovin E. Antimicrobial and antioxidant properties of rosemary and sage (Rosmarinus officinalis L. and Sal*via* officinalis L., Lamiaceae) essential oils. J Agric Food Chem 2007; 55(19): 7879-85.
[http://dx.doi.org/10.1021/jf0715323] [PMID: 17708648]

[13] Wedge DE, Tabanca N, Sampson BJ, *et al.* Antifungal and insecticidal activity of two Juniperus essential oils. Nat Prod Commun 2009; 4(1): 1934578X0900400.
[http://dx.doi.org/10.1177/1934578X0900400127] [PMID: 19370889]

[14] Iacobellis NS, Lo Cantore P, Capasso F, Senatore F. Antibacterial activity of *Cuminum cyminum* L. and *Carum carvi* L. essential oils. J Agric Food Chem 2005; 53(1): 57-61.
[http://dx.doi.org/10.1021/jf0487351] [PMID: 15631509]

[15] Arruda TA, Antunes RMP, Catão RMR, *et al.* Preliminary study of the antimicrobial activity of Mentha x villosa Hudson essential oil, rotundifolone and its analogues. Rev Bras Farmacogn 2006; 16(3): 307-11.
[http://dx.doi.org/10.1590/S0102-695X2006000300005]

[16] Kacem R, Meraihi Z. Effects of essential oil extracted from *Nigella sativa* (L.) seeds and its main components on human neutrophil elastase activity. Yakugaku Zasshi 2006; 126(4): 301-5.
[http://dx.doi.org/10.1248/yakushi.126.301] [PMID: 16596021]

[17] De Vincenzi M, Stammati A, De Vincenzi A, Silano M. Constituents of aromatic plants: carvacrol. Fitoterapia 2004; 75(7-8): 801-4.
[http://dx.doi.org/10.1016/j.fitote.2004.05.002] [PMID: 15567271]

[18] Jenner PM, Hagan EC, Taylor JM, Cook EL, Fitzhugh OG. Food flavourings and compounds of related structure I. Acute oral toxicity. Food Cosmet Toxicol 1964; 2: 327-43. [http://dx.doi.org/10.1016/S0015-6264(64)80192-9]

[19] Fenaroli G. Fenaroli's Handbook of Flavor Ingredients. 4th ed., Boca Raton, FL, USA: CRC 2001.

[20] Raina VK, Kumar A, Srivastava SK, Syamsundar KV, Kahol AP. Essential oil composition of 'kewda' (*Pandanus odoratissimus*) from India. Flavour Fragrance J 2004; 19(5): 434-6. [http://dx.doi.org/10.1002/ffj.1331]

[21] Harrathi J, Hosni K, Karray-Bouraoui N, *et al.* Effect of salt stress on growth, fatty acids and essential oils in safflower (Carthamus tinctorius L.). Naunyn Schmiedebergs Arch Pharmacol 2012; 34: 129-37.

[22] de Sousa DP, Quintans L Jr, de Almeida RN. Evolution of the Anticonvulsant Activity of α-Terpineol. Pharm Biol 2007; 45(1): 69-70. [http://dx.doi.org/10.1080/13880200601028388]

[23] Quintans-Júnior LJ, Oliveira MGB, Santana MF, *et al.* α-Terpineol reduces nociceptive behavior in mice. Pharm Biol 2011; 49(6): 583-6. [http://dx.doi.org/10.3109/13880209.2010.529616] [PMID: 21385090]

[24] Ribeiro TP, Porto DL, Menezes CP, *et al.* Unravelling the cardiovascular effects induced by α-terpineol: A role for the nitric oxide–cGMP pathway. Clin Exp Pharmacol Physiol 2010; 37(8): 811-6. [http://dx.doi.org/10.1111/j.1440-1681.2010.05383.x] [PMID: 20374260]

[25] Vila R, Santana AI, Pérez-Rosés R, *et al.* Composition and biological activity of the essential oil from leaves of Plinia cerrocampanensis, a new source of α-bisabolol. Bioresour Technol 2010; 101(7): 2510-4. [http://dx.doi.org/10.1016/j.biortech.2009.11.021] [PMID: 20015638]

[26] Leite GO, Leite LHI, Sampaio RS, *et al.* (−)-α-Bisabolol attenuates visceral nociception and inflammation in mice. Fitoterapia 2011; 82(2): 208-11. [http://dx.doi.org/10.1016/j.fitote.2010.09.012] [PMID: 20875845]

[27] Silva MTM, Ribeiro FPRA, Medeiros MAMB, *et al.* The vasorelaxant effect of p-cymene in rat aorta involves potassium channels. ScientificWorldJournal 2015; 2015: 1-6. [http://dx.doi.org/10.1155/2015/458080] [PMID: 25667938]

[28] Peskar BM, Ehrlich K, Peskar BA. Interaction of cyclooxygenase-2 inhibitors and salicylate in gastric mucosal damage. Eur J Pharmacol 2002; 434(1-2): 65-70. [http://dx.doi.org/10.1016/S0014-2999(01)01524-2] [PMID: 11755167]

[29] Craveiro AA, Andrade CHS, Matos FJA, Alencar JW, Dantas TNC. Fixed and volatile constituents of *Croton aff. nepetifolius.* J Nat Prod 1980; 43(6): 756-7. [http://dx.doi.org/10.1021/np50012a010] [PMID: 20707400]

[30] Chainy GBN, Manna SK, Chaturvedi MM, Aggarwal BB. Anethole blocks both early and late cellular responses transduced by tumor necrosis factor: effect on NF-κB, AP-1, JNK, MAPKK and apoptosis. Oncogene 2000; 19(25): 2943-50. [http://dx.doi.org/10.1038/sj.onc.1203614] [PMID: 10871845]

[31] Ghelardini C, Galeotti N, Di Cesare Mannelli L, Mazzanti G, Bartolini A. Local anaesthetic activity of β-caryophyllene. Farmaco 2001; 56(5-7): 387-9. [http://dx.doi.org/10.1016/S0014-827X(01)01092-8] [PMID: 11482764]

[32] Ertas A, Yigitkan S, Orhan IE. A Focused review on cognitive improvement by the genus *salvia* l. (sage)—from ethnopharmacology to clinical evidence. Pharmaceuticals 2023; 16(2): 171. [http://dx.doi.org/10.3390/ph16020171] [PMID: 37259321]

[33] Kamatou GPP, Van Zyl RL, Van Vuuren SF, *et al.* Seasonal variation in essential oil composition, oil toxicity and the biological activity of solvent extracts of three South African *Salvia species.* S Afr J Bot 2008; 74(2): 230-7.

[http://dx.doi.org/10.1016/j.sajb.2007.08.002]

[34] Kamatou GPP, Makunga NP, Ramogola WPN, Viljoen AM. South African Sal*via* species: A review of biological activities and phytochemistry. J Ethnopharmacol 2008; 119(3): 664-72. [http://dx.doi.org/10.1016/j.jep.2008.06.030] [PMID: 18640254]

[35] Böszörményi A, Héthelyi É, Farkas Á, *et al.* Chemical and genetic relationships among sage (Sal*via* officinalis L.) cultivars and Judean sage (Sal*via* judaica Boiss.). J Agric Food Chem 2009; 57(11): 4663-7. [http://dx.doi.org/10.1021/jf9005092] [PMID: 19449812]

[36] Hamidpour M, Hamidpour R, Hamidpour S, Shahlari M. Chemistry, pharmacology, and medicinal property of sage (sal*via*) to prevent and cure illnesses such as obesity, diabetes, depression, dementia, lupus, autism, heart disease, and cancer. J Tradit Complement Med 2014; 4(2): 82-8. [http://dx.doi.org/10.4103/2225-4110.130373] [PMID: 24860730]

[37] Ryu S, Lee C, Choi S. *In vitro* cytotoxicity of tanshinones from Sal*via* miltiorrhiza. Planta Med 1997; 63(4): 339-42. [http://dx.doi.org/10.1055/s-2006-957696] [PMID: 9270379]

[38] Longaray Delamare AP, Moschen-Pistorello IT, Artico L, Atti-Serafini L, Echeverrigaray S. Antibacterial activity of the essential oils of Sal*via* officinalis L. and Sal*via* triloba L. cultivated in South Brazil. Food Chem 2007; 100(2): 603-8. [http://dx.doi.org/10.1016/j.foodchem.2005.09.078]

[39] Loizzo MR, Tundis R, Menichini F, Saab AM, Statti GA, Menichini F. Cytotoxic activity of essential oils from labiatae and lauraceae families against *In vitro* human tumor models. Anticancer Res 2007; 27(5A): 3293-9. [PMID: 17970073]

[40] Loizzo MR, Saab AM, Tundis R, *et al. In vitro* inhibitory activities of plants used in Lebanon traditional medicine against angiotensin converting enzyme (ACE) and digestive enzymes related to diabetes. J Ethnopharmacol 2008; 119(1): 109-16. [http://dx.doi.org/10.1016/j.jep.2008.06.003] [PMID: 18601990]

[41] Kelen M, Tepe B. Chemical composition, antioxidant and antimicrobial properties of the essential oils of three Sal*via* species from Turkish flora. Bioresour Technol 2008; 99(10): 4096-104. [http://dx.doi.org/10.1016/j.biortech.2007.09.002] [PMID: 17936619]

[42] Ulubelen A, Öksüz S, Kolak U, *et al.* Diterpenoids from the roots of Sal*via* bracteata. Phytochemistry 1999; 52(8): 1455-9. [http://dx.doi.org/10.1016/S0031-9422(99)00453-7]

[43] Kilic T, Dirmenci T, Satil F, *et al.* Fatty acid compositions of seed oils of three Turkish Sal*via* species and biological activities. Chem Nat Compd 2005; 41(3): 276-9. [http://dx.doi.org/10.1007/s10600-005-0128-5]

[44] Ozen HC, Toker Z, Ertekin AS. Essential oil composition of two Sal*via* species from Turkey. AFS. Adv Food Sci 2004; 26: 32-4.

[45] Amiri H. Quantitative and qualitative changes of essential oil of Sal*via* bracteata Bank et Sol. In different growth stages. DARU-J Faculty Pharma 2007; 15: 79-82.

[46] Sefidkon' F, Hooshidary F, Jamzad Z. Chemical variation in the essential oil of Sal*via* bracteata Banks & Soland from Iran. J Essent Oil-Bear Plants 2007; 10(4): 265-72. [http://dx.doi.org/10.1080/0972060X.2007.10643552]

[47] Cardile V, Russo A, Formisano C, *et al.* Essential oils of Salvia bracteata and Salvia rubifolia from Lebanon: Chemical composition, antimicrobial activity and inhibitory effect on human melanoma cells. J Ethnopharmacol 2009; 126(2): 265-72. [http://dx.doi.org/10.1016/j.jep.2009.08.034]

[48] Tenore GC, Ciampaglia R, Arnold NA, *et al.* Antimicrobial and antioxidant properties of the essential

oil of Salvia lanigera from Cyprus. Food Chem Toxicol 2011; 49(1): 238-43. [http://dx.doi.org/10.1016/j.fct.2010.10.022] [PMID: 20977923]

[49] Russo A, Formisano C, Rigano D, *et al.* Chemical composition and anticancer activity of essential oils of Mediterranean sage (Salvia officinalis L.) grown in different environmental conditions. Food Chem Toxicol 2013; 55: 42-7. [http://dx.doi.org/10.1016/j.fct.2012.12.036] [PMID: 23291326]

[50] Hooper M. Herbs and Medicinal Plants. London: Kingfisher 1984; p. 125.

[51] Dragland S, Senoo H, Wake K, Holte K, Blomhoff R. Several culinary and medicinal herbs are important sources of dietary antioxidants. J Nutr 2003; 133(5): 1286-90. [http://dx.doi.org/10.1093/jn/133.5.1286] [PMID: 12730411]

[52] Ravindran PN, Geetha S, Pillai K. Under-utilized herbs and spices,In Woodhead Publishing Series in Food Science, Technology and Nutrition. Handbook of Herbs and Spices. Woodhead Publishing 2004.

[53] Lugasi A, Hóvári J, Hagymási K, Jakóczi I, Blázovics A. Antioxidant properties of a mixture of Lamiaceae plants intended to use as a food additive. Acta Aliment 2006; 35(1): 85-97. [http://dx.doi.org/10.1556/AAlim.35.2006.1.10]

[54] Vendittia A, Biancoa A, Frezzab C, *et al.* Essential oil composition, polar compounds, glandular trichomes and biological activity of Hyssopus officinalis subsp. aristatus (Godr.) Nyman from central Italy. Industrial crops and products. 2015 Dec 23; 77: 353-63.

[55] Lawles J. The Encyclopedia of Essential Oils. London, UK: Thorsons 2001.

[56] Steinmetz MD, Tognetti P, Morgue M, Jouglard J, And Millet Y. Sur la toxicitéde certaines huiles essentielles du commerce: Essence d'hysope et essence desauge. Plantes Méd. Phytothér 1980; 14: 34-45.

[57] Jankovský M, Landa T. Genus Hyssopus L. - recent knowledge: A review. Hortic Sci 2002; 29(3): 119-23. [http://dx.doi.org/10.17221/4474-HORTSCI]

[58] Gorunovic MS, Bogavac PM, Chalchat JC, Chabard JL. Essential oil of hyssopus officinalis of montenegro origin. J Essent Oil Res 1995; 7(1): 39-43. [http://dx.doi.org/10.1080/10412905.1995.9698459]

[59] Schulz G, Stahl-Biskup E. Essential oils and glycosidic bound volatiles from leaves, stems, flowers and roots of *Hyssopus officinalis* L. (lamiaceae). Flavour Fragrance J 1991; 6(1): 69-73. [http://dx.doi.org/10.1002/ffj.2730060109]

[60] Leung AY, Foster S. Encyclopedia of common natural ingredients used in Food, Drugs, and Cosmetics. New York, USA: John Wiley & Sons 2003.

[61] ISO. Oil of Hyssop Hyssopus officinalis L Ssp Officinalis. 2nd ed.., Geneva, Switzerland: International Organisation for Standardization 2007.

[62] Gilani AH, Shah AJ, Zubair A, *et al.* Chemical composition and mechanisms underlying the spasmolytic and bronchodilatory properties of the essential oil of Nepeta cataria L. J Ethnopharmacol 2009; 121(3): 405-11. [http://dx.doi.org/10.1016/j.jep.2008.11.004] [PMID: 19041706]

[63] Formisano C, Rigano D, Senatore F. Chemical constituents and biological activities of *Nepeta* species. Chem Biodivers 2011; 8(10): 1783-818. [http://dx.doi.org/10.1002/cbdv.201000191] [PMID: 22006710]

[64] Sakurai K, Ikeda K, And Mori K. Both (4as, 7S, 7ar)-(+)-nepetalactone and itsantipode are powerful attractants for cats. Agric Biol Chem 1988; 52(9): 2369-71.

[65] Birkett MA, Hassanali A, Hoglund S, Pettersson J, Pickett JA. Repellent activity of catmint, Nepeta cataria, and iridoid nepetalactone isomers against Afro-tropical mosquitoes, ixodid ticks and red poultry mites. Phytochemistry 2011; 72(1): 109-14.

[http://dx.doi.org/10.1016/j.phytochem.2010.09.016] [PMID: 21056438]

[66] Zomorodian K, Saharkhiz MJ, Rahimi MJ, Shariatifard S, Pakshir K, Khashei R. Chemical composition and antimicrobial activities of essential oil of *nepeta cataria L.* Against common causes of oral infections. J Dent 2013; 10(4): 329-37. [PMID: 24396352]

[67] Grbic-Ljaljevic M, Stupar M, Vukojevic J, *et al.* Antifungal activity of Nepeta rtanjensis essential oil. J Serb Chem Soc 2008; 73(10): 961-5. [http://dx.doi.org/10.2298/JSC0810961G]

[68] Nestorović J, Mišić D, Šiler B, *et al.* Nepetalactone content in shoot cultures of three endemic *Nepeta species* and the evaluation of their antimicrobial activity. Fitoterapia 2010; 81(6): 621-6. [http://dx.doi.org/10.1016/j.fitote.2010.03.007] [PMID: 20307630]

[69] Kobaisy M, Tellez MR, Dayan FE, *et al.* Composition and phytotoxic activity of Nepetapannonica L. Essential oil. J Essent Oil Res 2005; 17(6): 704-7. [http://dx.doi.org/10.1080/10412905.2005.9699037]

[70] Dmitrovi'c S. Essential oils of two *Nepeta species* inhibitgrowth and induce oxidative stress in ragweed shoots *In vitro*. Acta Physiol Plant 2015; 37: 1-15.

[71] Nestorovi'c Z. Allelopathic potential of essential oil of Nepeta rtanjensis? Allelopathy J 2016; 37(2): 207-19.

[72] Rigano D, Arnold NA, Conforti F, *et al.* Characterisation of the essential oil of *Nepeta glomerata* Montbret et Aucher ex Bentham from Lebanon and its biological activities. Nat Prod Res 2011; 25(6): 614-26. [http://dx.doi.org/10.1080/14786419.2010.488623] [PMID: 21409723]

[73] Tsuruoka T, Bekh-Ochir D, Kato F, *et al.* The essential oil of Mongolian *Nepeta sibirica* : A single component and its biological activities. J Essent Oil Res 2012; 24(6): 555-9. [http://dx.doi.org/10.1080/10412905.2012.729925]

[74] Kahkeshani N, Razzaghirad Y, Ostad SN, *et al.* Cytotoxic, acetylcholinesterase inhibitor and antioxidant activity of Nepetamenthoides Boiss & Buhse essential oil. J Essent. J Essent Oil-Bear Plants 2014; 17(4): 544-52. [http://dx.doi.org/10.1080/0972060X.2014.929040]

[75] Shakeri A, Khakdan F, Soheili V, Sahebkar A, Rassam G, And Asili J. Chemicalcomposition, antibacterial activity, and cytotoxicity of essential oil from Nepeta ucrainica L. Spp KopetdaghensisInd Crop Prod 2014; 58: 315-21. [http://dx.doi.org/10.1016/j.indcrop.2014.04.009]

[76] Kumar V, Mathela CS, Tewari G, Singh D. Antifungal activity of Nepeta elliptica Royle ex Benth. oil and its major constituent (7R)-trans,trans-nepetalactone: A comparative study. Ind Crops Prod 2014; 55: 70-4. [http://dx.doi.org/10.1016/j.indcrop.2014.02.003]

[77] Mišić D, Šiler B, Gašić U, *et al.* Simultaneous UHPLC/DAD/(+/-)HESI-MS/MS analysis of phenolic acids and nepetalactones in methanol extracts of Nepeta species: a possible application in chemotaxonomic studies. Phytochem Anal 2015; 26(1): 72-85. [http://dx.doi.org/10.1002/pca.2538] [PMID: 25431035]

[78] Sharma A, And Cannoo DS. Phytochemical composition of essential oilsisolated from different species of genus Nepeta of Labiatae family: A review. Pharmacophore 2013; 4(6): 181-211.

[79] Stojanović G, Radulović N, Lazarević J, Miladinović D, Đoković D. Antimicrobial activity of Nepeta rtanjensis essential oil. J Essent Oil Res 2005; 17(5): 587-9. [http://dx.doi.org/10.1080/10412905.2005.9699004]

[80] Gkinis G, Tzakou O, Iliopoulou D, Roussis V. Chemical composition andbiological activity of Nepeta parnassica oils and isolated nepetalactones. Z Naturforsch C J Biosci 2003; 58(9-10): 681-6.

[http://dx.doi.org/10.1515/znc-2003-9-1015]

[81] Skori'ca M, Gligorijevi'cb N. Cytotoxic activity of Nepeta rtanjensis Dikli'c & Milojevi'c essential oiland its mode of action. Ind Crops Prod 2017; 100: 163-70. [http://dx.doi.org/10.1016/j.indcrop.2017.02.027]

[82] Zomorodian K, Saharkhiz MJ, Shariati S, Pakshir K, Rahimi MJ, Khashei R. Chemical composition and antimicrobial activities of essential oils from Nepeta cataria L. Against common causes of food-borne infections. ISRN Pharm 2012; 2012(1–6): 1-6. [http://dx.doi.org/10.5402/2012/591953] [PMID: 22779012]

[83] Nedorostova L, Kloucek P, Kokoska L, Stolcova M, Pulkrabek J. Antimicrobial properties of selected essential oils in vapour phase against foodborne bacteria. Food Control 2009; 20(2): 157-60. [http://dx.doi.org/10.1016/j.foodcont.2008.03.007]

[84] Mothana RA. Chemical composition, antimicrobial and antioxidant activities of the essential oil of Nepeta deflersiana growing in Yemen. Rec Nat Prod 2012; 6(2): 189-93.

[85] Salehi P, Sonboli A, Allahyari L. Antibacterial and antioxidant properties of the essential oil and various extracts of Nepeta ispahanica from Iran. J Essent Oil-Bear Plants 2007; 10(4): 324-31. [http://dx.doi.org/10.1080/0972060X.2007.10643563]

[86] Alim A, Goze I, Cetin A, Atas AD, Cetinus SA, Vural N. Chemical composition and *In vitro* antimicrobial and antioxidant activities of the essential oil of Nepeta nuda L. Subsp Albiflora (Boiss.) Gams. Afr J Microbiol Res 2009; 3(8): 463-7.

[87] El-moaty HIA. Essential oil and iridoide glycosides of Nepeta septemcrenata Erenb. J Nat Prod 2010; 3: 103-11.

[88] Bisht D, Padalia R, Singh L, Pande V, Lal P, Mathela C. Constituents and antimicrobial activity of the essential oils of six Himalayan Nepeta species. J Serb Chem Soc 2010; 75(6): 739-47. [http://dx.doi.org/10.2298/JSC091106052B]

[89] Mollova S, Dzhurmanski A, Fidan H, *et al.* Chemical composition of essential oils from *nepeta transcaucasica* grossh. and *nepeta cataria* L. ACS Omega 2023; 8(17): 15441-9. [http://dx.doi.org/10.1021/acsomega.3c00704] [PMID: 37151483]

[90] Saggoo MIS, Srivastava DK, Grewal P. Meiotic studies in 14 species of the Nepeta L. (Lamiaceae) from Cold Desert regions of Lahaul-spiti and adjoining areas of Northwest-Himalaya, India. Cytologia (Tokyo) 2011; 76(3): 231-6. [http://dx.doi.org/10.1508/cytologia.76.231]

[91] Joshi RK, Barbalho SM, Soulimani R. Chemical Constituents and Biological Activities of Genus Nepeta (Lamiaceae) from India and Western Himalaya: A Review. Int J Pharmacogn Chinese Med 2021; 5(1): 000219. [http://dx.doi.org/10.23880/ipcm-16000219]

[92] Asgarpanah J, Sarabian S, Ziarati P. Essential oil of *Nepeta* genus (Lamiaceae) from Iran: a review. J Essent Oil Res 2014; 26(1): 1-12. [http://dx.doi.org/10.1080/10412905.2013.851040]

[93] Hassan-Abdallah A, Merito A, Hassan S, *et al.* Medicinal plants and their uses by the people in the Region of Randa, Djibouti. J Ethnopharmacol 2013; 148(2): 701-13. [http://dx.doi.org/10.1016/j.jep.2013.05.033] [PMID: 23707214]

[94] Mamadalieva NZ, Akramov DK, Ovidi E, *et al.* Aromatic medicinal plants of the lamiaceae family from uzbekistan: Ethnopharmacology, essential oils composition, and biological activities. Medicines 2017; 4(1): 8.

[95] Hussain A I, Anwar F, Chatha S A S, Jabbar A, Mahboob S, Nigam P S. Essential oil: Antiproliferative, antioxidant and antibacterial activities. Brazilian J Microbiol 2010; 41: 1070e1107.

[96] Karaman S, Digrak M, Ravid U, Ilcim A. Antibacterial and antifungal activity of the essential oils of

Thymus revolutus Celak from Turkey. J Ethnopharmacol 2001; 76(2): 183-6. [http://dx.doi.org/10.1016/S0378-8741(01)00238-0] [PMID: 11390134]

[97] Maksimović Z, Stojanović D, Šoštarić I, Dajić Z, Ristić M. Composition and radical-scavenging activity of *Thymus glabrescens* Willd. (Lamiaceae) essential oil. J Sci Food Agric 2008; 88(11): 2036-41. [http://dx.doi.org/10.1002/jsfa.3311]

[98] Rota MC, Herrera A, Martínez RM, Sotomayor JA, Jordán MJ. Antimicrobial activity and chemical composition of Thymus vulgaris, Thymus zygis and Thymus hyemalis essential oils. Food Control 2008; 19(7): 681-7. [http://dx.doi.org/10.1016/j.foodcont.2007.07.007]

[99] de Carvalho RJ, de Souza GT, Honório VG, *et al.* Comparative inhibitory effects of Thymus vulgaris L. essential oil against Staphylococcus aureus, Listeria monocytogenes and mesophilic starter co-culture in cheese-mimicking models. Food Microbiol 2015; 52: 59-65. [http://dx.doi.org/10.1016/j.fm.2015.07.003] [PMID: 26338117]

[100] Pekmezovic M, Rajkovic K, Barac A, Senerović L, Arsic Arsenijevic V. Development of kinetic model for testing antifungal effect of Thymus vulgaris L. and Cinnamomum cassia L. essential oils on Aspergillus flavus spores and application for optimization of synergistic effect. Biochem Eng J 2015; 99: 131-7. [http://dx.doi.org/10.1016/j.bej.2015.03.024]

[101] Ferreira LE, Benincasa BI, Fachin AL, *et al.* Thymus vulgaris L. essential oil and its main component thymol: Anthelmintic effects against Haemonchus contortus from sheep. Vet Parasitol 2016; 228: 70-6. [http://dx.doi.org/10.1016/j.vetpar.2016.08.011] [PMID: 27692335]

[102] Pacifico S, Piccolella S, Papale F, Nocera P, Lettieri A, Catauro M. A polyphenol complex from Thymus vulgaris L. plants cultivated in the Campania Region (Italy): New perspectives against neuroblastoma. J Funct Foods 2016; 20: 253-66. [http://dx.doi.org/10.1016/j.jff.2015.11.008]

[103] Pereira E, Barros L, Antonio AL, Cabo Verde S, Santos-Buelga C, Ferreira ICFR. Infusions from Thymus vulgaris L. treated at different gamma radiation doses: Effects on antioxidant activity and phenolic composition. Lebensm Wiss Technol 2016; 74: 34-9. [http://dx.doi.org/10.1016/j.lwt.2016.07.027]

[104] Le Floc'h E, Boulous L. Flore De Tunisie, Catalogue SynonymiqueCommente. In: Floc'h L, Ed. Montpellier, France 2008; p. 461.

[105] Al-Asmari AK, Athar MT, Al-Faraidy AA, Almuhaiza MS. Chemical composition of essential oil of *Thymus vulgaris* collected from Saudi Arabianmarket. Asian Pac J Trop Biomed 2017; 149.

[106] Kovač J, Šimunović K, Wu Z, *et al.* Antibiotic resistance modulation and modes of action of (-)-α-pinene in Campylobacter jejuni. PLoS One 2015; 10(4): e0122871. [http://dx.doi.org/10.1371/journal.pone.0122871] [PMID: 25830640]

[107] Rufino AT, Ribeiro M, Judas F, *et al.* Anti-inflammatory and chondroprotective activity of (+)-α-pinene: structural and enantiomeric selectivity. J Nat Prod 2014; 77(2): 264-9. [http://dx.doi.org/10.1021/np400828x] [PMID: 24455984]

[108] Vallianou I, Hadzopoulou-Cladaras M. Camphene, a plant derived monoterpene, exerts its hypolipidemic action by affecting SREBP- 1 and MTP expression. PLoS One 2016; 11(1): e0147117. [http://dx.doi.org/10.1371/journal.pone.0147117] [PMID: 26784701]

[109] Kim S, Choi Y, Choi S, Choi Y, Park T. Dietary camphene attenuates hepatic steatosis and insulin resistance in mice. Obesity (Silver Spring) 2014; 22(2): 408-17. [http://dx.doi.org/10.1002/oby.20554] [PMID: 23818423]

[110] Ciftci O, Ozdemir I, Tanyildizi S, Yildiz S, Oguzturk H. Antioxidative effects of curcumin, β-myrcene

and 1,8-cineole against 2,3,7,8-tetrachlorodibenzo- *p* -dioxin-induced oxidative stress in rats liver. Toxicol Ind Health 2011; 27(5): 447-53.
[http://dx.doi.org/10.1177/0748233710388452] [PMID: 21245202]

[111] Bonamin F, Moraes TM, dos Santos RC, *et al.* The effect of a minor constituent of essential oil from Citrus aurantium: The role of β-myrcene in preventing peptic ulcer disease. Chem Biol Interact 2014; 212: 11-9.
[http://dx.doi.org/10.1016/j.cbi.2014.01.009] [PMID: 24480520]

[112] Lee JH, Lee K, Lee DH, Shin SY, Yong Y, Lee YH. Anti-invasive effect of β-myrcene, a component of the essential oil from Pinus koraiensis cones, in metastatic MDA-MB-231 human breast cancer cells. J Korean Soc Appl Biol Chem 2015; 58(4): 563-9.
[http://dx.doi.org/10.1007/s13765-015-0081-3]

[113] Aazza S, Lyoussi B, Miguel MG. Antioxidant and antiacetylcholinesterase activities of some commercial essential oils and their major compounds. Molecules 2011; 16(9): 7672-90.
[http://dx.doi.org/10.3390/molecules16097672] [PMID: 21900869]

[114] Ocete MA, Risco S, Zarzuelo A, Jimenez J. Pharmacological activity of the essential oil of Bupleurum gibraltaricum: Anti-inflammatory activity and effects on isolated rat uteri. J Ethnopharmacol 1989; 25(3): 305-13.
[http://dx.doi.org/10.1016/0378-8741(89)90036-6] [PMID: 2747263]

[115] Romeo FV, De Luca S, Piscopo A, Poiana M. Antimicrobial effect of some essential oils. J Essent Oil Res 2008; 20(4): 373-9.
[http://dx.doi.org/10.1080/10412905.2008.9700034]

[116] de Oliveira TM, de Carvalho RBF, da Costa IHF, *et al.* Evaluation of *p* -cymene, a natural antioxidant. Pharm Biol 2015; 53(3): 423-8.
[http://dx.doi.org/10.3109/13880209.2014.923003] [PMID: 25471840]

[117] Barbosa, R.L., Santos, J.H., Cunha, P.S., Quintans-Júnior LJ, Bonjardim LR, de Souza Araújo AA. Vasorelaxant activity of p-cymene in superior mesenteric artery of rats. The FASEB J. 27(S1): lb599-lb599.
[http://dx.doi.org/10.1096/fasebj.27.1_supplement.lb599]

[118] Masoum S, Mehran M, Ghaheri S. Identification of potential antioxidant compounds in the essential oil of thyme by gas chromatography with mass spectrometry and multivariate calibration techniques. J Sep Sci 2015; 38(3): 410-7.
[http://dx.doi.org/10.1002/jssc.201400745] [PMID: 25403421]

[119] Park SN, Lim YK, Freire MO, Cho E, Jin D, Kook JK. Antimicrobial effect of linalool and α-terpineol against periodontopathic and cariogenic bacteria. Anaerobe 2012; 18(3): 369-72.
[http://dx.doi.org/10.1016/j.anaerobe.2012.04.001] [PMID: 22537719]

[120] Kavoosi G, Dadfar SMM, Purfard AM. Mechanical, physical, antioxidant, and antimicrobial properties of gelatin films incorporated with thymol for potential use as nano wound dressing. J Food Sci 2013; 78(2): E244-50.
[http://dx.doi.org/10.1111/1750-3841.12015] [PMID: 23317304]

[121] Dahham S, Tabana Y, Iqbal M, *et al.* The anticancer, antioxidant and antimicrobial properties of the sesquiterpene b-caryophyllene from the essential oil of Aquilaria crassna. Molecules 2015; 20(7): 11808-29.
[http://dx.doi.org/10.3390/molecules200711808] [PMID: 26132906]

[122] Govindarajan M, Benelli G. α-Humulene and β-elemene from Syzygium zeylanicum (Myrtaceae) essential oil: highly effective and eco-friendly larvicides against Anopheles subpictus, Aedes albopictus, and Culex tritaeniorhynchus (Diptera: Culicidae). Parasitol Res 2016; 115(7): 2771-8.
[http://dx.doi.org/10.1007/s00436-016-5025-2] [PMID: 27026503]

[123] Hanusov'a V, Sk'alov'a L, Ambroz M, Kr'alov'a V, Langhansov'a L, Matouskov'a P. The effect of Myrica rubra essential oil and its components a-humulene and trans-nerolidol on adhesion and

apoptosis of colorectal cancer cells. Cancer Cell Microenviron 2015; 2: e1058.

[124] Nikoli'ca M. Jasmina Glamo˘clijaa, Isabel C.F.R. Ferreirab, Ricardo C. Calhelhab,Ângela Fernandesb, Tatjana Markovi'cc, Dejan Markovi'cd, Abdulhamed Giwelie,Marina Sokovi'c (2014) Chemical composition, antimicrobial, antioxidant and antitumor activity of Thymus serpyllum L., *Thymus algeriensis* Boiss. and Reut andThymus vulgaris L. essential oils. Ind Crops Prod 2014; 52: 183-90.

[125] Hazzit M, Baaliouamer A, Veríssimo AR, Faleiro ML, Miguel MG. Chemical composition and biological activities of Algerian Thymus oils. Food Chem 2009; 116(3): 714-21. [http://dx.doi.org/10.1016/j.foodchem.2009.03.018]

[126] Alia IBEH. Maher Chaouachib, Radhia Bahrib, Ikbal Chaiebc,Mohamed Boussaïda, Fethia Harzallah-Skhiri (2015)Chemical composition and antioxidant, antibacterial, allelopathic andinsecticidal activities of essential oil of *Thymus algeriensis* Boiss. etReut. Ind Crops Prod 2015; 77: 631-9. [http://dx.doi.org/10.1016/j.indcrop.2015.09.046]

[127] Hussain AI, Anwar F, Nigam PS, *et al.* Antibacterial activity of some Lamiaceae essential oils using resazurin as an indicator of cell growth. Lebensm Wiss Technol 2011; 44(4): 1199-206. [http://dx.doi.org/10.1016/j.lwt.2010.10.005]

[128] Barbosa LN, Rall VLM, Fernandes AAH, Ushimaru PI, da Silva Probst I, Fernandes A Jr. Essential oils against foodborne pathogens and spoilage bacteria in minced meat. Foodborne Pathog Dis 2009; 6(6): 725-8.
[http://dx.doi.org/10.1089/fpd.2009.0282] [PMID: 19580445]

[129] Fratianni F, De Martino L, Melone A, De Feo V, Coppola R, Nazzaro F. Preservation of chicken breast meat treated with thyme and balm essential oils. J Food Sci 2010; 75(8): M528-35. [http://dx.doi.org/10.1111/j.1750-3841.2010.01791.x] [PMID: 21535509]

[130] Kofidis G, Bosabalidis A, Kokkini S. Seasonal variations of essential oils in alinalool-rich chemotype of Mentha spicata grown wild in Greece. J Essent Oil Res 2004; 16(5): 469-72. [http://dx.doi.org/10.1080/10412905.2004.9698773]

[131] Celiktas OY, Kocabas EEH, Bedir E, Sukan FV, Ozek T, Baser KHC. Antimicrobial activities of methanol extracts and essential oils of Rosmarinus officinalis, depending on location and seasonal variations. Food Chem 2007; 100(2): 553-9.
[http://dx.doi.org/10.1016/j.foodchem.2005.10.011]

[132] Trivino MG, Johnson CB. Season has a major effect on the essential oilyield response to nutrient supply in Origanum majorana. J Hortic Sci Biotechnol 2000; 75(5): 520-7. [http://dx.doi.org/10.1080/14620316.2000.11511278]

[133] Nezhadali A, Nabavi M, Rajabian M, Akbarpour M, Pourali P, Amini F. Chemical variation of leaf essential oil at different stages of plant growth and*In vitro* antibacterial activity of Thymus vulgaris Lamiaceae, from Iran.Beni-Suef U. J Basic Appl Sci 2014; 3(2): 87-92.

[134] McKay DL, Blumberg JB. A Review of the bioactivity and potential health benefits of chamomile tea (*Matricaria recutita* L.). Phytother Res 2006; 20(7): 519-30. [http://dx.doi.org/10.1002/ptr.1900] [PMID: 16628544]

[135] Markus Lange B, Croteau R. Genetic engineering of essential oil production in mint. Curr Opin Plant Biol 1999; 2(2): 139-44.
[http://dx.doi.org/10.1016/S1369-5266(99)80028-4] [PMID: 10322195]

[136] Naigre R, Kalck P, Roques C, Roux I, Michel G. Comparison of antimicrobial properties of monoterpenes and their carbonylated products. Planta Med 1996; 62(3): 275-7. [http://dx.doi.org/10.1055/s-2006-957877] [PMID: 8693045]

[137] Flamini G, Cioni PL, Puleio R, Morelli I, Panizzi L. Antimicrobial activity of the essential oil ofCalamintha nepeta and its constituent pulegone against bacteria and fungi. Phytother Res 1999; 13(4): 349-51.
[http://dx.doi.org/10.1002/(SICI)1099-1573(199906)13:4<349::AID-PTR446>3.0.CO;2-Z] [PMID:

10404547]

[138] Al-Bayati FA. Isolation and identification of antimicrobial compound from Mentha longifolia L. leaves grown wild in Iraq. Ann Clin Microbiol Antimicrob 2009; 8(1): 20. [http://dx.doi.org/10.1186/1476-0711-8-20] [PMID: 19523224]

[139] Mimica-Dukić N, Bozin B, Soković M, Mihajlović B, Matavulj M. Antimicrobial and antioxidant activities of three *Mentha species* essential oils. Planta Med 2003; 69(5): 413-9. [http://dx.doi.org/10.1055/s-2003-39704] [PMID: 12802721]

[140] Gulluce M, Sahin F, Sokmen M, *et al.* Antimicrobial and antioxidant properties of the essential oils and methanol extract from Mentha longifolia L. ssp. longifolia. Food Chem 2007; 103(4): 1449-56. [http://dx.doi.org/10.1016/j.foodchem.2006.10.061]

[141] Puangpronp D, Sittiwet C. Antimicrobial properties of Cinnamomumverum aqueous extract. Asian Journal of Biological Sciences 2009; 2(2): 49-53. [http://dx.doi.org/10.3923/ajbs.2009.49.53]

[142] Nickavar B, Alinaghi A, Kamalinejad M. Evaluation of the antioxidant prop-erties of five Mentha species. Iran J Pharm Res 2008; 7(3): 203-9.

[143] Lorenzi H, Matos FJA. Plantas Medicinais no Brasil: Nativas e ExóticasCultivadas. Nova Odessa, SP: Instituto Plantarum 2002; pp. 246-51.

[144] Cowan MM. Plant products as antimicrobial agents. Clin Microbiol Rev 1999; 12(4): 564-82. [http://dx.doi.org/10.1128/CMR.12.4.564] [PMID: 10515903]

[145] İşcan G, Kiri̇mer N, Kürkcüoğlu M, Demi̇rci̇ F, Demirci F. Antimicrobial screening of Mentha piperita essential oils. J Agric Food Chem 2002; 50(14): 3943-6. [http://dx.doi.org/10.1021/jf011476k] [PMID: 12083863]

[146] Moreno L, Bello R, Primo-Yúfera E, Esplugues J. Pharmacological properties of the methanol extract from Mentha suaveolens Ehrh. Phytother Res 2002; 16(Suppl. 1): S10-3. [http://dx.doi.org/10.1002/ptr.744] [PMID: 11933132]

[147] Barrosa AS. Selene Maia de Moraisa, Pablito Augusto Travassos Ferreiraa, Ícaro Gusmão Pinto Vieirab, Afrânio Aragão Craveiroc, Raquel Oliveira dos Santos Fontenelled,Jane Eire Silva Alencar de Menezesa,b, Francisco Walber Ferreira da Silvaa,Halisson Araújo de Sousa Chemical composition and functional properties of essential oils from Mentha species. Ind Crops Prod 2015; 76: 557-64.

[148] Economou KD, Oreopoulou V, Thomopoulos CD. Antioxidant activity of some plant extracts of the family labiatae. J Am Oil Chem Soc 1991; 68(2): 109-13. [http://dx.doi.org/10.1007/BF02662329]

[149] Kaur C, Kapoor HC. Anti-oxidant activity and total phenolic content of some Asian vegetables. Int J Food Sci Technol 2002; 37(2): 153-61. [http://dx.doi.org/10.1046/j.1365-2621.2002.00552.x]

[150] Daferera DJ, Ziogas BN, Polissiou MG. The effectiveness of plant essential oils on the growth of Botrytis cinerea, Fusarium sp. and Clavibacter michiganensis subsp. michiganensis. Crop Prot 2003; 22(1): 39-44. [http://dx.doi.org/10.1016/S0261-2194(02)00095-9]

[151] Gruenwald J, Brendler T, Jaenicke C. PDR for Herbal Medicines. Montvale, NJ: Medical Economic Company Inc. 2000.

[152] Agnihotri VK, Agarwal SG, Dhar PL, *et al.* Essential oil composition ofMentha pulegium L. growing wild in the north-western Himalayas India. Flavour Fragrance J 2005; 20(6): 607-10. [http://dx.doi.org/10.1002/ffj.1497]

[153] Aghel N, Yamini Y, Hadjiakhoondi A, Pourmortazavi SM. Supercritical carbon dioxide extraction of Mentha pulegium L. essential oil. Talanta 2004; 62(2): 407-11. [http://dx.doi.org/10.1016/j.talanta.2003.08.011] [PMID: 18969310]

[154] Petrakis EA, Kimbaris AC, Pappas CS, Tarantilis PA, Polissiou MG. Quantitative determination of pulegone in pennyroyal oil by FT-IR spectroscopy. J Agric Food Chem 2009; 57(21): 10044-8. [http://dx.doi.org/10.1021/jf9026052] [PMID: 19817373]

[155] Müller-Riebau FJ, Berger BM, Yegen O, Cakir C. Seasonal variations in the chemical compositions of essential oils of selected aromatic plants growing wild in Turkey. J Agric Food Chem 1997; 45(12): 4821-5.
[http://dx.doi.org/10.1021/jf970110y]

[156] Reis-Vasco EMC, Coelho JAP, Palavra AMF. Comparison of pennyroyal oils obtained by supercritical CO2 extraction and hydrodistillation. Flavour Fragrance J 1999; 14(3): 156-60. [http://dx.doi.org/10.1002/(SICI)1099-1026(199905/06)14:3<156::AID-FFJ793>3.0.CO;2-J]

[157] Teixeira B, Marques A, Ramos C, *et al.* European pennyroyal (Mentha pulegium) from Portugal: Chemical composition of essential oil and antioxidant and antimicrobial properties of extracts and essential oil. Ind Crops Prod 2012; 36(1): 81-7.
[http://dx.doi.org/10.1016/j.indcrop.2011.08.011]

[158] Zargari A. Herbal Medicines. Tehran University Publications; 1990.

[159] Newall CA. Herbal Medicines. In: Anderson LA, Philipson JD, Eds. A Guide for Health Care Professional. London: The Pharmaceutical Press 1996; p. 208.

[160] Mahboubi M, Haghi G. Antimicrobial activity and chemical composition of Mentha pulegium L. essential oil. J Ethnopharmacol 2008; 119(2): 325-7.
[http://dx.doi.org/10.1016/j.jep.2008.07.023] [PMID: 18703127]

[161] Arranz E, Mes J, Wichers H J, Jaime L, Mendiola J A, Reglero G, *et al.* Anti-inflammatory activity of the basolateral fraction of Caco-2 cells exposed to a rosemary supercritical extract. J Funct Foods 2015; 13: 384e390.
[http://dx.doi.org/10.1016/j.jff.2015.01.015]

[162] Babovic N, Djilas S, Jadranin M, Vajs V, Ivanovic J, Petrovic S, *et al.* Supercritical carbon dioxide extraction of antioxidant fractions from selected Lamiaceae herbs and their antioxidant capacity. Innov Food Sci Emerg Technol 2010; 11(1): 98-107.
[http://dx.doi.org/10.1016/j.ifset.2009.08.013]

[163] Teixeira B, Marques A, Ramos C, Neng N R, Nogueira J M F, Saraiva J A, *et al.* Chemical composition and antibacterial and antioxidant properties of commercial essential oils. Ind Crops Prod 2013; 43: 587-95.
[http://dx.doi.org/10.1016/j.indcrop.2012.07.069]

[164] Ribeiro-Santos R, Carvalho-Costa D, Cavaleiro C, *et al.* A novel insight on an ancient aromatic plant: The rosemary (Rosmarinus officinalis L.). Trends Food Sci Technol 2015; 45(2): 355-68.
[http://dx.doi.org/10.1016/j.tifs.2015.07.015]

[165] Mohamed AA., Alotaibi BM. Essential oils of some medicinal plants and their biological activities: a mini review. J.Umm Al-Qura Univ. Appll. Sci. 2023. 9: 40–49.
[http://dx.doi.org/10.1007/s43994-022-00018-1]

[166] Ghasemzadeh Rahbardar M, Hosseinzadeh H. Effects of rosmarinic acid on nervous system disorders: an updated review. Naunyn Schmiedebergs Arch Pharmacol 2020; 393(10): 1779-95.
[http://dx.doi.org/10.1007/s00210-020-01935-w] [PMID: 32725282]

[167] Amaral G P, Carvalho N R, Barcelos R P, Dobrachinski F, Portella R D L, Silva M H, *et al.* Protective action of ethanolic extract of Rosmarinus officinalis L. in gastric ulcer prevention induced by ethanol in rats. Food Chem Toxicol 2013; 55: 48-55.

[168] Barreto H M, Silva Filho E C, Lima E D O, Coutinho H D M. Chemical composition and possible use as adjuvant of the antibiotic therapy of the essential oil of Rosmarinus officinalis L. Ind Crops Prod 2014; 59: 290e294.

[169] Holmes P. Rosemary oil. Int J Aromather 1999; 9(2): 62-e66.

[170] aPeter KV. Introduction to herbs and species. In: Peter KV, Ed. Handbook of herbs and spices. IntechOpen 2004.bRozman T. Antimicrobial activity of rosemary extracts (Rosmarinus officinalis L.) against different species of Listeria. Acta Agricult Slovenica 2009; 93(1): 51-8.

[171] Sasikumar B. Rosemary. In: Peter KV, Ed. Handbook of herbs and spices. 2012; pp. 452-68. [http://dx.doi.org/10.1533/9780857095671.452]

[172] Haloui M, Louedec L, Michel J B, Lyoussi B. Experimental diuretic effects of Rosmarinus officinalis and Centaurium erythraea. J Ethnopharmacol 2000; 71: 465-72. [http://dx.doi.org/10.1016/S0378-8741(00)00184-7]

[173] Afonso MS, de O Silva AM, Carvalho EBT, *et al.* Phenolic compounds from Rosemary (Rosmarinus officinalis L.) attenuate oxidative stress and reduce blood cholesterol concentrations in diet-induced hypercholesterolemic rats. Nutr Metab (Lond) 2013; 10(1): 19. [http://dx.doi.org/10.1186/1743-7075-10-19] [PMID: 23374457]

[174] Bakirel T, Bakirel U, Keles¸ O U, Ulgen S G, Yardibi H. *In vivo* assessment of antidiabetic and antioxidant activities of rosemary (Rosmarinus officinalis) in alloxan-diabetic rabbits. J Ethnopharmacol 2008; 116(1): 64-73.

[175] United States Department of Agriculture, Agricultural Research Services USDA. 2015. Available from:http://ndb.nal.usda.gov/ndb/foods/show/256

[176] Goldbeck JC, do Nascimento JE, Jacob RG, Fiorentini ÂM, da Silva WP. Bioactivity of essential oils from Eucalyptus globulus and Eucalyptus urograndis against planktonic cells and biofilms of Streptococcus mutans. Ind Crops Prod 2014; 60: 304-9. [http://dx.doi.org/10.1016/j.indcrop.2014.05.030]

[177] Ishnava KB, Chauhan JB, Barad MB. Anticariogenic and phytochemical evaluation of Eucalyptus globules Labill. Saudi J Biol Sci 2013; 20(1): 69-74. [http://dx.doi.org/10.1016/j.sjbs.2012.11.003] [PMID: 23961222]

[178] Bachir RG, Benali M. Antibacterial activity of the essential oils from the leaves of *Eucalyptus globulus* against *Escherichia coli* and *Staphylococcus aureus.* Asian Pac J Trop Biomed 2012; 2(9): 739-42. [http://dx.doi.org/10.1016/S2221-1691(12)60220-2] [PMID: 23570005]

[179] Elliot WR, Jones D. The Encyclopaedia of Australian plants. AbeBooks 1986.The Encyclopaedia of Australian plants.

[180] Northern Australia. 2nd ed. Brooker MIH, Kleinig DA. Field guide to EucalyptsMelbourne, Australia: Bloomings Books 2004; 3.

[181] Singh HP, Kaur S, Negi K, *et al.* Assessment of *In vitro* antioxidant activity of essential oil of Eucalyptus citriodora (lemon-scented Eucalypt; Myrtaceae) and its major constituents. Lebensm Wiss Technol 2012; 48(2): 237-41. [http://dx.doi.org/10.1016/j.lwt.2012.03.019]

[182] Batish DR, Singh HP, Kohli RK, Kaur S. Eucalyptus essential oil as a natural pesticide. For Ecol Manage 2008; 256(12): 2166-74. [http://dx.doi.org/10.1016/j.foreco.2008.08.008]

[183] Habila N, Agbaji A S, Ladan Z, Bello I A, Haruna E, Dakare M A, *et al.* Evaluation of *In vitro* activity of essential oils against Trypanosoma brucei brucei and Trypanosoma evansi. J Parasitol Res 2010; 2012: 534601. [http://dx.doi.org/10.1155/2010/534601]

[184] Ramezani H, Singh HP, Batish DR, Kohli RK. Antifungal activity of the volatile oil of Eucalyptus citriodora. Fitoterapia 2002; 73(3): 261-2. [http://dx.doi.org/10.1016/S0367-326X(02)00065-5] [PMID: 12048022]

[185] Singh H P, Batish D R, Setia N, Kohli R K. Herbicidal activity of volatile oils from Eucalyptus citriodora against Parthenium hysterophorus. Annals Appl Biol 2005; 146: 89-94. [http://dx.doi.org/10.1111/j.1744-7348.2005.04018.x]

[186] Pascual ME, Slowing K, Carretero E, Sánchez Mata D, Villar A. Lippia: traditional uses, chemistry and pharmacology: A review. J Ethnopharmacol 2001; 76(3): 201-14. [http://dx.doi.org/10.1016/S0378-8741(01)00234-3] [PMID: 11448540]

[187] de Albuquerque UP, de Medeiros PM, de Almeida ALS, *et al.* Medicinal plants of the caatinga (semi-arid) vegetation of NE Brazil: A quantitative approach. J Ethnopharmacol 2007; 114(3): 325-54. [http://dx.doi.org/10.1016/j.jep.2007.08.017] [PMID: 17900836]

[188] Rosana PCF, Diogo S. Cytotoxic effect of leaf essential oil of Lippia gracilis Schauer (Verbenaceae). Phytomedicine 2013; 20: 615-21.

[189] Lorenzi H, Matos FJA. Plantas Medicinais no Brasil: Nativas e Exóticas. 2nd ed., Instituto Plantarum, Nova Odessa 2008.

[190] Pessoa ODL, de Carvalho CBM, Silvestre JOVL, *et al.* Antibacterial activity of the essential oil from Lippia aff. gracillis. Fitoterapia 2005; 76(7-8): 712-4. [http://dx.doi.org/10.1016/j.fitote.2005.07.004] [PMID: 16233961]

[191] Silva WJ, Dória GAA, Maia RT, *et al.* Effects of essential oils on Aedes aegypti larvae: Alternatives to environmentally safe insecticides. Bioresour Technol 2008; 99(8): 3251-5. [http://dx.doi.org/10.1016/j.biortech.2007.05.064] [PMID: 17662602]

[192] Mendes SS, Bomfim RR, Jesus HCR, *et al.* Evaluation of the analgesic and anti-inflammatory effects of the essential oil of Lippia gracilis leaves. J Ethnopharmacol 2010; 129(3): 391-7. [http://dx.doi.org/10.1016/j.jep.2010.04.005] [PMID: 20420889]

[193] Teles TV, Bonfim RR, Alves PB, *et al.* Composition and evaluation of the lethality of Lippia gracilis essential oil to adults of Biomphalaria glabrata and larvae of Artemia salina. Afr J Biotechnol 2010; 9: 8800-4.

[194] Guimarães AG, Gomes SVF, Moraes VRS, *et al.* Phytochemical characterization and antinociceptive effect of Lippia gracilis Schauer. J Nat Med 2012; 66(3): 428-34. [http://dx.doi.org/10.1007/s11418-011-0601-3] [PMID: 22146971]

[195] Han X, Rodriguez D, Parker TL. Biological activities of frankincense essential oil in human dermal fibroblasts. Biochim Open 2017; 4: 31-5. [http://dx.doi.org/10.1016/j.biopen.2017.01.003] [PMID: 29450138]

[196] Dozmorov MG, Yang Q, Wu W, *et al.* Differential effects of selective frankincense (Ru Xiang) essential oil versus non-selective sandalwood (Tan Xiang) essential oil on cultured bladder cancer cells: a microarray and bioinformatics study. Chin Med 2014; 9(1): 18. [http://dx.doi.org/10.1186/1749-8546-9-18] [PMID: 25006348]

[197] Matsuo AL, Figueiredo CR, Arruda DC, *et al.* α-Pinene isolated from Schinus terebinthifolius Raddi (Anacardiaceae) induces apoptosis and confers antimetastatic protection in a melanoma model. Biochem Biophys Res Commun 2011; 411(2): 449-54. [http://dx.doi.org/10.1016/j.bbrc.2011.06.176] [PMID: 21756878]

[198] Chen W, Liu Y, Li M, Mao J, Zhang L, Huang R, *et al.* Anti-tumor effect of a-pinene on human hepatoma cell lines through inducing G2/M cell cycle arrest. J Pharmacol Sci 2015; 127: 332. [http://dx.doi.org/10.1016/j.jphs.2015.01.008]

[199] Gaware V, Nagare R, Dhamak KB, *et al.* Aromatherapy: Art or science. Int J Biomed Res 2013; 4(2): 74-83. [http://dx.doi.org/10.7439/ijbr.v4i2.231]

[200] Mohammadi F, Faghih Zadeh S, Nemati E, Ahmadi F. Effect of progressive muscle relaxation on vital sign of MI patients. Clinical trial. J Semnan Univ Med Sci 2006; 7: 189-95.

[201] Baba shahi A. The effect of aromatherapy massage and massage therapy on anxiety of patients before surgery: A clinical trial. J Evid-Based Care 2012; 2: 20-7.

[202] Bikmoradi A, Seifi Z, Poorolajal J, Araghchian M, Safiaryan R, Oshvandi K. Effect of inhalation aromatherapy with lavender essential oil on stress and vital signs in patients undergoing coronary artery bypass surgery: a single-blinded randomized clinical trial. Complement Ther Med 2014. [PMID: 26051567]

[203] Emami A, Ahi A. Medical botany. Iran University of Medical Sciences and Health Services 2008.

[204] Koulivand PH, Khaleghi Ghadiri M, Gorji A. Lavender and the nervous system. Evid-Based Complement Altern Med 2013. [http://dx.doi.org/10.1155/2013/681304]

[205] Mahmoudi B. Essential oils. 1st ed. Tehran: Noor Danesh 2002; pp. 3-56.

[206] Kheirkhah M. Effect of aromatherapy with essential damask rose oil on anxiety of the active phase of labor nulliparous women. J Urmia Nurs Midwifery Faculty 2013; 11.

[207] Katalin V. Chemical composition and antimicrobial activities of essential oils of four lines of Origanum vulgare subsp. hirtum (link) Ietswaart grown in Hungary. Nat Prod Comm 2007; 2(11): 1155-8.

[208] Kirtikar KR, Basu BD. Indian medicinal plants. In: Blatter E, Caius JF, Mhaskar SK, Eds. Bishen Singh and Mahendra Pal Sing. Dehradun 1985; 3: p. 250.

[209] Maisonneuve SA. Sainte-Ruffine. European Pharmacopoeia 1975.

[210] Farooqi AA, Sreeramu BS. Cultivation of Medicinal and Aromatic Crops. Universities Press, India 2004.

[211] Asgary S, Zarfeshany A, Javanmard S. Potent health effects of pomegranate. Adv Biomed Res 2014; 3(1): 100. [http://dx.doi.org/10.4103/2277-9175.129371] [PMID: 24800189]

[212] Achraf A, Hamdi C, Turki M, *et al.* Natural pomegranate juice reduces inflammation, muscle damage and increase platelets blood levels in active healthy Tunisian aged men. Alex J Med 2018; 54(1): 45-8. [http://dx.doi.org/10.1016/j.ajme.2017.03.005]

[213] Aviram M, Rosenblat M, Gaitini D, *et al.* Pomegranate juice consumption for 3 years by patients with carotid artery stenosis reduces common carotid intima-media thickness, blood pressure and LDL oxidation. Clin Nutr 2004; 23(3): 423-33. [http://dx.doi.org/10.1016/j.clnu.2003.10.002] [PMID: 15158307]

[214] Heber D, Seeram NP, Wyatt H, *et al.* Safety and antioxidant activity of a pomegranate ellagitannin-enriched polyphenol dietary supplement in overweight individuals with increased waist size. J Agric Food Chem 2007; 55(24): 10050-4. [http://dx.doi.org/10.1021/jf071689v] [PMID: 17966977]

[215] Renaud S, de Lorgeril M. Wine, alcohol, platelets, and the French paradox for coronary heart disease. Lancet 1992; 339(8808): 1523-6. [http://dx.doi.org/10.1016/0140-6736(92)91277-F] [PMID: 1351198]

[216] Dubick MA, Omaye ST. Evidence for grape, wine and tea polyphenols as modulators of atherosclerosis and ischemic heart disease in humans. Journal of Nutraceuticals, Functional & Medical Foods 2001; 3(3): 67-93. [http://dx.doi.org/10.1300/J133v03n03_04]

[217] Nardini M, Natella F, Scaccini C. Role of dietary polyphenols in platelet aggregation. A review of the supplementation studies. Platelets 2007; 18(3): 224-43. [http://dx.doi.org/10.1080/09537100601078083] [PMID: 17497435]

[218] Vitrac X, Monti J-P, Vercauteren J, Deffieux G, Mérillon JM. Direct liquid chromatographic analysis

of resveratrol derivatives and flavanonols in wines with absorbance and fluorescence detection. Anal Chim Acta 2002; 458(1): 103-10.
[http://dx.doi.org/10.1016/S0003-2670(01)01498-2]

[219] Luqman S, Rizvi SI. Protection of lipid peroxidation and carbonyl formation in proteins by capsaicin in human erythrocytes subjected to oxidative stress. Phytother Res 2006; 20(4): 303-6.
[http://dx.doi.org/10.1002/ptr.1861] [PMID: 16557614]

[220] Pandey KB, Mishra N, Rizvi SI. Protective role of myricetin on markers of oxidative stress in human erythrocytes subjected to oxidative stress. Nat Prod Commun 2009; 4(2): 1934578X0900400.
[http://dx.doi.org/10.1177/1934578X0900400211] [PMID: 19370927]

[221] Scalbert A, Manach C, Morand C, Rémésy C, Jiménez L. Dietary polyphenols and the prevention of diseases. Crit Rev Food Sci Nutr 2005; 45(4): 287-306.
[http://dx.doi.org/10.1080/1040869059096] [PMID: 16047496]

[222] Siervo M, Lara J, Ogbonmwan I, Mathers JC. Inorganic nitrate and beetroot juice supplementation reduces blood pressure in adults: a systematic review and meta-analysis. J Nutr 2013; 143(6): 818-26.
[http://dx.doi.org/10.3945/jn.112.170233] [PMID: 23596162]

[223] Bailey SJ, Vanhatalo A, Winyard PG, Jones AM. The nitrate-nitrite-nitric oxide pathway: Its role in human exercise physiology. Eur J Sport Sci 2012; 12(4): 309-20.
[http://dx.doi.org/10.1080/17461391.2011.635705]

[224] Ferguson SK, Hirai DM, Copp SW, *et al.* Impact of dietary nitrate supplementation *via* beetroot juice on exercising muscle vascular control in rats. J Physiol 2013; 591(2): 547-57.
[http://dx.doi.org/10.1113/jphysiol.2012.243121] [PMID: 23070702]

[225] Larsen FJ. Dietary inorganic nitrate improves mitochondrial efficiency in humans. Cell Metab 2011; 12(2): 149-59.

[226] Bescós R, Sureda A, Tur JA, Pons A. The effect of nitric-oxide-related supplements on human performance. Sports Med 2012; 42(2): 99-117.
[http://dx.doi.org/10.2165/11596860-000000000-00000] [PMID: 22260513]

[227] Leikert JF, Räthel TR, Wohlfart P, Cheynier V, Vollmar AM, Dirsch VM. Red wine polyphenols enhance endothelial nitric oxide synthase expression and subsequent nitric oxide release from endothelial cells. Circulation 2002; 106(13): 1614-7.
[http://dx.doi.org/10.1161/01.CIR.0000034445.31543.43] [PMID: 12270851]

[228] Gruenwald J, Freder J, Armbruester N. Cinnamon and Health. Crit Rev Food Sci Nutr 2010; 50(9): 822-34.
[http://dx.doi.org/10.1080/10408390902773052] [PMID: 20924865]

[229] Leach MJ, Kumar S. Cinnamon for diabetes mellitus. Cochrane Database Syst Rev 2012; 2012(9): CD007170.
[http://dx.doi.org/10.1002/14651858.CD007170] [PMID: 22972104]

[230] Keshvari M, Asgary S, Jafarian-Dehkordi A, Najafi S, Ghoreyshi-Yazdi SM. Preventive effect of cinnamon essential oil on lipid oxidation of vegetable oil. ARYA Atheroscler 2013; 9(5): 280-6.
[PMID: 24302936]

[231] Shreaz S, Bhatia R, Khan N, *et al.* Spice oil cinnamaldehyde exhibits potent anticandidal activity against fluconazole resistant clinical isolates. Fitoterapia 2011; 82(7): 1012-20.
[http://dx.doi.org/10.1016/j.fitote.2011.06.004] [PMID: 21708228]

[232] Liao JC, Deng JS, Chiu CS, *et al.* Anti-inflammatory activities of Cinnamomum cassia constituents *In vitro* and *In vivo*. Evid Based Complement Alternat Med 2012; 2012: 1-12.
[http://dx.doi.org/10.1155/2012/429320] [PMID: 22536283]

[233] Kim BH, Lee YG, Lee J, Lee JY, Cho JY. Regulatory effect of cinnamaldehyde on monocyte/macrophage-mediated inflammatory responses. Mediators Inflamm 2010; 2010: 1-9.
[http://dx.doi.org/10.1155/2010/529359] [PMID: 20467561]

[234] El-Bassossy HM, Fahmy A, Badawy D. Cinnamaldehyde protects from the hypertension associated with diabetes. Food Chem Toxicol 2011; 49(11): 3007-12.
[http://dx.doi.org/10.1016/j.fct.2011.07.060] [PMID: 21840367]

[235] Sharifi-Rad J, Quispe C, Herrera-Bravo J, *et al.* *Glycyrrhiza* genus: Enlightening phytochemical components for pharmacological and health-promoting abilities. Oxid Med Cell Longev 2021; 2021: 1-20.
[http://dx.doi.org/10.1155/2021/7571132] [PMID: 34349875]

[236] Shakeri A. Identification and biological activity of the volatile compounds of Glycyrrhiza triphylla Fisch. & C.A. Mey Microbial Pathogenesis 2017; 109: 39-44.
[http://dx.doi.org/10.1016/j.micpath.2017.05.022] [PMID: 28526637]

[237] Jaiswal N, Verma Y, Misra P. Elicitation enhanced the production of bioactive compound and biomass accumulation in callus cultures of Glycyrrhiza glabra L. *In vitro* Cellular & Developmental Biology – Plant, DO- Res Square 2021.
[http://dx.doi.org/10.21203/rs.3.rs-162959/v1]

[238] Buchbauer G. Biological activities of essential oils. Handbook of Essential Oils:Science, Technology and Applications. CRC Press, Taylor and Francis Group 2010.

[239] Akhmedzhanova VI, Bessonova IA, Yunusov SY. The roots of Dictamnus angustifolius. Chem Nat Compd 1978; 14: 404-6.

[240] Hu C, Han J, Zhao J, Song G, Li Y, Yin D. Limonoidsfrom Dictamnus angustifolius. J Integr Plant Biol 1989; 31: 453-8.

[241] Sun JB, Qu W, Xiong Y, Liang JY. Quinoline alkaloids and sesquiterpenes from the roots of Dictamnus angustifolius. Biochem Syst Ecol 2013; 50: 62-4.
[http://dx.doi.org/10.1016/j.bse.2013.03.036]

[242] Wu TS, Li CY, Leu YL, Hu CQ. Limonoids and alkaloids of the root bark of Dictamnus angustifolius. Phytochemistry 1999; 50(3): 509-12.
[http://dx.doi.org/10.1016/S0031-9422(98)00519-6]

[243] Sun J. Xinzhi Wang b, Pei Wang c, Linzhen Lia, Wei Quan, Jingyu Liang Antimicrobial, antioxidant and cytotoxic properties of essential oil from Dictamnus angustifolius. J Ethnopharmacol 2015; 159: 296-300.
[http://dx.doi.org/10.1016/j.jep.2014.06.055] [PMID: 24997390]

CHAPTER 3

Essential Oil Biochemistry

Manoj Kumar Tripathi[1], **Rahul M. Srivastava**[2], **Muzaffar Hasan**[1,*], **Chirag Maheshwari**[1,3] and **Rajpal S. Jadam**[1]

[1] *ICAR-Central Institute of Agricultural Engineering, Navi Bagh, Bhopal, Madhya Pradesh-462038, India*

[2] *Maulana Azad National Institute of Agricultural Engineering, Bhopal, Madhya Pradesh, India*

[3] *ICAR-Indian Agricultural Research Institute, Pusa, New Delhi-110012, India*

Abstract: Essential oils which are complex blends of volatile compounds particularly present in a copious amount in aromatic plants, and are mainly composed of terpenes biochemically generated through the mevalonate pathway. In natural conditions, essential oils play a significant role in the defense mechanism of plants as antibacterial, antiviral, antifungal, insecticides and protect from herbivores by reducing their taste for such plants. Because of their chemical constituents, essential oil holds various biological activities such as antioxidants, antimicrobial, anti-inflammatory, *etc.* which finds important applications in food, cosmetic, agriculture, industrial, and medical fields. This chapter covers the chemical constituents and chemistry of essential oils on the one hand and their biological activities on the other hand.

Keywords: Biological activities, Chemical composition, Essential oil chemistry.

1. INTRODUCTION

Essential oils are volatile, natural, complex compounds characterized by a strong odour and are formed by aromatic plants as secondary metabolites. They are usually obtained by steam or hydro-distillation first developed in the Middle Ages by Arabs. Known for their antiseptic, *i.e.*, bactericidal, virucidal and fungicidal, and medicinal properties and their fragrance, they are used in embalment, preservation of foods and as antimicrobial, analgesic, sedative, anti-inflammatory, spasmolytic and locally anesthetic remedies. Up to the present day, these characteristics have not changed much except that more is now known about some of their mechanisms of action, particularly at the antimicrobial level. In nature, essential oils play an important role in the protection of plants as antibacterial, antiviral, antifungal, insecticides and against herbivores by reducing

* **Corresponding author Muzaffar Hasan:** ICAR-Central Institute of Agricultural Engineering, Navi Bagh, Bhopal, Madhya Pradesh-462038, India; E-mail: muzaffarhassan88@gmail.com

Pradeep Kumar Shukla, Ajeet Kumar Srivastav, Deepti Chopra, Shikha Agnihotry, Pragati Misra and Jyoti Singh (Eds.)

their appetite for such plants. They also may attract some insects to favor the dispersion of pollen and seeds, or repel undesirable others. Essential oils are extracted from various aromatic plants generally localized in temperate to warm countries like Mediterranean and tropical countries, where they represent an important part of the traditional pharmacopoeia. They are liquid, volatile, limpid and rarely coloured, lipid soluble and soluble in organic solvents with a generally lower density than that of water. They can be synthesized by all plant organs, *i.e.*, buds, flowers, leaves, stems, twigs, seeds, fruits, roots, wood, or bark, and are stored in secretory cells, cavities, canals, epidermic cells or glandular trichomes. Essential oils have been largely employed for their properties already observed in nature, *i.e.*, for their antibacterial, antifungal, and insecticidal activities. At present, approximately 3000 essential oils are known, 300 of which are commercially important, especially for the pharmaceutical, agronomic, food, sanitary, cosmetic, and perfume industries. Essential oils or some of their components are used in perfumes and make-up products, in sanitary products, in dentistry, in agriculture, as food preservers and additives, and as natural remedies. For example, d-limonene, geranyl acetate, or d-carvone are employed in perfumes, creams, soaps, as flavour additives for food, as fragrances for household cleaning products and as industrial solvents. Moreover, essential oils are used in massage as mixtures with vegetal oil or in baths but most frequently in aromatherapy. Some essential oils appear to exhibit particular medicinal properties that have been claimed to cure one or another organ dysfunction or systemic disorder [1, 2]. Chemical composition essential oils are very complex natural mixtures which can contain about 20–60 components at quite different concentrations. They are characterized by two or three major components at fairly high concentrations (20–70%) compared to others components present in trace amounts. For example, carvacrol (30%) and thymol (27%) are the major components of the *Origanum compactum* essential oil, linalol (68%) of the *Coriandrum sativum* essential oil, a- and b-thuyone (57%) and camphor (24%) of the Artemisia herba-alba essential oil, 1,8-cineole (50%) of the *Cinnamomum camphora* essential oil, a-phellandrene (36%) and limonene (31%) of leaf and carvone (58%) and limonene (37%) of seed *Anethum graveolens* essential oil, menthol (59%) and menthone (19%) of *Mentha piperita* (=Mentha · piperita) essential oil. Generally, these major components determine the biological properties of the essential oils. The components include two groups of distinct biosynthetical origin [3-5]. The main group is composed of terpenes and terpenoids and the other of aromatic and aliphatic constituents, all characterized by low molecular weight. It is known that plants produce essential oils as secondary metabolites in response to physiological stress, pathogen attack, and ecological factors. Moreover, in nature, essential oils are recognised as defence compounds and attractors of pollinators, facilitating the reproduction of vegetal species. The environmental variations, in turn, are also important in a plant's ability to produce these compounds. Considering all of these factors, the main problems related to the cultivation of aromatic plants are due to variations that occur in quantitative and qualitative changes in the essential oils production. The main factors involved in the biosynthesis of essential oils from medicinal and aromatic plants are discussed in this chapter. In order to optimize its commercial exploitation, the different factors involved in the production of essential oils must be taken into account, since the induction of its substance synthesis could affect the specific compounds of interest and their economic applications, as well as affecting the standard amount of produced oil.

2. CHEMICAL CHARACTERISTICS OF ESSENTIAL OILS

The designation *essential oil* originated from Aristotle's era, because of the idea of life-essential elements — fire, air, earth and water. In this case, the fifth element was considered the soul or the spirit of life. Distillation and evaporation were the processes of removing the soil from the plant or essential oils. Nowadays, these oils are also known as volatile oils, but far from being the soul, essential oils are a complexity of aroma's composition. Those constituents of essential oils are generally derived from phenylpropanoid routes [6]. The studies of those routes have disclosed the relevance of the aspect of physiology regulation, but certainly isoprenoid exemplifies the major group of secondary metabolites in herbs, which exhibit extremely vast varieties of chemical structures and biochemical functions. Since primary metabolites exist in all plant cells that are qualified by division, secondary metabolites are there exclusively by accident and are not essential for that herb. In contrariety to primary metabolites, secondary compounds vary extensively in their occurrence in those herbs and some may appear only in a unique or a few species [7]. Due to the connection of terpenoids in many pharmacological properties and their great value added especially for pharmaceutical, cosmetic, and food industries, the isoprenoid route has been a spotlight for most related articles. Essential oils are nearly always rotational and have a high refractory index; they are sparingly soluble in water, usually less dense than water and liquid at room temperature, but there is some exception, as trans-anethole (anise camphor) from the oil of anise (*Pimpinella anisum L.*), and they may be classified using different criteria: consistency, origin and chemical nature. As stated by their consistency, essential oils are classified as essences, balsams, or resins. Depending on their origin, essential oils are natural, artificial, or synthetic. Essential oils are aromatic chemical compounds that come from plant's glands. Due to their volatility, flavour, and toxicity, this class of compounds also plays significant aspects in the defence's herbs, communication between plants and pollinator attractiveness [6, 8]. A lot of herbs can be viewed as being composed of a basic unit called isoprene or isopentane. Terms such as isoprenoid or terpenoid are employed concurrently. Many terpenoids are assembled of carbon atoms from acyclic disposition to a cyclic disposition by different chemical reactions, like condensation, addition, cyclisation, deletion, or rearrangements to be transformed into a basic unit, and generally, are very extensively diffused throughout the total plant kingdom. These compounds comprise a structurally varied class that can be splitted into main and minor terpenoids [8, 9]. Biosynthesis of terpenes can occur in a distinct sector of the herb, such as bark, flowers, fruits, leaves, roots, rhizomes, seeds, and wood, and have all been described to concentrate them in different herbs. Terpenes that are the main metabolites include carotenes, regulators of growth, proteins, quinones, polyprenols, and sterol, substitutes of terpenes with an alcohol functional group [9]. These constituents are indispensable for preserving the membrane to keep the entirety of its structure, also for protection against light, and securing the maintenance of its biological functionality. Terpenes are a large class of chemical compounds, classified by molecular weight, being monoterpenes, sesquiterpenes, diterpenes, seterterpenes, triterpenes, tetraterpenes and phytosterols amongst others [6]. Monoterpenes are the major contributor of most important essential oils in nature. Since the monoterpenes ($C_{10}H_{16}$) are small molecules with two isoprene units, such as menthol and linalool, and they are lipophilic; they are promptly consumed through the skin. Synthetic compounds can be used to break down the problems coming across with herbal products by creating actions for the construction of such molecules, regardless of the original species. Indeed, ways have been developed for most of the natural molecules, but, given their commonly complex spatial arrangements, industrial production is not practicable for the majority of examples [6, 8, 9]. Characteristically, the plant's secondary metabolites are cumulated and stored in relatively large quantities, which can be explained by their role as chemical signals or defence compounds. Terpenes are built up from the union of two carbon units with five members each by condensation, isopentenyl diphosphate, synonym isopentenyl pyrophosphate (IPP) and dimethylallyldiphosphate synonym dimethylallyl pyrophosphate (DMAPP), with different modes of structure formation, number of unsaturated bonds and type of linker groups. Not all terpenoids have a composition of their structure in the repetition of five carbon atoms, as can be habitual of them, considering that they are formed usually from isoprene as the forming matrix [6]. Terpenes consisting of more than five isoprene structures appear in all herbs, and simpler terpenes (C_{10}–C_{25}) are mainly restricted in the phylogeny classification to vascular plants/higher plants, synonym Tracheophyta, while sesquiterpenes have been found broadly in division Bryophyta and in the kingdom Fungi. Monoterpenoids are colourless, distilled by steam, and liquids insoluble in water with a typical scent, with a range of boiling points of 140 until 180 °C. Some of them have shown potentiality as insect plague management because they simply provide herbs with defences against insects that feed on it. Many terpenes also operate as insects captivate, being green and innocuous to humans and other animals [6]. More than a thousand sesquiterpenes are known today. Sesquiterpenes are the biggest category of terpenoids with broad molecular structure and are constituted of three isoprene matrixes, that is, they are composed with 15 carbon atoms, such as farnesol, guaiazulene, bisabolol and become from medicinal plants in distilleries equipments, in the bitter-tasting substances and essential oils in a lot of herbs. Diterpenes are formed by 20 carbon atoms by their condensation of four isoprene residues, such as taxol, gibberellins, phytol, and fusicocsin. Like sesquiterpenes, we know a thousand or more C_{20} compounds in this category, which fit into 20 main typical skeletons. Triterpenes are categorised based on the linear composition or number of cyclic compounds actual. Triterpenes relate to an inharmonious compilation of chemical compounds, which are considered to be acquired from squalene; the C_{30} is non cyclic component by types of rings and ligands. Pentacyclic triterpenes are usually distributed in vascular plants, occurring as glycosides with sugar ligands (saponins) or without sugar ligands (aglycones) [6]. Two routes have been extensively studied, leading to these precursors, through the mevalonate (typically known as MVA route; C6] and the 1-deoxyxylulose-D-5-phosphate (coded as the DXP route) pathways. The DXP compound, also known as the 2-C-methyl- D-erythritol-4-phosphate or methylerythritol phosphate (coded as the MEP route), occurs in plant plastids (chloroplasts) and by bacteria, while the MVA track different sources such as fungus, in the herb's cytosol and in some animals. In the mevalonic acid route, the key enzyme is 3-hydroxy-3-methylglutaryl coenzyme A reductase (HMG-CoA reductase, coded as HMGR). HMGR assemble the initial sequence of the MVA route by converting HMG-CoA to MVA using NADPH as coenzyme [6, 8]. The synthesis of mevalonic acid is illustrated in Fig. (**1**). In higher plants, the condensation of the basic C5 units, isopentenyl diphosphate (coded as IPP) and dimethylallyldiphosphate (coded as DMAPP), is catalysed by the enzyme prenyltransferases (Fig. **2**), which builds the chain of prenyldiphosphate, designated as the original source for each category of terpenoids: geranyl diphosphate (coded as GPP; C10), farnesyl diphosphate (coded as FPP; C15) and geranylgeranyl diphosphate (coded as GGPP), respectively for the monoterpenes, sesquiterpenes and diterpenes [6, 8].

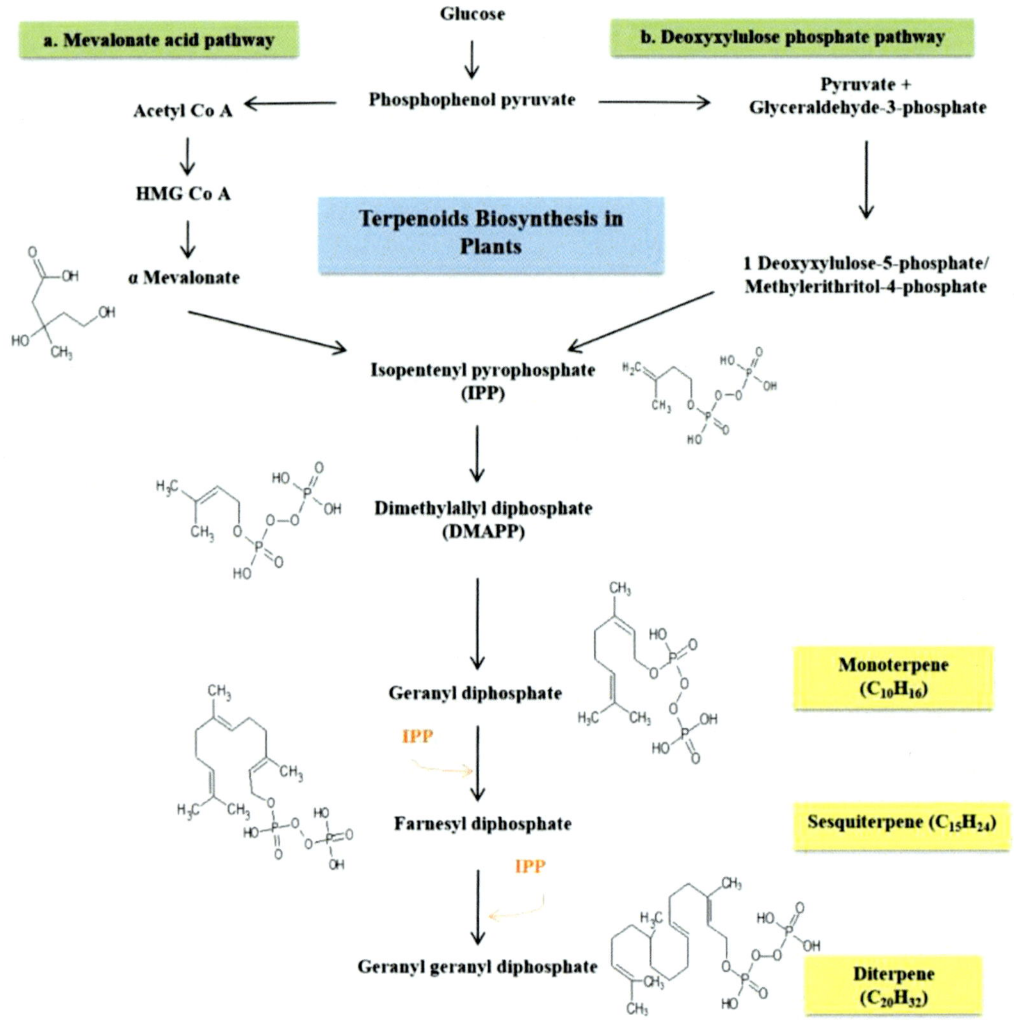

Fig. (1). Terpenoids biosynthesis pathway in Plants (a.) Mevalonate acid pathway. (b.) Deoxyxylulose phosphate pathway.

3. CHEMICAL COMPOSITION AND CONGENERIC GROUPS

In addition to the key chemical markers for the technical flavor effect, an essential oil found on the market will normally contain many other chemical constituents, some having little or no flavor function. However, the chemical constituents of essential oils are not infinite in structural variation. Because they are derived from higher plants, these constituents are formed *via* one of four or five major biosynthetic pathways: lipoxygenase, oxidation of lipids, shikimic acid, isoprenoid (terpenoid), and photosynthetic pathways. In ripening vegetables, lipoxygenases oxidize polyunsaturated fatty acids, eventually yielding low-molecular-weight aldehydes (2-hexenal), alcohols (2,6-nonadienol), and esters, many exhibiting flavoring properties. Plant amino acids phenylalanine and tyrosine are formed *via* the shikimic acid pathway and can subsequently be deaminated, oxidized, and reduced to yield important aromatic substances such as cinnamaldehyde and eugenol. The vast majority of constituents detected in commercially *via*ble essential oils are terpenes [*e.g.*, hydrocarbons (limonene), alcohols (menthol), aldehydes (citral), ketones (carvone), acids, and esters (geranyl acetate)] that are formed *via* the isoprene pathway [10]. Since all of these pathways operate in plants, albeit to different extents depending on the species, season, and growth environment, many of the same chemical constituents are present in a wide variety of essential oils. A consequence of having a limited number of plant biosynthetic pathways is that the structural variation of chemical constituents in an essential oil is limited. Essential oils typically contain 5–10 distinct chemical classes or congeneric groups. Some congeneric groups, such as aliphatic terpene hydrocarbons, contain upwards of 100 chemically identified constituents. In some essential oils, a single constituent (*e.g.*, citral in lemongrass oil) or a congeneric group of constituents (*e.g.*, hydroxyallylbenzene derivatives; eugenol, eugenyl acetate, *etc*., in clove bud oil) comprise the majority of the mass of the essential oil. In others, no single congeneric group predominates. For instance, although eight congeneric groups comprise >98% of the composition of the oil of *mentha piperita* (peppermint oil), >95% of the oil is accounted for by three chemical groups—[1] terpene aliphatic and aromatic hydrocarbons, [2] terpene alicyclic secondary alcohols, ketones, and related esters, and [3] terpene 2-isopropylidene substituted cyclohexanone derivatives and related substances. The formation and members of a congeneric group are chosen based on a combination of structural features and known biochemical fate. Substances with a common carbon-skeletal structure and functional groups that participate in common pathways of metabolism are assigned to the same congeneric group. For instance, menthyl acetate hydrolyzes prior to absorption to yield menthol, which is absorbed and is inconvertible with menthone in fluid compartments (*e.g.*, blood). Menthol is either conjugated with glucuronic acid and excreted in the urine or undergoes further hydroxylation mainly at C8 to yield a diol that is also excreted, either free or conjugated. Despite the fact that menthyl acetate is an ester, menthol is an alcohol, menthone a ketone, and 3,8-menthanediol diol; they are structurally and metabolically related (Fig. **1**). Therefore, are members of the same congeneric group. In the case of *Mentha piperita*, the three principal congeneric groups listed above have different metabolic options and possess different organ-specific toxic potential. The congeneric group of terpenes, aliphatic and aromatic hydrocarbons is represented mainly by limonene and myrcene. The second and most predominant congeneric group is the alicyclic secondary alcohols, ketones, and related esters that include *d*-menthol, menthone, isomenthone, and menthyl acetate. Although the third congeneric group contains alicyclic ketones similar in structure to menthone, it is metabolically quite different in that it contains an exocyclic isopropylidene substituent that undergoes hydroxylation principally at the C9 position, followed by ring closure and dehydration to yield a heteroaromatic furan ring of increased toxic potential. In the absence of a C4–C8 double bond, neither menthone nor isomenthone can participate in this intoxication pathway. Hence, they are assigned to a different congeneric group. The presence of a limited number of congeneric groups in an essential oil is critical to the organization of constituents and subsequent safety evaluation of the oil itself.Members of each congeneric group exhibit common structural features and participate in common pathways of pharmacokinetics and metabolism and exhibit similar toxicologic potential. If the mass of the essential oil (>95%) can be adequately characterized chemically and the constituents assigned to well-defined congeneric groups, the safety evaluation of the essential oil can be reduced to [1] a safety evaluation of each of the congeneric groups comprising the essential oil; and [2] a "sum of the parts" evaluation of all congeneric groups to account for any chemical or biological interactions between congeneric groups in the essential oil under conditions of intended use. Validation of such an approach lies in the stepwise comparison of the dose and toxic effects for each key congeneric group with similar equivalent doses and toxic effects exhibited by the entire essential oil. Potential interactions between congeneric groups can, to some extent, be analyzed by an in-depth comparison of the biochemical and toxicologic properties of different congeneric groups in the essential oil. For some representative essential oils that have been the subject of toxicology studies, a comparison of data for the congeneric groups in the essential oil with data on the essential oil itself (congeneric groups together) is a basis for analyzing the presence or absence of interactions. Therefore, the impact of interaction between congeneric groups is minimal if the levels of and endpoints of toxicity of congeneric groups (*e.g.*, tertiary terpene alcohols) are similar to those of the essential oil (*e.g.*, coriander oil). Since composition plays such a critical role in the evaluation, analytical identification requirements are also critical to the evaluation. Complete chemical characterization of the essential oil may be difficult or economically unfeasible based on the small volume of essential oil used as a flavor ingredient. In these few cases, mainly for low-volume essential oils, the unknown fraction may be appreciable and a large number of chemical constituents will not be identified. However, if the intake of the essential oil is low or significantly less than its intake from the consumption of food (*e.g.*, thyme) from which the essential oil is derived (*e.g.*, thyme oil), there should be no significant concern for safety under the conditions of intended use. For those cases in which the chemical characterization of the essential oil is limited but the volume of intake is more significant, it may be necessary to perform additional analytical work to decrease the number of unidentified constituents or, in other cases, to perform selected toxicity studies on the essential oil itself. A principal goal of the safety evaluation of essential oils is that no congeneric groups that have significant human intake should go unevaluated.

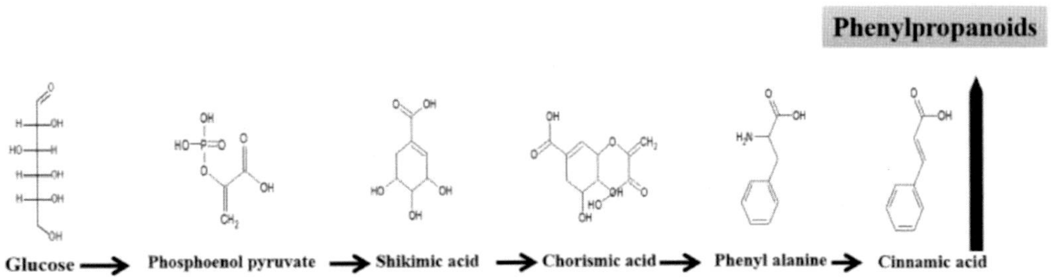

Fig. (2). Shikimic acid pathway.

3.1. Chemistry of Essential oils

Essential oils are chemically and physically differed from fatty acids, because essential oils have volatile organic compounds, whereas fatty acids contain glycerides. Presence of high volatile compounds enables the extraction of essential oils through hydro distillation and other distillation processes.

Essential oils are composed of different chemical compounds and classified in two classes:

1. Terepens/Terpenoids
2. Phenylpropanoids

3.1.1. Terpenes/Terpenoids-

Terpenes formed by the condensation of isoprene molecules. Isoprene is a four carbons compounds chemically named 2-methyl-1, 3-butadiene, which have two unsaturated double bonds and therefore many times called isoprenoids. Terpenoids are more complex than terpenes [11]. Terpenoids have cyclic or linear structure, degree of unsaturation, substitutions, and oxygenated compounds in its structure. More than 30,000 terpenoids have been isolated from living organisms like plants, animals, and microorganisms [12].

- In 1880, Kekule scientists first time gave the name Terpene with $C_{10}H_{16}$ compound.

- In 1887, Wallach (an assistant of Kekule) hypothetically purposed thatterpenes constructed *via* two or more isoprene units; later in 1970 he got Nobel Prize.
- In 1947, Robinson gave "isoprene rule" suggesting that isoprene units should be connected to each other in "Head-to-Tail fashion". (Received Nobel Prize).
- In 1950, Ruzicka purposed "biogenetic isoprene rule" suggested that terpenoids derived from an aliphatic precursors like geraniol for the formation of monoterpenes.

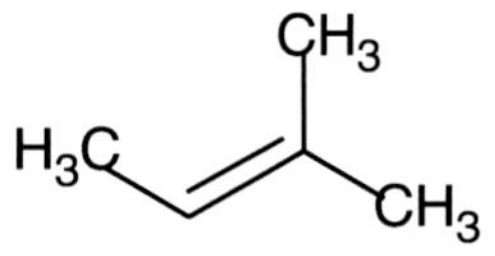

Isoprene

Isoprene units connect to each other in one direction like head-to--to-tail fashion. Branched side of the molecule referred as a head of the molecule and the opposite side referred as tail of the molecule. Biosynthesis pathways of terpenes and terpenoids also follows the same pattern of joining. Terpenes are diverse volatile organic compounds (VOCs) which can be classified on a structural and functional basis. Terpenes are classified mainly on the basis of the number of isoprene units (Table **1**).

Table 1. Classification of Terpenes.

No. of isoprene unit	Class	Formula
1	Hemiterpenes	C_5H_8
2	Monoterpene	$C_{10}H_{16}$
3	Sesquiterpene	$C_{15}H_{24}$
4	Diterpene	$C_{20}H_{32}$
5	Sesterpene	$C_{25}H_{40}$
6	Troterpene	$C_{30}H_{48}$
8	Tetraterpene	$C_{40}H_{64}$
n	Polyterpene	$(C_5H_8)_n$

Terpenes and terpenoids are synthesized in plants through two different pathways, mevalonate acid pathways occur in cytosol, whereas deoxyxylulose phosphate pathways runs in the chloroplast of the plant cell (Fig. **1**). Both pathways formed the universal precursor, IPP (Isopentenyl pyrophosphate) and DMAPP (Dimethyl allyl diphosphate) for terpenes and terpenoids derivatives (Fig. **1**) [13].

3.1.2. Phenylpropanoids

Phenylpropanoids have one or more C6 or C 3 units in their structure. Generally, benzene ring (C6) occurs in phenylpropanoids. Phenylpropanoids mainly synthesized through shikimic acid pathway in plants and cinnamic acid acts as a precursor (Fig. **2**) [11, 14].

4. BIOLOGICAL ACTIVITY OF ESSENTIAL OIL

Since ancient times, plant materials has been utilized in many traditional folk medicines due to their healing properties. With the advancement of science, we have come to know the constituents of essential oil (Tables **2** & **3**; Figs. **2** & **3**), the reason behind their healing properties. In nature, plants are attacked by a number of biotic stress (pathogens such as bacteria, fungi, viruses, and insects), here in these conditions essential oil provides a protection mechanism to the plant by playing various functional roles such as antibacterial, antivirals, antifungals, insecticides and many times these oils protect the plant against herbivores by reducing their appetite for such plants. Essential oil attractants pollinator, and seed dispersion agents through their fragrance effects. Essential oil has secured a major place in medicine and preservatives to impart flavor and aroma to food consumed by humen due to the presence of numerous biological activities. Many previous studies have confirmed that essential oils are indeed effective against a variety of organisms which includes bacteria [15], virus [16], fungi, protozoa [17] parasites [18], insects [19]. This will improve our knowledge regarding the biological activity of essential oil and allow us to develop new applications in human health, agriculture, and the environment.

Table 2. Some important essential oils with chemical constituents.

Limonene- Limonene is widespread monoterpene in essential oils, which have lemon-like odor in essential oil [20].
Pinene- Pinene is also a monoterpene, mainly found in pines. Pinenes have two isoforms in nature, α and β pinenes. A pinene is mainly used in perfume industry because of its pine odor [21].
Myrecne- Myrecene is monoterpene hydrocarbon. Only β isoforms of myrecene are found in nature. Myrecene has a fresh citrus odor.
Zingiberene- Zingiberene is an open chain sesquiterpene and gives a unique odor to ginger.
Linalool- Linalool is an open chain alcoholic hydrocarbon which provides light and fresh lemon odor to plants.
Geraniol- Geraniol is an open chain alcoholic hydrocarbon which mainly found in geranioum plant species. In nature, two isoforms are found, *the cis* forms known as nerol [21].
Geranial- Geranial is an open chain hydrocarbon with an aldehyde groups.

(Table 2) cont.....

Menthol- Menthol is a cyclic hydrocarbon which has a hydroxyl groups in its ring structure. Menthol is mainly found in Mentha plant species [22].
Citronellol- Citronellol is an open chain alcoholic hydrocarbon, responsible for rose type flavors [21].
Patchoulol- Patchoulol is a cyclic hydrocarbon which has a hydroxyl groups in its structure. Patchoulol mainly gives a unique flavor to patchouli oil.
Thymol- Thymol is a monoterpene phenolic compound, generally used in fragrance and household products [21].
Linalyl acetate- An esteric compound, mainly found in Lavender plant species [22].
Carotol- Mainly found in Carrot.
Cinnemaldehyde- Cinnemaldehyde is an aldehyde with a phenyl group, mainly found in cinnamon, used as a fragrance and sweetener [23].
Eugenol- Eugenol is mainly found in clove [24].
Eucalyptol- Eucalyptol is also known as 1, 8- Cineole, which mainly found in Eucalyptus plant species [25].
Diallyl sulfide- This compound is mainly found in garlic. This sulfur containing compound is responsible for the pungent smell of garlic [26].
S-alk(en)ylcystiene sulfoxide- This compound is mainly found in onion and responsible for onion pungent smell and flavour of onion-based products [27].

Table 3. Important trade essential oils with chemical constituents [13].

Trade Name	Species	Important Constituents
Cedarwood	*Juniperus mexicana* Schiede	Sesquiterpene hydrocarbons- (α-cedrene, thujopsene, cuperene); cedrol
Cypress	*Cupressus sempervirens* L.	Monoterpene hydrocarbons – (limonene, α-phellandrene, δ-3-carene)
Ginger	*Zingiber officinale*	Sesquiterpene hydrocarbons – (zingiberene, β-sesquiphellandrene)
Bergamot	*Citrus aurantium* L.	Monoterpene hydrocarbon (limonene); linalyl acetate
Lemon	*Citrus limon* (L.) Burman fil.	Monoterpene hydrocarbons (limonene, β-pinene, γ-terpinene)
Mandarin	*Citrus reticulata* Blanco	Monoterpene hydrocarbons (limonene, γ-terpinene)
Pepper	*Piper nigrum* L.	Monoterpene hydrocarbons (pinenes, sabinene, limonene, δ-3-carene); β-caryophyllene
Pine silvestris	*Pinus sylvestris* L.	Monoterpne hydrocarbons (pinenes, δ---carene, limonene, myrcene)
Sweet orange	*Citrus sinensis* (L.) Osbeck	Monoterpene hydrocarbons (limonene)
Turpentine	*Pinus* spp.	Monoterpene hydrocarbons (pinenes)

(Table 3) cont.....

Trade Name	Species	Important Constituents
Nutmeg	*Myristica fragrans* Houtt.	Monoterpene hydrocarbons (sabinene, pinenes); myristicine
Peppermint	*Mentha* × *piperita* L.	Menthol; menthone
Rose	*Rosa* × *damascena*Miller	Citronellol, geraniol, nerol; nonadecane
Rosewood	*Aniba rosaeodora* Ducke	Linalool
Thyme	*Thymus vulgaris* L	Monoterpene phenol (thymol); ρ-cymene, γ-terpinene
Cardamom	*Elettaria cardamomum* Maton	α-Terpenyl acetate; 1,8-cineole
Clary sage	*Salvia sclarea* L.	Linalyl acetate; linalool
Lavandin	*Lavandula angustifolia* Mill. × *L. latifolia*Medik. (*Lavandula intermedia*)	Linaly acetate; linalool, 1,8-cineole
Carrot seed	*Daucus carota* L.	Carotol
Coriander	*Coriandrum sativum* L.	Linalool
Geranium	*Pelargonium* spp.	Citronellol, geraniol
Neroli	*Citrus aurantium* L. subsp. *aurantium*	Linalool; linalyl acetate, β-pinene, limonene
Oregano	*Origanumonites* L	Monoterpene phenol (carvacrol); ρ-cymene, γ-terpinene
Palmarosa	*Cymbopogon martinii* (Roxb.) W. Wats	Geraniol
Patchouli	*Pogostemon cablin* (Blanco) Benth.	Patchoulol; bulnesene, α-guaiene
Lavender	*Lavandula latifolia* Medik.	Linalool; linalyl acetate, 1,8-cineole, camphor
Petitgrain	*Citrus aurantinum* L. subsp. *aurantinum*	Linaly acetate; Linalool
Wintergreen	*Gaultheria procumbens* L.,	Methyl salicylate
Ylang-ylang	*Cananga odorata* (Lam.) Hook. f. & Thomson	Benzyl acetate, germacrene geranyl acetate, ρ-cresyl methyl ether; linalool, (E, E, α-farnesene)
Cinnamon bark, Ceylon	*Cinnamomum zeylanicum* Nees	Cinnamaldehyde
Cumin	*Cuminum cyminum* L.	Cuminaldehyde, ρ-mentha- 1,3-dien-7-al; γ-terpinene, ρ-cymene
Lemongrass	*Cymbopogon flexuosus* (Nees ex Steud.) J. F. Watson	Geranial, neral
Caraway	*Carum carvi* L.	Carvone; limonene
Mugwort common	*Artemisia vulgaris* L.	α-Thujone, camphor; 1,8-cineole
Dill	*Anethum graveolens* L.	Carvone; limonene, α-phellandrene, dillapiole

(Table 3) cont.....

Trade Name	Species	Important Constituents
Pennyroyal	*Menthapulegium*L.	Pulegone, piperitenone, piperitone, isomentone, neoisomentone
Sage, Dalmatian	*Salvia officinalis* L.	α-Thujone, β-thujone, camphor; 1,8-cineole
Wormwood	*Artemisia absinthium* L.	β-Thujone, α-thujone; (Z)- epoxy-ocimene, sabinyl acetate, chrysanthenyl acetate, α-phellandrene
Eucalyptus	*Eucalyptus globulus*Labill.	1,8-Cineole; α-pinene
Laurel leaf	*Laurus nobilis* L.	1,8-Cineole
Anise seed	*Pimpinellaanisum* L.	(E)-Anethole
Clove buds	*Syzygium aromaticum* (L.) Merill et L. M. Perry	Eugenol, eugenyl acetate
Clove leaf	*Syzygium aromaticum* (L.) Merill et L. M. Perry	Eugenol; β-caryophyllene
Parsley seed	*Petroselinum crispum* (Mill.) Nym. Ex A. W. Hill	Myristicine, apiol; α-pinene, β-pinene
Chenopodium	Chenopodium	Ascaridole
Asafoetida	*Ferula assa-foetida* L.	R-2-Butyl-1-propenyl disulfide, 1-(1-methylthiopropenyl)-1-propenyl disulfide, 2-butyl-3-methyl-thioallyl disulfide
Buchu leaf	*Agathosma betulina* (Bergius) Pillans, *A. crenulata* (L.) Pillans	trans-p-Menthane-8-thiol-3-one and its S-acetate as characteristic minor components
Garlic	*Allium sativum* L.	Diallyl disulfide
Onion	*Allium cepa* L.	Methylpropyl disulfide, dipropyl disulfide, propenylpropyl disulfide, 2-hexyl-5-methyl-3(2 H)-furanone
Angelica root	*Angelica archangelica* L.	15-Pentadecanolide, 13-tridecanolide as characteristic minor components in addition to terpenoids and sesquiterpenoids
Celery seed	*Apium graveolens* L.	3-Butylphthalide and sedanenolide as characteristic components in addition to terpenoids (limonene and β-selinene)
Lovage root	*Levisticum officinale* Koch	3-Butylphthalide, ligustilide, ligusticum lactone

4.1. Essential Oils as Antibacterial Agents

Multidrug resistance becomes a leading cause of human death.This has prompted Pharma Industries to explore alternative new key molecules against bacterial strains. A number of previous studies had described the correlation between the chemical constituents and antibacterial activities of essential oils [28, 29]. Several types of essential oils and their major chemical constituents have been reported to possess a wide range of bacterial inhibitory potentials. Essential oil either inhibits the growth of bacteria (bacteriostatic) or destroys bacterial cells (bactericidal), nevertheless, it is difficult to distinguish these actions. Different essential oils have differences in their effectiveness against different target bacteria depending on their structure (Gram-positive and Gram-negative bacteria), this is due to their variable chemical composition. Lipophilic nature of essential oils, which makes them easy to pass through the cell wall and cytoplasmic membrane and increase the permeability of the membrane. Increase permeability of bacterial cell wall has been associated with cell viability due to many reasons such as loss of ions and reduction of membrane potential, the collapse of the proton pump, and depletion of the ATP pool [30, 31] had conducted a study on 52 plant oils to investigate antimicrobial activity against *Acinetobacter baumanii, Aeromonasveronii, biogroupsobria, Candida albicans, Enterococcus faecalis, Escherichia coli, Klebsiella pneumoniae, Pseudomonas aeruginosa, Salmonella enterica subsp. enterica serotype typhimurium, Serratia marcescens,* and *Staphylococcus aureus,* using an agar dilution method. This study concluded that Lemongrass, oregano, and bay inhibited all organisms at concentrations of ≤2·0% (v/v) [31, 32] reported the antibacterial potential of chia oil against four G+ve bacterial strains (*Bacillus megaterium, B. megaterium, B. mojavensis, and Clavibacter michiganensis*) and six G-ve bacterial strains (*Xanthomonas campestris Pammel, X. vesicatoria Doidge, Pseudomonas syringaepv. phaseolicola Van Hall, Escherichia coli Migula. P. savastanoiJanse,Burkholderia gladioli pv. agaricicolaYabuuch)i.* According to them, chia oil was effectively inhibiting the growth of Gram-positive (G+ve) bacterial strains more than Gram-negative (G-ve). This study also confirms the fact that essential oils differ in their effectiveness against different target bacteria. [33], reported that clove and oregano oils were capable of damaging the cell membranes of gram-negative bacteria (*E. coli*) more effectively than those of gram-positive bacteria. Tea tree oil was effective against gram-positive bacteria and gram-negative bacteria causing respiration inhibition and increasing cytoplasmic membrane permeability along with potassium ion leakage [34].

4.2. Essential Oils as Antifungal Agents

Over the past two decades, the frequency of invasive mycoses due to opportunistic fungal pathogens has increased significantly, directly associated with excessive morbidity and mortality. Patient populations which include individuals undergoing solid organ and blood and marrow (BMT) transplantation and major surgery and those with AIDS, neoplastic disease, immunosuppressive therapy, advanced age, and premature birth are more prone to the development of serious fungal infections, [35, 36], studied the antifungal activity of *Thymus schimperi* Ronniger essential oil against a wide spectrum of pathogenic fungal which includes *Penicillium chrysogenum*, *Verticillium sp.*, *Aspergillus tubingensis*, *Aspergillus minutus*, *Beauveria bassiana* and *Microsporum gypseum*. The study strongly concluded that most of the isolated fungi were resistant to amphotericin B and itraconazole, whereas T. schimperi essential oil showed antifungal activity against all tested fungal isolates. Anise oil were shown antifungal activity against the filamentous fungus, Mucormucedo by hyphal morphological changes such as swollen hyphae at the tips [37] Thymol, a major component of thyme essential oil, were shown a great fungicidal activity against *Aspergillus flavus*, through the ROS scavenging [38]. Other essential oils, such as cinnamon oil, linalool, and xanthorrizol, were also shown to possess biofilm inhibition properties. [39], demonstrated that cinnamon oil exhibits higher antifungal activity compared to basil and peppermint. Essential oil (EO) of flowers from *Tagetesminuta* L.A possessed a good antifungal activity against *Candida lipolityca*, *Candida parapsilosis*, *Trichosporo nasahii* and *Sphacelomaam pelinum* [40, 41], studied the antifungal properties of 12 essential oils (tea tree, laurel, anise, basil, bergamot, lavender, mint, oregano, grapefruit, rosemary, winter savory on *C. glabrata* which is an opportunistic pathogen, associated with endocarditis, meningitis and 28 disseminated diseases and with complicated vaginitis. The study concluded that oregano and winter savory are the two most effective essential oils, inducing growth inhibition and cell damage of *C. glabrata* strains, through his study confirmed that tea tree oil (*Melaleuca alternifolia*) has both inhibitory and fungicidal activity against dermatophytes (n = 106] and filamentous fungi (n = 78]. MICs for all fungi ranged from 0.004% to 0.25% and minimum fungicidal concentrations (MFCs) ranged from <0.03% to 8.0% [42].

4.3. Essential Oils as Antioxidant Agents

Molecular alterations at the proteins, amino acids, unsaturated lipids, and DNA levels due to oxidative stress can lead to many health issues such as aging, arteriosclerosis, cancer, Alzheimer's disease, parkinson's disease, diabetes and asthma. 'Oxidative stress' refers to an imbalance between free radical production and their removal by the body's antioxidant system, which is present in almost all cells [43, 44]. External supplement of antioxidants are the best possible way to cure the imbalance. [45] studied the radical scavenging and antioxidant properties assayed for seven essential oils which includes basil, cinnamon, clove, nutmeg, oregano and thyme. Studys concluded that all seven oil have the antioxidant and radical scavenging activity where clove oil has the highest [45]. Oregano essential oil were proved to be a good source of natural antioxidants with the major components are thymol (45%) and carvacrol (37.4%) and has a potential application in food and pharmaceutical industries, as an alternative to synthetic antioxidants [46]. Essential oils from *Aloysia triphylla* and *Minthostachys mollis* have shown antioxidant potential and radical scavenging [47, 48] investigated the antioxidant properties of L. mairei EOs *in vitro* using: the DPPH assay and reducing power determination. The obtained results showed that both EOs exhibited antioxidant activity across the two testing methods [48]. Many studies in the past have come to a conclusion that high content of thephenol, carvacrol leads to high antioxidant/reducing power activities of essential oils [49, 50].

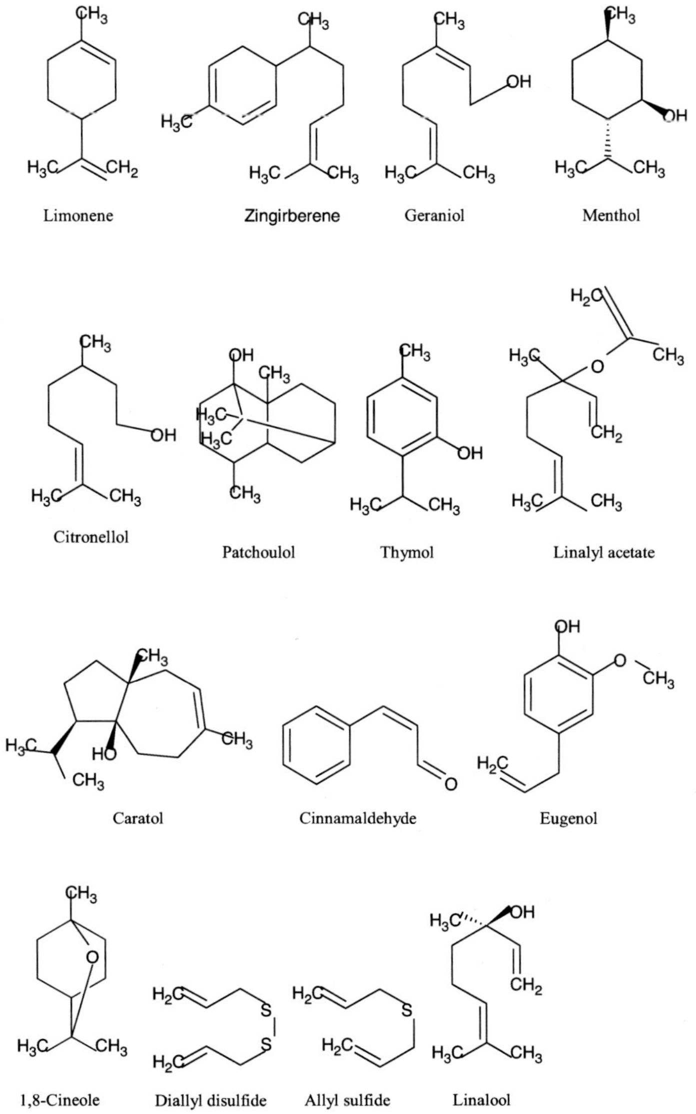

Fig. (3). Structures of some important chemical compounds of essential oils.

4.4. Other Activities of Essential Oil

Other than major identified function of essential oil such as antibacterial agents, antifungal agents, and antioxidant agents, much research has also supported various other functions of essential oil. Antimutagenic activity, anticarcinogenic [51, 52], Anthelmintic Activity [53], allelopathic agents [54, 55], antiangiogenic agent [56, 57], food preservative [58, 59]. With the advancement of science, essential oils have been characterized with many more functions. But still a lot more to understand regarding the functional characteristics of essential oil which have direct impact from environmental factors such as pH, ionic strength, temperature, and water activity on efficacy.

5. ESSENTIAL OIL PREPARATION TECHNIQUES

Plant-based volatile oils with strong aromatic components extracted from oil 'sacs' in flowers, seeds, leaves, stems, roots, wood, and bark are known as essential oils. The essential oils are used in body oils, hair rinses, cosmetic lotions, detergents, soaps, perfumes and room sprays, toilet products, pharmaceuticals, confectionery, food products, soft drinks, distilled alcoholic beverages (hard drinks) and insecticides, [60]. These are plant secondary metabolites comprising complex mixtures of volatile organic compounds like phenols, aldehydes, alcohols, esters and ketones [61]. Chemically, they are hydrophobic and lower density oils soluble in organic solvents. Their extraction yields depend on the species and part of plant used for the extraction [62]. According to plant organs, age, soil configuration, climate change, and stages of plant life, quality, quantity, and composition of extracted essential oils can be transformed [63]. Characteristics and constituents required in the botanical extract are the major factors of choosing the manufacturing methods and techniques used to extract essential oils.

Extraction techniques can be divided into two categories: classical methods and innovative methods. There are several by-the number methods of extraction behavior of essential oils.

5.1. Classical Extraction Techniques

The conventional technologies applied for processing essential oils are of ample significance and are still commonplace in copious parts of the globe. Maceration, Cold Pressing, Hydro distillation (HD), Steam distillation (SD), Solvent extraction, Enfleurage, Soxhlet extraction and are the traditional and generally used methods.

5.1.1. Maceration

Maceration gives more of an "infused oil" rather than an "essential oil". The plant matter is soaked in vegetable oil, heated and strained to a point it can be used for massage.

5.1.2. Cold Pressing

This process is applied for carrier oils and essential oils. In this procedure, the oil present in the outer layer of the plant is separated by scrubbing. The rinds are separated from the fruit, followed by grounding or chopping and then pressing. Then to squeeze the whole plant is pressed, the material is taken out from the pulp and releasing essential oil from the pouches. This method, appropriate to extract the oil from plants, involves simple pressing of the rind at about 120°F. The essential oil is separated from the material by centrifugation.This method is used to extract the essential oils from citrus rinds such as orange, lemon, grapefruit, and bergamot.

5.1.3. Hydrodistillation (HD)

This is a conventional method to isolate essential oils from aromatic and medicinal plants. The first plant extract used and purified by this method was rose. Isotropic distillation is the principle of this extraction method. The setup consists of a condenser and a decanter to collect the condensate and to separate essential oils from water, respectively. In this technique, the processes begin with immersing the plant materials directly into water or other solvent inside the alembic (vessel), and the whole mixture is boiled. Then the essential oils are evaporated by heating the mixture of water and plant materials, followed by the liquefaction of the vapours in a condenser.

For powders (*i.e.*, spice powder, ground wood, *etc.*) and very tough materials like roots, wood, or nuts, hydro distillation seems to be efficient. This method is capable of protecting essential oils to be extracted at a certain degree without being overheated, as the oils are surrounded by water. The key benefit of this technique is the ability to isolate plant materials below 100°C [62].

5.1.4. Steam Distillation (SD)

Steam distillation is one of the early and formally accepted techniques for the isolation of essential oils from plant materials. It is a type of distillation (separation or extraction process) applied to the temperature-sensitive plants such as natural aromatic compounds. According to the studies by this technique, 93%

of essential oils are extracted and the remaining 7% can be further extracted by other methods [64].

The principle of this method is the collective vapour pressure is equal to the ambient pressure at about 100 °C, so the volatile components with boiling points ranging from 150 to 300 °C can be evaporated at a temperature close to that of water. The technique benefits in carrying out the extraction of essential oil under pressure depending upon the oils extraction difficulty. In essence, the process starts with the heating of the plant material with steam which is supplied from the steam generator. Heat is the key factor for determining the efficiency of the plant material structures break down and burst and release of aromatic components or essential oils. The plant materials are charged with steam in the alembic (Gourd shaped distillation apparatus) without maceration in water. The injected steam passes through the plant from the base of the alembic to the top. This steam works as a medium to breakdown the pores of the raw material and releases the essential oil from it. The system produces a mixture of vapour and the desired essential oil. Then this vapour is condensed and further the essential oil is collected.

To evaluate the antioxidant properties of a component 2, 2-diphenyl-1-picryl hydrazyl (DPPH) in the study, Steam distillation extraction method gave a higher yield of antioxidant components than the oils extracted by hydro distillation [65].

5.1.5. Solvent Extraction

This is also known as liquid–liquid extraction or partitioning method used for the separation of essential oils from the plant extract based on the difference in their solubility. This technique is useful to extract oil from fragile or delicate flower materials which cannot be extracted by heat or steam supplied. Solvents obtained by this method are acetone, vegetable oil, petroleum ether, biodiesel, hexane, methanol, and ethanol. Firstly, the plant samples are mixed with solvents to be extracted by mildly heating the mixture, and the process is followed by filtration and evaporation of the solvents. From the concentrate, pure alcohol is used to extract the oil to dissolve the essential oil into it, the alcohol is mixed with the filtrate mixture, and thereafter it is distilled at low temperature. The oil remains and alcohol vaporizes.

5.1.6. Enfleurage

It is a rigorous and traditional way of extracting essential oil from flowers. Uniform deposition of fat over flower petals is the key step in this process. Fats get absorbed by essential oils, and then alcohol separates and extracts the oils from the fat.

5.1.7. Soxhlet Extraction

Soxhlet extractions consist of use of solid-liquid contact for the removal of one or several compounds from a solid by dissolution into a refluxing liquid phase. Soxhlet extraction is used for the compound having desired limited solubility in a solvent, and the impurity is insoluble in that solvent. It allows efficiently recycling of small amounts of solvent to dissolve a larger amount of material in an unmonitored and unmanaged operation.

In a soxhlet device, the solid matrix is gradually filled with the extracting liquid phase which is placed in a cavity and condensation of vapour from a distillation flask occurs. A siphon pulls the contents of the cavity back into the distillation flask, when the liquid reaches the present level, thus carrying the extracted analytes into the bulk liquid. This procedure is repeated until an almost complete extraction is achieved. The most substantial benefit of this technique is that the sample is repeatedly brought into contact with fresh portions of the solvent. This procedure avoids the possibility of the solvent becoming saturated with the extractable material and enhances the removal of the analytes from the matrix.

Advantages: These systems are broad range techniques, they can be applied to a variety of different plants possessing similar physio-chemical properties. The apparatuses applied for the procedures are cheap in comparison with the other modified techniques.

Disadvantages: The further modification of extraction techniques is due to various disadvantages of conventional methods which encourage essential oils to undergo chemical alterations like hydrolysis, isomerization, and oxidation. These processes involve high temperatures and affect the quality of essential oils, at the same time prolonging the extraction period.

5.2. Innovative Extraction Techniques

It is important that extraction methods should maintain the chemical composition and natural proportion of essential oils at its original state. For obtaining natural extracts with new techniques for similar or better quality products, the parameters under consideration are reduced extraction time, energy consumption, solvent use, and CO_2 emissions.

Supercritical Fluid Extraction, Microwave-Assisted Hydrodistillation (MAHD), Subcritical Extraction Liquid, and Solvent Free Microwave Extraction are the effective and modified methods.

5.2.1. Supercritical Fluid Extraction

The supercritical fluid state mainly depends on two factors that are the fluid critical pressure (Pc) and critical temperature (Tc), respectively. Fluids with these critical parameters reveal very remarkable properties like high diffusivity, low viscosity, and density closer to liquids [62]. The principle behind the supercritical fluid extraction method comprises the use and recycling of fluid in repeated steps of compression/decompression. Supercritical solvent used for the extraction of essential oils is carbon dioxide due to its numerous attractive properties: (i) easily reach the critical point (low critical pressure (Pc) = 72.9 atm, and temperature (Tc) = 31.2°C); (ii) its polarity is similar to pentane which makes it suitable for extraction of lipophilic compounds [66].

This technique is beneficial as CO_2 is relatively non-toxic, noncorrosive, non-flammable, safe, available in high purity at relatively low cost and is easily removed from the extract. Although this technique is costly and it is handled by trained professionals only. Supercritical extracts are substantiated as of superior quality, with better functional and biological activities.

5.2.2. Microwave-Assisted Hydrodistillation (MAHD)

Microwave-assisted hydro distillation is utilizing a microwave oven in the extraction process. The efficiency of microwave assisted hydro distillation largely depends on the dielectric constant of water and the sample. The principle of heating in Microwave-assisted hydro distillation is governed by two phenomenons: ionic conduction and dipole rotation, which in most cases occurs simultaneously, and it's direct impact on polar materials/solvents. In separation and extraction processes, this method is efficient to reduce both the extraction time and the volume of solvent required, it also minimizes the impact of CO_2 in the atmosphere by emitting less in environment. It is a useful technique to develop various types of materials for industrial materials under an extensive array of conditions.

5.2.3. Subcritical Extraction

Water and CO_2 are the fluids that can be used to extract essential oils using this method. The subcritical state of the fluid compromises several superior features like lower viscosity, lower density, and enhanced diffusivity between gas and liquids. This extraction technique is considered as the best substitute approach to enable a fast essential oil isolation process, which conducts at a low working temperature.

5.2.4. Solvent Free Microwave Extraction

SFME combines two techniques which are heating plant samples using microwave technology followed by dry distillation in the absence of any solvent which operates at a certain atmospheric pressure. This technique aids the isolation of essential oils from spices, aromatic herbs, and dry seeds. Several advantages of SFME have been reported like obtaining essential oils with high yield and selectivity, shorter extraction time, and environmentally friendly process.

Advantages: These are innovative methods that take less time, less amount of sample, and energy to extract the essential oils.

Disadvantages: These methods require critical sample preparation, costly and précised to operate.

5.3. Chromatographic Separation Techniques for Essential Oil

Essential oils are combinations of volatile components from different chemical classes, for their separation effective and available technology is one of the methodological goals. Essential oils have positive health effects with novel characteristics like antioxidant, antibacterial, and antifungal activities. Chromatographic methods are the best techniques to study the qualitative and quantitative composition of essential oils. An exhaustive study of hydro distillation, supercritical fluid extraction, ultrasound and microwave-assisted extraction, solid-phase micro extraction, pressurized liquid extraction, pressurized hot water extraction, liquid–liquid extraction, liquid-phase micro extraction, matrix solid-phase dispersion, and gas chromatography (one- and two-dimensional) hyphenated with mass spectrometry for the extraction through various plant species and analysis of essential oils has been provided in this chapter.

5.3.1. Thin Layer Chromatography

Thin-layer chromatography (TLC) is a widely used chromatographic technique, and its modern method such as HPTLC (High Pressure Thin-layer chromatography) can be advantageously used. Some of the advantages of TLC are its simplicity, cost effective, and simultaneous analysis of a large number of samples. In both analytical and preparative procedures, thin-layer chromatography is effectively used in a very wide range of applications of essential oils. Thin-layer chromatography has the ability to separate mixtures of substances of similar structure and the flexibility of a variety of methods of detection.

5.3.2. Analytical TLC

Analytical TLC has been used to analyze components such as flavonoids, phenolic acids, or coumarone. For the characterization of plant materials and determination of specific pharmacological activities, these classes of components are essential. In combination with special spray reagents TLC can provide valuable information about the type of essential oils. Visualization reagents are numerous, *e.g.*, vanillin/o-phosphoric acid, anisaldehyde or p-dimethylamino-benzal-dehyde-sulfuric acid, sulfuric acid, resorcin-sulfuricor phosphoric acid, aluminium chloride or hydroxyl-amine. This chromatographic method is rapid and easy; performed without the need of large instrumental equipment.

5.3.3. Liquid Chromatography

It is a common method for the chromatographic profiling and separation of essential oils using liquid column chromatography and high-performance liquids. Liquid column chromatography method is applied to the analytical and preparative fractionation of numerous types of oils. Essential oils were fractionated on silica columns using a mobile phase of solvent (methanol, ethanol. chloroform, benzene, *etc.*), with refractive index detection. Fractions were separated, collected, concentrated, and analyzed directly by spectrometry. The HPLC method is used to determine oils mixtures having a different functional group from plant essential oils. The oil sample is diluted with solvent and the constituents are separated on a C18 column using an acetonitrile (ACN)/water gradient. The constituents derivatives are identified using HPLC with ultra violet detector (UV), flame ionization detector (FID), photo diode detector (PD), and mass spectrometry (MS) detection.

5.3.4. Gas Chromatography

GC-MS applies advancements in both the separation technique and improvements in mass spectrometry detection along with enhanced data handling tools are relevant to the essential oil area. GC-MS (gas chromatography coupled to mass spectrometry) is only one of several possibilities: GC-FID (flame ionization detector) is widespread, and other detectors include TCD (thermal conductivity detector), ECD (electron capture detector), FPD (flame photometric detector), IRD (infrared detector) and so on.

5.3.5. IR Spectrophotometry

Fourier Transformed Infrared Spectroscopy (FTIR) is constructed on the absorption of infrared radiation by the essential oils. Through the detection of the characteristic vibrations of the chemical bonds, it makes it possible to carry out the analysis of the chemical functions present in the oils. FTIR allowed us to identify volatile compounds and indicated that the functional groups of the essential oils are C-H (Alkene), C-H (aromatic), and C=C.

5.3.6. NMR Spectroscopy

NMR spectroscopy basically used for the non-separated identification of the individual constituents of complex mixtures of essential oils. Computer-aided analysis of the carbon-13 NMR spectrum of the complex mixture, which allows the identification of the main components of essential oils. The excellent visual spacing of the signals enables oil samples to be analysed without preliminary separation of their components. Moreover, information relating to the molecular structure of the oil constituents can be ascertained from the measured chemical shifts.

6. PHOTO TOXICITY

Some essential oils contain photoactive molecules like furocoumarins. For instance, *Citrus bergamia* (*Citrus aurantium ssp. bergamia*) essential oil contains psoralens which bind to DNA under ultraviolet A light exposure producing mono- and biadducts that are cytotoxic and highly mutagenic [67]. However, in the dark, this oil is not cytotoxic or mutagenic by itself. Researchershave shown that Fusanusspicatuswood essential oil was not phototoxic but was very cytotoxic. In other words, cytotoxicity seems rather antagonistic to phototoxicity. In the case of cytotoxicity, essential oils damage the cellular and organelle membranes and can act as prooxidants on proteins and DNA with the production of reactive oxygen species (ROS), and light exposures do not add much to the overall reaction. In the case of phototoxicity, essential oils penetrate the cell without damaging the membranes or proteins and DNA. Radical reactions by excitation of certain molecules and energy transfer with production of oxygen singlet occur when cells are exposed to activated light. This may cause damage to cellular macromolecules and in some cases the formation of covalent adducts to DNA, proteins, and membrane lipids. Clearly, cytotoxicity or phototoxicity depends on the type of molecules present in the essential oils and their compartmentation in the cell, producing different types of radicals with or without light exposure. However, such an antagonism is not quite a strict rule.

7. PROCESSING OF ESSENTIAL OILSS FOR FLAVOR FUNCTIONS

Because essential oils are a product of nature, environmental and genetic factors will impact the chemical composition of the plant. Factors such as species and subspecies, geographical location, harvest time, plant parts, and method of isolation all affect the chemical composition of the crude material separated from the plant. The variability of the composition of crude essential oil as isolated from nature has been the subject of much research and development since plant and oil yields are major economic factors in crop production. However, the crude essential oil that arrives at the flavour processing plant is not normally used as such. The crude oil is often subjected to a number of processes that are intended to increase purity and to produce a product with the intended flavour characteristics. Some essential oils may be distilled and cooled to remove natural waxes and improve clarity, while others are distilled more than once (*i.e.*, rectified) to remove undesirable fractions or to increase the relative content of certain chemical constituents. Some oils are dry or vacuum distilled. Normally, at some point during processing, the essential oil is evaluated for its technical function as a flavour. This evaluation typically involves the analysis (normally by gas chromatography (GC) or liquid chromatography) of the composition of the essential oil for chemical constituents that are markers for the desired technical flavour effect. For an essential oil such as cardamom oil, levels of target constituents such as terpinyl acetate, 1, 8-cineole, and limonene are markers for technical viability as a flavouring substance. Based on this initial assessment, the crude essential oil may be blended with other sources of the same oil or chemical constituents isolated from the oil to reach target ranges for key constituent markers that reflect flavour function. The mixture may then be further rectified by distillation. Each step of the process is driven by a flavor function. Therefore, the chemical composition of the product to be marketed may be significantly different from that of the crude oil. Moreover, the chemical composition of the processed essential oil is more consistent than that of the crude batches of oil isolated from various plant harvests. The range of concentrations for individual constituents and for groups of structurally related constituents in an essential oil are dictated, in large part, by the requirement that target levels of flavor marker constituents must be maintained.

CONCLUSION

The array of biological and pharmacological effects of EOs may be explicated by their diversity of chemical compounds, with varying amount and percentage. These chemical entities have capacity to permeate cells and tissues, reach biological targets, and execute the pharmacological replication due to their lipophilic profiles. A diverse union of volatile plant components make-up essential oils. Terpenes, phenols, aldehydes, ketones, and esters are a few of the intricate cumulations of innumerable organic chemicals that make up essential oils. The aroma, is reliant on the chemical architecture of essential oils, which is predicated on the enzymatic makeup of the plant species. Chemical background of essential oils is categorised on four aspects: i) principal biosynthetic precursor; ii) carbon atom size/number; iii) parent carbon skeleton/backbone; and iv) nature of oxidation by electronegative atoms. The three major biosynthetic groups of essential oil include, i) terpenes; ii) phenylpropanoids iii) isothiocyanates and they are mainly derived by major biosynthetic pathways comprising a) mevalonate and methylerythritol phosphate pathway; b) shikimate pathway; and c) glucosinolate pathways.

The intricate biochemistry of essential oils is enormously consequential in biological and aromatic contexts. Every EO has a unique chemical composition that incorporates potent biological capabilities in additament to influencing its unique aroma. Assessing the many therapeutic applications of EOs, ranging from aromatherapy to possible medical utilization, requires a construal of their biochemistry. It withal entails considering elements that might affect the chemical makeup of essential oils, such as plant species, extraction techniques, and environmental circumstances. With perpetuated investigation, the intricacy of essential oils is being revealed, and it is becoming more and more clear how paramount they are to many businesses and how they may be utilized in healthcare. Future revelations and ingenious uses might result from the perpetuated investigation and comprehension of their intricate biological makeup.

REFERENCES

[1] Silva MJ, Malek NA, Hodge CC, *et al.* Improved quantitative detection of 11 urinary phthalate metabolites in humans using liquid chromatography-atmospheric pressure chemical ionization tandem mass spectrometry. J Chromatogr B Analyt Technol Biomed Life Sci 2003; 789(2): 393-404. [http://dx.doi.org/10.1016/S1570-0232(03)00164-8] [PMID: 12742130]

[2] Hajhashemi V, Ghannadi A, Sharif B. Anti-inflammatory and analgesic properties of the leaf extracts and essential oil of Lavandula angustifolia Mill. J Ethnopharmacol 2003; 89(1): 67-71. [http://dx.doi.org/10.1016/S0378-8741(03)00234-4] [PMID: 14522434]

[3] Croteau R, Kutchan TM, Lewis NG. Natural products (secondary metabolites). Biochemistry and molecular biology of plants. 2000; 24: 1250-319.

[4] Betts AK, Ball JH, McCaughey JH. Near-surface climate in the boreal forest. J Geophys Res 2001; 106(D24): 33529-41. [http://dx.doi.org/10.1029/2001JD900047]

[5] Pichersky E, Noel JP, Dudareva N. Biosynthesis of plant volatiles: nature's diversity and ingenuity. Science 2006; 311(5762): 808-11. [http://dx.doi.org/10.1126/science.1118510] [PMID: 16469917]

[6] Sadasivam S, Thayumanayan B. Molecular host plant resistance to pests. CRC Press 2003. [http://dx.doi.org/10.1201/9780203912386]

[7] Krings U, Berger RG. Biotechnological production of flavours and fragrances. Appl Microbiol Biotechnol 1998; 49(1): 1-8. [http://dx.doi.org/10.1007/s002530051129] [PMID: 9487704]

[8] Muñoz-Bertomeu J, Sales E, Ros R, Arrillaga I, Segura J. Up-regulation of an N-terminal truncated 3-hydroxy-3-methylglutaryl CoA reductase enhances production of essential oils and sterols in transgenic *Lavandula latifolia.* Plant Biotechnol J 2007; 5(6): 746-58. [http://dx.doi.org/10.1111/j.1467-7652.2007.00286.x] [PMID: 17714440]

[9] Daviet L, Schalk M. Biotechnology in plant essential oil production: Progress and perspective in

metabolic engineering of the terpene pathway. Flavour Fragrance J 2010; 25(3): 123-7. [http://dx.doi.org/10.1002/ffj.1981]

[10] Roe FJC, Field WEH. Chronic toxicity of essential oils and certain other products of natural origin. Food Cosmet Toxicol 1965; 3(2): 311-23. [http://dx.doi.org/10.1016/S0015-6264(65)80090-6] [PMID: 5859246]

[11] Zuzarte M, Vale-Silva L, Gonçalves MJ, *et al.* Antifungal activity of phenolic-rich Lavandula multifida L. essential oil. Eur J Clin Microbiol Infect Dis 2012; 31(7): 1359-66. [http://dx.doi.org/10.1007/s10096-011-1450-4] [PMID: 22020493]

[12] Mann JM, Gostin L, Gruskin S, Brennan T, Lazzarini Z, Fineberg HV. Health and human rights. Health Hum Rights 1994; 1(1): 6-23. [http://dx.doi.org/10.2307/4065260] [PMID: 10395709]

[13] Zuzarte M, Salgueiro L. Essential oils chemistry. In: de Sousa D, Ed. Bioactive Essential Oils and Cancer. Cham: Springer 2015. [http://dx.doi.org/10.1007/978-3-319-19144-7_2]

[14] Tisserand R, Young R. Essential oil safety: A guide for health care professionals. Elsevier 2013.

[15] Jiang N, Liu X, Yang J, Li Z, Pan J, Zhu X. Regulation of copper homeostasis by Cuf1 associates with its subcellular localization in the pathogenic yeast Cryptococcus neoformans H99. FEMS Yeast Res 2011; 11(5): 440-8. [http://dx.doi.org/10.1111/j.1567-1364.2011.00733.x] [PMID: 21489137]

[16] Duschatzky CB, Possetto ML, Talarico LB, *et al.* Evaluation of chemical and antiviral properties of essential oils from South American plants. Antivir Chem Chemother 2005; 16(4): 247-51. [http://dx.doi.org/10.1177/095632020501600404] [PMID: 16130522]

[17] Monzote L, Stamberg W, Patel A, *et al.* Synthetic chromanol derivatives and their interaction with complex III in mitochondria from bovine, yeast, and Leishmania. Chem Res Toxicol 2011; 24(10): 1678-85. [http://dx.doi.org/10.1021/tx200233c] [PMID: 21809846]

[18] Priestley K, Debayle E, McKenzie D, Pilidou S. Upper mantle structure of eastern Asia from multimode surface waveform tomography. J Geophys Res Solid Earth 2006; 111: B10.

[19] Tahghighi M, Brown JA, Breen LJ, Kane R, Hegney D, Rees CS. A comparison of nurse shift workers' and non-shift workers' psychological functioning and resilience. J Adv Nurs 2019; 75(11): 2570-8. [http://dx.doi.org/10.1111/jan.14023] [PMID: 30957259]

[20] Kim HJ, Kim NC, Wang YD, *et al.* Mutations in prion-like domains in hnRNPA2B1 and hnRNPA1 cause multisystem proteinopathy and ALS. Nature 2013; 495(7442): 467-73. [http://dx.doi.org/10.1038/nature11922] [PMID: 23455423]

[21] Bauer KP, Garbe D, Surburg H. Single Fragrance and Flavor Materials. Wiley 2001. [http://dx.doi.org/10.1002/3527600205.ch2]

[22] Kamatou GPP, Vermaak I, Viljoen AM, Lawrence BM. Menthol: A simple monoterpene with remarkable biological properties. Phytochemistry 2013; 96: 15-25. [http://dx.doi.org/10.1016/j.phytochem.2013.08.005] [PMID: 24054028]

[23] Ooi EE, Goh KT, Gubler DJ. Dengue prevention and 35 years of vector control in Singapore. Emerg Infect Dis 2006; 12(6): 887-93. [http://dx.doi.org/10.3201/eid1206.051210] [PMID: 16707042]

[24] Jirovetz L, Buchbauer G, Stoilova I, Stoyanova A, Krastanov A, Schmidt E. Chemical composition and antioxidant properties of clove leaf essential oil. J Agric Food Chem 2006; 54(17): 6303-7. [http://dx.doi.org/10.1021/jf060608c] [PMID: 16910723]

[25] Hunter CA, Anderson HL. What is Cooperativity? Angew Chem Int Ed 2009; 48(41): 7488-99.

[http://dx.doi.org/10.1002/anie.200902490] [PMID: 19746372]

[26] Baser KHC, Demirci F. Chemistry of essential oils. In: Berger RG, Ed. Flavours and Fragrances: Chemistry, Bioprocessing and Sustainability. New York: Springer 2007; pp. 43-86.

[27] Hasan MK, Ali MR, Saha CK, Alam MM, Hossain MM. Assessment of paddy harvesting practices of Southern Delta Region in Bangladesh. Progress Agric 2019; 30: 57-64. [http://dx.doi.org/10.3329/pa.v30i0.41558]

[28] Rosato A, Tenori L, Cascante M, De Atauri Carulla PR, Martins dos Santos VAP, Saccenti E. From correlation to causation: analysis of metabolomics data using systems biology approaches. Metabolomics 2018; 14(4): 37. [http://dx.doi.org/10.1007/s11306-018-1335-y] [PMID: 29503602]

[29] Inouye S, Takizawa T, Yamaguchi H. Antibacterial activity of essential oils and their major constituents against respiratory tract pathogens by gaseous contact. J Antimicrob Chemother 2001; 47(5): 565-73. [http://dx.doi.org/10.1093/jac/47.5.565] [PMID: 11328766]

[30] Bakkali F, Averbeck S, Averbeck D, Idaomar M. Biological effects of essential oils--a review. Food Chem Toxicol 2008; 46(2): 446-75.

[31] Hammer KA, Carson CF, Riley TV. Antimicrobial activity of essential oils and other plant extracts. J Appl Microbiol 1999; 86(6): 985-90. [http://dx.doi.org/10.1046/j.1365-2672.1999.00780.x] [PMID: 10438227]

[32] Elshafie HS, Aliberti L, Amato M, De Feo V, Camele I. Chemical composition and antimicrobial activity of chia (Sal*via* hispanica L.) essential oil. Eur Food Res Technol 2018; 244(9): 1675-82. [http://dx.doi.org/10.1007/s00217-018-3080-x]

[33] Rhayour K, Bouchikhi T, Tantaoui-Elaraki A, Sendide K, Remmal A. The mechanism of bactericidal action of oregano and clove essential oils and of their phenolic major components on Escherichia coli and Bacillus subtilis. J Essent Oil Res 2003; 15(5): 356-62. [http://dx.doi.org/10.1080/10412905.2003.9698611]

[34] Cox KH, Rai R, Distler M, Daugherty JR, Coffman JA, Cooper TG. Saccharomyces cerevisiae GATA sequences function as TATA elements during nitrogen catabolite repression and when Gln3p is excluded from the nucleus by overproduction of Ure2p. J Biol Chem 2000; 275(23): 17611-8. [http://dx.doi.org/10.1074/jbc.M001648200] [PMID: 10748041]

[35] Pfaller MA, Diekema DJ. Rare and emerging opportunistic fungal pathogens: concern for resistance beyond Candida albicans and Aspergillus fumigatus. J Clin Microbiol 2004; 42(10): 4419-31. [http://dx.doi.org/10.1128/JCM.42.10.4419-4431.2004] [PMID: 15472288]

[36] Pagiotti R, Angelini P, Rubini A, Tirillini B, Granetti B, Venanzoni R. Identification and characterisation of human pathogenic filamentous fungi and susceptibility to *Thymus schimperi* essential oil. Mycoses 2011; 54(5): e364-76. [http://dx.doi.org/10.1111/j.1439-0507.2010.01926.x] [PMID: 20633233]

[37] Yutani M, Hashimoto Y, Ogita A, Kubo I, Tanaka T, Fujita K. Morphological changes of the filamentous fungus Mucor mucedo and inhibition of chitin synthase activity induced by anethole. Phytother Res 2011; 25(11): 1707-13. [http://dx.doi.org/10.1002/ptr.3579] [PMID: 21721062]

[38] Shen BQ, Yu XC, Zhi Y, *et al.* Detection of single nanoparticles using the dissipative interaction in a high-Q microcavity. Phys Rev Appl 2016; 5(2): 024011. [http://dx.doi.org/10.1103/PhysRevApplied.5.024011]

[39] Liao M, Xie XM. Cadmium release in contaminated soils due to organic acids. Pedosphere 2004; 14(2): 223-8.

[40] de Oliveira DH, Abib PB, Giacomini RX, *et al.* Antioxidant and antifungal activities of the flowers' essential oil of *Tagetes minuta*, (*Z*)-tagetone and thiotagetone. J Essent Oil Res 2019; 31(2): 160-9.

[http://dx.doi.org/10.1080/10412905.2018.1519465]

[41] Massa N, Cantamessa S, Novello G, *et al.* Antifungal activity of essential oils against azole-resistant and azole-susceptible vaginal *Candida glabrata* strains. Can J Microbiol 2018; 64(10): 647-63. [http://dx.doi.org/10.1139/cjm-2018-0082] [PMID: 29746162]

[42] Hammer KA, Carson CF, Riley TV. *In vitro* activity of Melaleuca alternifolia (tea tree) oil against dermatophytes and other filamentous fungi. J Antimicrob Chemother 2002; 50(2): 195-9. [http://dx.doi.org/10.1093/jac/dkf112] [PMID: 12161399]

[43] Halliwell B, Gutteridge JMC. Role of free radicals and catalytic metal ions in human disease: An overview. Methods Enzymol 1990; 186: 1-85. [http://dx.doi.org/10.1016/0076-6879(90)86093-B] [PMID: 2172697]

[44] Abdollahi M, Mostafalou S, Pournourmohammadi S, Shadnia S. Oxidative stress and cholinesterase inhibition in saliva and plasma of rats following subchronic exposure to malathion. Comp Biochem Physiol C Toxicol Pharmacol 2004; 137(1): 29-34. [http://dx.doi.org/10.1016/j.cca.2003.11.002] [PMID: 14984701]

[45] Tomaino A, Cimino F, Zimbalatti V, *et al.* Influence of heating on antioxidant activity and the chemical composition of some spice essential oils. Food Chem 2005; 89(4): 549-54. [http://dx.doi.org/10.1016/j.foodchem.2004.03.011]

[46] Stanojevic LP, Stanojevic JS, Cvetkovic DJ, Ilic DP. Antioxidant activity of oregano essential oil (Origanum vulgare L.). Biol NYSSANA 2016; 2

[47] Olmedo R, Ribotta P, Grosso NR. Antioxidant activity of essential oils extracted from Aloysiatriphylla and Minthostachysmollis that improve the oxidative stability of sunflower oil under accelerated storage conditions. Eur J Lipid Sci Technol 2018; 120(8): 1700374. [http://dx.doi.org/10.1002/ejlt.201700374]

[48] El Hamdaoui A, Msanda F, Boubaker H, *et al.* Essential oil composition, antioxidant and antibacterial activities of wild and cultivated Lavandula mairei Humbert. Biochem Syst Ecol 2018; 76: 1-7. [http://dx.doi.org/10.1016/j.bse.2017.11.004]

[49] Polatoğlu K, Karakoç ÖC, Gören N. Phytotoxic, DPPH scavenging, insecticidal activities and essential oil composition of Achillea vermicularis, A. teretifolia and proposed chemotypes of A. biebersteinii (Asteraceae). Ind Crops Prod 2013; 51: 35-45. [http://dx.doi.org/10.1016/j.indcrop.2013.08.052]

[50] Tepe B, Daferera D, Sokmen A, Sokmen M, Polissiou M. Antimicrobial and antioxidant activities of the essential oil and various extracts of Salvia tomentosa Miller (Lamiaceae). Food Chem 2005; 90(3): 333-40. [http://dx.doi.org/10.1016/j.foodchem.2003.09.013]

[51] Blowman K, Magalhães M, Lemos MFL, Cabral C, Pires IM. Anticancer properties of essential oils and other natural products. Evid Based Complement Alternat Med 2018; 2018: 1-12. [http://dx.doi.org/10.1155/2018/3149362] [PMID: 29765461]

[52] Aruna K, Sivaramakrishnan VM. Anticarcinogenic effects of the essential oils from cumin, poppy and basil. Phytother Res 1996; 10(7): 577-80. [http://dx.doi.org/10.1002/(SICI)1099-1573(199611)10:7<577::AID-PTR906>3.0.CO;2-Q]

[53] Pessoa LM, Morais SM, Bevilaqua CML, Luciano JHS. Anthelmintic activity of essential oil of Ocimum gratissimum Linn. and eugenol against Haemonchus contortus. Vet Parasitol 2002; 109(1-2): 59-63. [http://dx.doi.org/10.1016/S0304-4017(02)00253-4] [PMID: 12383625]

[54] Scrivanti LR, Zunino MP, Zygadlo JA. Tagetes minuta and Schinus areira essential oils as allelopathic agents. Biochem Syst Ecol 2003; 31(6): 563-72. [http://dx.doi.org/10.1016/S0305-1978(02)00202-8]

[55] Dudai N, Poljakoff-Mayber A, Mayer AM, Putievsky E, Lerner HR. Essential oils as allelochemicals

and their potential use as bioherbicides. J Chem Ecol 1999; 25(5): 1079-89.
[http://dx.doi.org/10.1023/A:1020881825669]

[56] Kıyan HT, Demirci B, Başer KHC, Demirci F. The *in vivo* evaluation of anti-angiogenic effects of *Hypericum* essential oils using the chorioallantoic membrane assay. Pharm Biol 2014; 52(1): 44-50.
[http://dx.doi.org/10.3109/13880209.2013.810647] [PMID: 24044783]

[57] Kamble SS, Gacche RN. "Evaluation of anti-breast cancer, anti-angiogenic and antioxidant properties of selected medicinal plants". Eur J Integr Med 2019; 25: 13-9.
[http://dx.doi.org/10.1016/j.eujim.2018.11.006]

[58] Calo JR, Crandall PG, O'Bryan CA, Ricke SC. Essential oils as antimicrobials in food systems – A review. Food Control 2015; 54: 111-9.
[http://dx.doi.org/10.1016/j.foodcont.2014.12.040]

[59] Ribeiro-Santos R, Andrade M, Melo NR, Sanches-Silva A. Use of essential oils in active food packaging: Recent advances and future trends. Trends Food Sci Technol 2017; 61: 132-40.
[http://dx.doi.org/10.1016/j.tifs.2016.11.021]

[60] Tongnuanchan P, Benjakul S. Essential oils: Esxtraction, bioactivities, and their uses for food preservation. J Food Sci 2014; 79(7): R1231-49.
[http://dx.doi.org/10.1111/1750-3841.12492] [PMID: 24888440]

[61] Bilia AR, Guccione C, Isacchi B, Righeschi C, Firenzuoli F, Bergonzi MC. Essential oils loaded in nanosystems: A developing strategy for a successful therapeutic approach. Evid Based Complement Alternat Med 2014; 2014: 1-14.
[http://dx.doi.org/10.1155/2014/651593] [PMID: 24971152]

[52] Asbahani AE, Miladi K, Badri W, *et al.* Essential oils: From extraction to encapsulation. Int J Pharm 2015; 483(1-2): 220-43.
[http://dx.doi.org/10.1016/j.ijpharm.2014.12.069] [PMID: 25683145]

[63] Angioni A, Barra A, Coroneo V, Dessi S, Cabras P. Chemical composition, seasonal variability, and antifungal activity of Lavandula stoechas L. ssp. stoechas essential oils from stem/leaves and flowers. J Agric Food Chem 2006; 54(12): 4364-70.
[http://dx.doi.org/10.1021/jf0603329] [PMID: 16756368]

[64] Masango P. Cleaner production of essential oils by steam distillation. J Clean Prod 2005; 13(8): 833-9.
[http://dx.doi.org/10.1016/j.jclepro.2004.02.039]

[65] Yıldırım V. A parametric study on the natural frequencies of unidirectional composite conical springs. Commun Numer Methods Eng 2004; 20(3): 207-27.
[http://dx.doi.org/10.1002/cnm.661]

[66] Ghannadi A, Bagherinejad M, Abedi D, Jalali M, Absalan B, Sadeghi N. Antibacterial activity and composition of essential oils from Pelargonium graveolens L'Her and Vitex agnus-castus L. Iran J Microbiol 2012; 4(4): 171-6.
[PMID: 23205247]

[67] Averbeck D, Averbeck S, Dubertret L, Young AR, Morlière P. Genotoxicity of bergapten and bergamot oil in Saccharomyces cerevisiae. J Photochem Photobiol B 1990; 7(2-4): 209-29.
[http://dx.doi.org/10.1016/1011-1344(90)85158-S] [PMID: 2128325]

CHAPTER 4

Essential Oils' Biosynthesis and their Application

Sandeep Negi[1,*], **Ajeet Kumar Srivastav**[2,3] and **Lakshmi Bala**[2]

[1] *Photobiology Laboratory, Systems Toxicology and Health Risk Assessment Group CSIR-Indian Institute of Toxicology Research Vishvigyan Bhavan 31, P.O. Box No. 80, M.G. Marg Lucknow-226001, India*

[2] *Department of Biochemistry, Babu Banrasi Das University, Lucknow, India*

[3] *Redcliffe Hygiene Private Limited, Gurugram, India*

Abstract: Essential oils are natural plant products that have a wide range of applications in various fields like medicine, flavors, fragrance, *etc*. Their wide range of uses benefits people by exhibiting a variety of diverse properties like anti-allergic, anti-inflammatory, antiviral, antibacterial, insect repellent, anticancer, anti-oxidant, and many more. They are also crucial to plants in terms of function. They are aromatic and are present in plants inside specialized cells or glands. Their biosynthesis occurs in the leaves and is present inside them until flowering. After the flowering of the plant, these oils get transferred to the flowers. These essential oils can be extracted using a variety of techniques, including solvent applications, steam distillation, and more. The quality and amount of essential oils in plants are affected by a variety of circumstances. These factors include the development stage of plants, the effect of UV radiation, the effect of Arbuscular mycorrhizal fungi, the effect of light quality, the effect of salt stress, and the effect of fertilizers.

Keywords: Anticancer, Anti-oxidant, Arbuscular mycorrhizal fungi, Essential oils, UV radiations.

1. INTRODUCTION

Natural plant compounds called essential oils are used in a variety of industries, including medicine, flavoring, and scent. Their wide range of uses benefits humans by exhibiting a variety of diverse properties, such as anti-allergic, anti-cancer, anti-inflammatory, antiviral, antibacterial, antimicrobial, insect repellent, anti-oxidant, and many others, in addition to being beneficial to the plant itself [1, 2]. They have an aromatic character and are found in the specialized cells or

* **Corresponding author Sandeep Negi:** Photobiology Laboratory, Systems Toxicology and Health Risk Assessment Group CSIR-Indian Institute of Toxicology Research Vishvigyan Bhavan 31, P.O. Box No. 80, M.G. Marg Lucknow-226001, India; E-mail: lakshmi266@gmail.com

Pradeep Kumar Shukla, Ajeet Kumar Srivastav, Deepti Chopra, Shikha Agnihotry, Pragati Misra and Jyoti Singh (Eds.)

glands of plants. They play a crucial part in the plant's defense mechanisms. Their increased concentration protects plants from predators and pests while also acting as an attractant for pollinators [3]. Volatile organic compounds extracted from various parts of the plant have distinct therapeutic and energetic properties. In addition, these are highly complex substances that are both highly potent and extremely precise in action. Essential oils are typically not treated as oils because they don't contain any fatty substances. They are derived from an essence rich in natural flavors and active ingredients that are secreted by various plant parts. These beneficial liquids are produced by distilling or pressing secretory organs [4].

2. AROMATIC PLANTS' ESSENTIAL OIL-SECRETING CELLS

Essential oils became very popular due to the significance of their medicinal value, culinary, and fragrant properties, as well as various other biological applications [5]. Plants contain specialized secretory structures that are responsible for their production. After being created in plants, these essential oils are occasionally released by conical-papillate cells, non-specialized cells, glandular trichomes, osmophores, ducts, and cavities [6]. The architecture of these cells can be examined with contemporary tools including light microscopy, scanning, and transmission electron microscopy [7].

2.1. Osmophores

The word "Osmophores" comes from the words "Osmo," which means "smell," and "phore," which means "to carry."This term was first used in 1962 to designate a floral tissue enclosed area that is specifically designed for scent emission. Osmophores are regions of floral tissue that are enclosed and are considered responsible for the emission of odor. These are also referred to as floral fragrance glands, a specialized group of cells that are distributed on the sepals and petals of flowers to attract insect pollinators [7]. Except for the eighteen species of Stanhopea and Sievekingia, having Osmophores along with epidermal cells which are morphologically different from the adjacent cells, they are composed of multilayered glandular epithelium with homogeneous cell layers [8, 9]. Large amounts of storage compounds like starch are found in the mesophyll of these cells. Most epidermis cells don't have these deposits. This makes a difference between the layer of production and the layer of emissions [9]. More than 200 species of flowers have conical-papillate cells on their petals, and Osmophore cells resemble these cells [10], which include Stanhopea, Rosa x hybrid, *Galanthus nivalis*, Orchidaceae, Araceae and *Arabidopsis thaliana* (Brassicaceae) [11]. Conical-papillate shape contributes to light reflection and offers a very large surface area for evaporation. In *Antirrhinum majus*, the MIXTA gene, which gives rise to the conical shape, has been cloned (Scrophulariaceae). Surprisingly, its overexpression in 35S is as follows: MIXTA *Nicotiana tabacum* (Solanaceae) causes ectopic trichome secretion across the plant, implying a link between conical-papillate cells and the differentiation of secreting trichomes [12]. Two characteristics that are possibly related to the production of fragrances are cytoplasmic lipid inclusions and plastoglobuli in amyloplasts. These characteristics demonstrated enough variation to be included due to their important properties. Plastoglobuli are found in the amyloplasts of both *Sievekingia* species and the majority of *Stanhopea* species. The Osmophores of *Galanthus nivalis* flowers exhibit polarised epidermal cell protoplasts, big cell nuclei, and huge vacuoles with diverse contents in the periphery region of the cells [13]. The Osmophores in *Stanhopea graveolens* and *Cycnoches chlorochilon* are located at the base of the labellum. The wrinkled surfaces of the Osmophores increased the surface area of the scent emission. Secretion remains are visible on the surface of the epidermis in *S. graveolens*, but not in *C. chlorochilon* [7].

2.2. Glandular Trichomes (GTs)

Trichomes, which are hairs found on the surface of plants, serve a variety of purposes, such as pest and insect control, heat retention, and moisture retention [14]. Plants contain trichomes of different varieties, and they occasionally have complex structures [15]. They can be classified into two different types (non-glandular as well as glandular trichomes) [16]. Glandular trichomes (GTs) are hairs found on the epidermis. These cells are specialized for the biosynthesis and release of specific secretory substances, such as nectar, mucilage, acyl lipids, digestive enzymes, and essential oils. These trichomes are abundant and exhibit a variety of morphologies throughout the plant kingdom. A mixture of chemicals is contained in or secreted by these trichomes. Plants have a large number of secreting trichomes with various morphologies. A large number of chemicals that are very helpful in the pesticide, pharmaceutical, and flavor or fragrance industries are secreted by GTs. Some crop species use these as well because they exhibit resistance to insects and pests [15]. There is a growing interest in learning about the chemical composition of glandular trichome exudates and taking advantage of their numerous applications today [20].

GTs are found in several monocotyledon plants, including Tradescantia, Dioscorea, and Sisyrinchium. GTs are more common in eudicots and are distinctive vegetative epidermal features of numerous families and genera, including Lamiaceae, Asteraceae, Sphaerosepalaceae, Caryophyllaceae, Cucurbitaceae, Fabaceae, Rosaceae, Sapindaceae, Saxifragaceae, and Cannabaceae [17]. Metcalfe and Chalk gave a more comprehensive list of the distributions of GTs in dicotyledons of various morphological categories [20].

GTs can be branching or unbranched, sessile, long or short, or both. A cluster of glandular cells is typically seen at the terminal of a stalk of one or more cells in length. A thick cuticle layer was frequently observed attached to fossil seed fern leaves, although it appears to be lacking from conifers [17, 18]. Apart from hydropotes and similar GTs in various Nymphaeales, GTs are absent in Amborella, Nymphaea, Illicium, Trimenia, and Austrobaileya [19].

GTs are frequently depicted as being randomly distributed across the surfaces of plants, however careful study reveals that this is not always the case. Peltate GTs, for example, appear more or less equally spaced in peppermint and are extremely rarely found in pairs or clusters. They are separated by a comparable number of epidermal cells but have predictable densities within distinct leaf regions [20]. Recent research has identified networks of transcription factors that seem to work in concert to either activate or inhibit the start and maturation of trichomes in protodermal cells [20].

3. BIOSYNTHESIS OF ESSENTIAL OILS

The majority of essential oils are found in and are produced in the leaves, where they remain until flowering. As the plant blooms, the essential oils move into the flowers, and some of them are used up in the fertilization process. Following fertilization, it gathers in the fruits and seeds or migrates to the leaves, bark, and roots [21, 22]. The makeup of essential oils changes as a plant ages. While immature plants primarily contain terpenic hydrocarbons and simpler molecules, reproductive organs primarily contain etheric oils richer in oxygenated chemicals. Ethereal oils have a variety of benefits, even though their function in the plant organism is still partially understood. Approximately 150 of the more than 3,000 essential oils that have been physically and chemically described are produced on an industrial scale [23 - 25].

3.1. Essential Oils' Chemical Composition

Essential oils are complex combinations (5000-7000 chemical constituents) with a predominance of mono and sesquitrpene ingredients, but also aromatic chemicals, commonly phenylpropane derivatives, and only rarely diterpenes. Terpenic chemicals can be hydrocarbons or oxygenated derivatives (oxygenated alcohols, alcohols, aldehydes, ketones, acids) or reaction products of these (esters, ethers). Terpenic compounds are plant-derived chemicals that enter the natural composition of molecular combinations that result in the creation of volatile (essential etheric) oils. The production of aromatic waters and essential oils necessitates the use of raw materials, plant products, and high quality. First and foremost, the plant material should be harvested with extreme caution so that it does not become contaminated with other plant species. Essential oils are found in a wide range of plant organs but are most typically found in flowers and leaves [25, 26].

Essential oils' chemical makeup is extremely diverse, and their primary constituents may belong to the aliphatic, aromatic, or terpenic series. Essential oils typically contain ternary, and very infrequently quaternary, compounds. Terpenes, aromatics, aldehydes, ketones, phenols, volatile acids, esters, and other substances make up volatile products. After harvesting, the plant material subject to hydrodynamics is not usually processed [27].

Except for cinnamon, lime flowers, and lavender flowers, which are used dry, fresh plants result in more pleasant odor solutions and stronger therapeutic efficacy. In the case of dry plants, decreased volatile urine is occasionally obtained as a result of morphological and chemical changes caused by air heating, or as a result of gram buildup, potentially by modification [28, 29]. Furthermore, the technological technique of extracting volatile oil has a significant impact on its composition and quality. Hydrodistillation produces physical and chemical processes that dramatically affect the content of the plant material and, as a result, the volatile oil released. Crushing, cutting, and grinding are methods used to reduce the size of vegetable products, which are chosen based on their origin and chemical content [30].

3.2. Extraction of Essential Oils

The ideal method for obtaining essential oils is one of the following:

- Pressing (a technique commonly used for extracting lemon peel oil).
- *Via* distillation in a stream of water vapor.
- By using supercritical fluids like carbonic anhydride under pressure or solvents like ether, petroleum, benzene, acetone, or toluene to extract fresh vegetable products.
- *Via* maceration or extraction from concentrated liquids acquired from the extraction of fragrances.

Depending on their distinctive qualities, several processes are used to extract essential oils for industrial use from a variety of aromatic plants. In actuality, the most popular techniques are:

- Steam distillation used to extract essential oils.
- Essential oil extraction using various solvents [31].

3.3. Essential Oils Extracted by Steam Distillation

It is a standard technique for obtaining volatile oil from the majority of aromatic plants. In this situation, hot water vapor helps remove and transport things, especially essential oils. The oil is volatilized when water vapors enter the vegetal mass during distillation, remove the olefin covering, and then combine with the oil. The water and oil vapor mixture enters the refrigerant (condensing vessel), where it condenses into a liquid composed solely of water and volatile oil. The volatile oil is simpler to deposit at the beginning above the water, therefore, this mixture enters the florentine vessel (separation vessel) where the separation occurs [32]. The following distillation processes are known, depending on how the raw material is added to the boiler:

1. It is useful for all essential oils that do not disintegrate at 100°C during distillation in water. Its 1:4 ratio makes the raw ingredient.
2. Water and water vapor distillation: it is used in essential oils when certain components dissolve in water, and the raw material is placed above the water. Direct fire or blind steam pipes are used to heat water from the boiler for vapor transformation. Thus, the volatile oil will be removed from the vapor that is being created.
3. Most oils are extracted *via* water vapor distillation. The technique entails passing water vapor, produced in special boilers at high temperatures and pressures, through vegetative masses put in particular baskets.

Water vapor distillation is the most prevalent process and is used in the majority of countries that produce essential oils [33].

3.4. Essential Oil Extraction using Various Solvents

It is one of the most ancient, well-known, and widely utilized techniques for manufacturing essential oils. The use of solvents is a time-consuming and costly procedure that is rarely used. This method is based on essential oils' capacity to dissolve in a variety of substances such as animal fats, vegetable oils, gasoline, petroleum ether, and so on. The extraction of essential oils is referred to as extraction, while non-volatile solvents such as fats are referred to as macerates. Solvent extraction is especially beneficial for oil extracted from flowers and species whose volatile oil degrades when exposed to high heat [34]. The method mentioned above is used in the processing of roses, lilacs, acacias, shrubs, and other plants. In the event of maceration, the raw item subjected to extraction is placed in the fat. If animal fat is used, it will remain at 40-60°C. The raw material will be kept in the solvent for 24-48 hours, depending on its qualities. Dissolvent is employed 6-15 times to remove a volatile oil. It alters after complete saturation [35].

4. FACTORS INFLUENCING ESSENTIAL OIL QUANTITY AND QUALITY IN PLANTS

Although secondary metabolites in aromatic and medicinal plants are often regulated by their genotypes, their production is also significantly influenced by environmental conditions. This means that the growth characteristics, essential oil yield, and chemical composition of these oils are all influenced by biotic and abiotic environmental conditions. The following sections go into great detail on a few of these factors [32, 34].

4.1. Developmental Stage of the Plant

The dependency of the synthesis and accumulation of oil on the developmental stage of the associated cells, tissues, organs, and plants is one of the most significant elements that determine the biosynthesis of essential oils. The developmental stages of the leaves, from the genesis to growth to full maturity to ultimate loss through senescence, which is fundamentally critical, vary amongst the plants that include the leaves as a source of commercially significant essential oil. Many aromatic plants in the Lamiaceae family as well as some Poaceae and Asteraceae species have shown a strong link between leaf development and oil biosynthesis and accumulation [36]. The content of the essential oil is influenced by the stage of development as well. The primary component of *C.flexuosus*, the citral, reaches its peak concentration on the twentieth day of growth [37]. Sal*via* officinalis has camphor, which is more concentrated with expanding leaves [38]. The concentration of the essential oil and its primary ingredient, menthol, peaks in Japanese mint during the beginning of the flower bud stage. Individual leaves, however, demonstrate a steady decline in oil percentage with increasing dry matter and leaf age. Up until the point of leaf maturity, the menthol concentration in the oil was raised; but, as it continued to age, it began to decline [39]. At the peak of flowering, the proportion of the main ingredient, artemisia ketone, exceeds 50% in *Artemisia annua* [40]. Menthone concentrations in young leaves are highest in *M. arvensis*, followed by menthol concentrations in older leaves [41, 42]. With the progression of leaf age, a similar progressive increase in monoterpene alcohols was seen in peppermint [41 - 43]. Tajidin *et al.* investigated the effects of the three maturity stages of lemongrass on the chemical composition of essential oil and citral contents and discovered that the maturity stage at harvest influenced the essential oil and citral contents of lemongrass [44]. Thyme (*Origanum syriacum* L.) demonstrated the effect of growth stages, such as pre-flowering and blooming, on essential oil output and composition. The plant's total oil yield was higher during the blooming period than during the pre-flowering stage. During the blossoming stage, increased quantities of volatile chemicals were detected. Carvacrol, gamma-terpinene, alpha-terpinene, and para-cymene were exceptions, with larger quantities discovered in the pre-flowering stage. Surprisingly, carvacrol, a structural isomer of thymol, has a larger quantity during the pre-flowering period. Rosa damascene has essential oil in all regions of the flower. In general, the essential oil output is highest when the petals form a cup shape and the stamens are bright yellow. The rate of essential oil biosynthesis is highest in the crown petals. Rose oil's composition varies greatly with the developmental stages of the flower. This is owing to the various rates at which different components are synthesized. Flowers have higher quantities of stearoptene, alpha-pinene, and myrcene in the early stages of development than the key alcohols citronellol, geraniol, and nerol. In later phases of development, the alcohol content quickly rises to around 60% [45]. The essential oil yield of *Salvia sclarea* was lower at the flowering bud stage, higher at the full bloom stage, and then rapidly reduced after maturation. The oil contained linalool (the primary ingredient), linalyl acetate, -Humulene, -cadinene, -caryophyllene, and sclareol, which increased in proportion over the maturation stages with no notable yield loss at the maturation stage. At full maturity, the output of essential oil and monoterpenes is reduced [46].

4.2. The Influence of UV Radiation

Ultraviolet light is significant because it encourages the formation of secondary metabolites in many circumstances. The UV-B band (280-315 nm) in the ultraviolet daylight spectrum is extremely changeable and worthy of special attention. The study found that UV-B radiation induced a 50% increase in essential oil production on a dry-weight basis in one chemotype of *Mentha spicata*, while the rise in the other chemotype was insignificant [47]. More extensive research on the production of essential oil from sweet basil (*Ocimum basilicum* L.) was conducted, with the action of ultraviolet light being of major importance. UV-B radiation had a favorable effect on 22 different essential oil components and increased with plant age [48]. A separate study found that UV-B radiation is required for the correct development and filling of oil glands in sweet basil [49]. Chang *et al.* discovered that exposing Ocimumbasilicum to supplemental UV-B light in the early morning in a controlled setting at room temperature resulted in shorter plants with higher dry mass, more axillary shoots, and thicker leaves [50]. In *Mentha piperita*, UV-B radiation raised the oil content to some level, but when the synthesis of menthone, menthofuran, and menthyl acetate increased, the concentration of menthol declined significantly. Along with modifications in leaf area, the plant's ability to lengthen its stem was considerably restricted [51]. The total essential oil content, particularly menthofuran and menthol, was significantly increased by the application of UV-A radiation (360 nm) during the day. Both the overall leaf area and the total phenols rose. However, when this plant was exposed to UV-A radiation at night, it developed a characteristic shade-avoidance condition with an extended stem, smaller leaves, and lower levels of menthol and essential oils [52]. The maximum essential oil yield was attained during flowering at high PAR (1150 mol m^2s^{-1}) and nearly ambient UV-B radiation (0.6 Wm), according to research on the effects of various UV-B radiation (280-315 nm) and photosynthetically active radiation (PAR, 400-700 nm) levels and ratios on the yield and pattern of peppermint essential oil. Without UV-B radiation and at low PAR (550 mol m^2s^{-1}), the menthol content fell and the menthone content increased, which significantly degraded the oil quality [53]. Additionally, *Cymbopogon flexuosus* has been examined to learn more about the impact of supplemental UV-B (sUV-B) radiation on the production and chemical make-up of its essential oil. exposure to solar ultraviolet B. A higher percentage of essential oil was found in the plant's aerial portions during the time intervals of 15 minutes, 30 minutes, and one hour. The percentage of subaerial portions containing essential oils did not vary much. Citral percentage in plants treated with UV light increased in comparison to the control, according to an examination of the essential oils from aerial parts. Higher percentages of neral and junipene were observed in subaerial portions of sUV-B-treated plants [54].

4.3. Effect of Light Quality

The chemical components of plants as well as the percentage of secondary metabolite accumulation in plant tissues can be affected by light quality and intensity. The quality of electromagnetic radiation influences the quantity and content of essential oils in aromatic plants [55]. The quality of incident light of different wavelength sections of the spectrum affects the manufacture of essential oil in the leaves of geranium (*Pelargonium spp*.). Irradiation with red light resulted in the production of essential oil using $^{14}CO_2$ as an externally provided main precursor [56]. The study on dill (*Anethum graveolens* L.) to investigate the influence of light quality on different wavelength regions, such as supplemental red, far-red, and blue light treatments, as well as end-of-the-day light treatments, revealed substantial changes in plant biomass output. The plants that were exposed to far-red light produced the most essential oil. As a result, plants exposed to 4 hours of red and far red light produced oil with higher phellandrene and less myristicin. The growth and essential oil yield of dill rose as the light level increased, and it was maximum under full sunlight [57, 58]. The effect of different light wavelengths on the manufacture of essential oil has also been studied in sage and thyme. When sage plants were exposed to 45% full sunshine, they produced essential oil with (+)-thujonone as the main component, and camphor in lower concentrations than plants grown in other amounts of sunlight.

Full sunlight produced the highest oil yield and proportion of thymol and myrcene in thyme [59]. To determine the impact of shade on the yield and chemical makeup of essential oil leaves, *Pothomorphe umbellata* (Piperaceae) nine-month-old seedlings were exposed to three levels of shadow (30%, 50%, and 70%), as well as full light. The plants harvested in the second year of development from which the highest essential oil concentration was noted were those that were cultivated in 30% shade. There were found to be 26 chemicals, with trans-nerolidolas being the main one [60]. Three significant *Mentha* species—*M. arvensis*, *M. citrata*, and *M. cardiac*—were grown for 60 cycles under short-day, normal-day, or long-day conditions before being examined for plant growth efficiency, essential oil biosynthesis, yield, and composition. Longer days resulted in the species' better growth, which led to *M. citrata* early flowering. The highest rate of essential oil biosynthesis and, consequently,the maximum output of essential oil were found in the short-day plants. This photoperiodic treatment also had an impact on the composition of the oil [61]. In a separate study, *Mentha aquatica* and Mentha x piperita were grown under varying radiation levels of 23%, 46%, and 100% to examine the influence of photoperiodic modulation. Leaf area, stem number, and total dry mass were all reduced in all plants exposed to the lowest quantity of radiation. Although the essential oil yield and percentages of menthol, menthone, linalool, and linalyl acetate in this oil fell as radiation levels declined, there was no discernible association between plant development and essential oil synthesis. The essential oil yield and growth of African basil, *Ocimum gratissimum* L., were studied in under-watered and water-stressed field conditions in full sunlight and a natural shade (26.7-44.2% full sunlight). Water stress reduced African basil plant height and overall leaf area more than in light or shade conditions. Shade increased the essential oil content, but water stress decreased the essential oil level under shade but increased it in full sunlight. Water stress was only noticed in plants grown in full sunshine. The results showed that when grown in a natural shadow, African basil produces relatively significant essential oil outputs per plant, despite water stress and poor vegetative growth [62].

4.4. Effect of Salt Stress

One of the most important environmental issues limiting crop yield on marginal agricultural soils in many arid and semi-arid parts of the world is salt stress. The effects of salt stress on the quantity and content of essential oils generated by various aromatic plants vary. The main negative impacts of salinity on plant development and yield are due to the osmotic effect, ion toxicity, and nutritional imbalance, which leads to reduced photosynthetic efficiency and stomatal closure [63]. In Egypt, a field trial on three species and four cultivars of basil to examine their behaviour in saline soil revealed that *O. basilicum*. Plant height and number of branches per plant were higher in Var. Siam queen and *O. tenuiflorum* than in *O. basilicum*. Var.genoveser and *O. tenuiflorum* yielded the highest fresh and dry weight values in both seasons. *O. basilicum*. var. Siam queen had the highest essential oil yield, whereas *O. basilicum*. var. Purpleruffle had the lowest essential oil yield [64]. The impacts of four salinity levels on dill revealed that as salinity rose, so did the mean production of essential oils. The dill plant is highly salt-tolerant, and it may thrive in environments with salinities of up to 12 dS/m NaCl [65]. When salinity was increased in a peppermint (*Mentha piperita* L.) experiment, the length and weight of the stems and roots, the internode length, the total biomass, and the yield and percentage of essential oil all decreased. The non-salinity environment produced the highest growth parameter, essential oil output, and percentage values. The commercial grade of the distilled essential oil was improved by an increase in menthone and a decrease in menthofuran with increasing salinity levels (Khorasaninejad *et al.*, 2010). It has been demonstrated that salt stress has an impact on the production, composition, and biosynthesis of shoot essential oil in *Mentha pulegium* L. Under salt stress, the production of essential oil increased by around 2.75 percent, and the proportion of menthone, the main component of the oil, was also impacted. Salt stress caused significant alterations in the number, size, and location of trichomes on both sides [66]. Water stress increased the content of antioxidant chemicals in basil leaf tissues, with the greatest concentration reported at a 25% irrigation intensity. The antioxidant components and antioxidant activity of basil extracts were reduced as the irrigation level was reduced to 12% [67].

4.5. Effect by the Presence of Arbuscular Mycorrhizal Fungi

Arbuscular mycorrhizal fungi (AMF) are undeniably an important part of the lower soil system due to their large established impact on the sustainability and yield of agricultural systems. Arbuscular mycorrhizal fungi are considered to colonize plants by first encouraging the development of secondary plant chemicals such as flavonoids, pathogenesis-related proteins, and phenolics in the roots of the host plant [68 - 70]. However, the buildup of secondary chemicals in mycorrhizal plants' aerial portions has been much less. Arbuscular mycorrhizal fungi were shown to increase the essential oil outputs of Origanum species. According to research on *Coriandrum*, *Anethum*, and *Foeniculum vulgare*, Arbuscular mycorrhizal fungi root colonization changed the chemical composition of the essential oils, which improved the quality of the essential oils [71]. Increased concentrations of artemisinin in mycorrhizal *Artemisia annua* leaves were shown to be connected with a higher density of glandular trichomes [72, 73]. The experiments conducted on three accessions of Artemisia annua to compare the efficacy of two arbuscular mycorrhizal fungi, *Glomus macrocarpum* (GM) and *Glomus fasciculatum* (GF), revealed that the synthesis of plant biomass, dry weight of shoot, nutrient status (P, Zn, and Fe) of the shoot, the concentration of essential oil, and artemisinin in leaves was significantly improved in comparison with non-inoculated plants. The interaction of the fungus and the plant altered the rate of growth, the concentration of nutrients, and the production of secondary metabolites in the plants. *Glomus macrocarpum* was less effective than *Glomus fasciculatum* at boosting the concentration of essential oils in the shoot. *Glomus fasciculatum* was superior to GM in two accessions for increasing artemisinin content [74]. Additionally, these two arbuscular mycorrhizal (AM) fungi significantly accelerated the development and concentration of the *Foeniculum vulgare* essential oil. In comparison to any of the components used alone, the inoculation of arbuscular mycorrhizal fungus into plants and the administration of phosphate fertilizer significantly boosted plant growth, phosphorus uptake, and essential oil content [71].

4.6. Impact of Fertilizers on Essential Oil

Fertilizer application typically impacts essential oil yield by increasing plant biomass yield per unit area; however, fertilizer also has a cultivar-specific effect. Two pot experiments were conducted in oregano plants in the seasons of 2006 and 2007 to investigate the influence of varied quantities of nitrogen fertilizer as ammonium sulfate on the fresh weight of the plant and essential oil. The yield of both herbs and essential oil was increased by watering the plants every seven days and adding 1.2 g of nitrogen to each container. According to reports, the Java citronella plant responds well to nitrogen fertilizer, with cultivars showing differences in oil yields (per hectare) of up to 36% and herbage content of up to 42% at the same nitrogen levels. Additionally, it has been shown that using several urea kinds on the same cultivar might alter the production of herbs [75]. The amount of nitrogen applied to lemongrass has been discovered to affect the amount of citral in the oil, however, sometimes lemongrass needs more potassium than nitrogen to generate the optimum oil [76]. Better flower and oil yield in Rosa damascena has been discovered to be correlated with levels of NPK in leaves at the bud development stage. In several regions, nitrogen application has increased rose flower yield [77].

The most valuable single micronutrient that raises essential oil yield is manganese, according to research. Magnesium administration generally enhances herb yield in geraniums, although oil concentration or composition has no discernible effects [78]. Chlorosis is created in the leaves of *C. winterianus* as a result of the iron shortage, which lowers herb yield and output. Their oil contents aren't much impacted, though [79]. When ferric and manganese sulfates are applied to palmarosa plants during the time of tillering and before the plant begins to flower, it has been discovered that both herbage and oil production dramatically increase [80].

Zn has been discovered to be necessary for the synthesis and accumulation of essential oils in Japanese mint [81]. The maximum overall oil percentage, as well as the highest khusimol and khusinol oil contents, were obtained with the Zn at 0.250 mg/L application to Khus-Khus and in the middle circumferential position [82]. When sufficient nitrogen and phosphate are present, Zn administered as zinc sulfate (2.5 kg/ha) to palmarosa herbs enhances the output of herb and oil [83]. Two field tests on chamomile revealed that foliar applications of Fe and Zn boosted flower and essential oil output in calcareous soils. In comparison to spraying at just one stage, using Fe+Zn spray at the stages of stem elongation and flowering exhibited greater favorable impacts on floral dry yield, essential oil percentage, and yield [84].

The results of an experiment with peppermint grown in Egypt's west Nile Delta under drip irrigation showed that a cobalt concentration of 15 ppm produced the highest yield of essential oils, the best yield of fresh and dry herbs, and improved uptake of both macronutrients (N, P, and K) and micronutrients (Mn, Zn, and Cu). At the highest cobalt concentration, the main components of the oil, including menthone and isomenthone, rose relative to a declining L-menthol level. In comparison to the control and other treatments, the low cobalt level yielded the highest L-menthol content. Thus, the relatively high percentage of menthol in peppermint oil suggests that peppermint essential oil with high commercial value could be successfully produced in recently reclaimed land in Egypt [85]. In well-fertilized plants, the addition of molybdenum and copper has boosted the yield of herbs and oils [86]. Alizadeh *et al.* investigated the effects of various complete fertilizer dosages on the yield, fresh and dry weight, and essential oil composition of *Satureja hortensis* L. The findings indicated that fertilizer use increased the fresh and dry weight of *S. hortensis*. Different fertilizer dosages have very little if any, impact on the composition of essential oils. However, following fertilizer application, certain constituent levels, such as carvacrol, -terpinene, and -terpinene, changed [87]. Ahmadian *et al.* experimented on *Cuminum cyminum* to investigate the effects of water stress and manure treatment on the percentage of oil and its primary components as well as the yield of these components. According to the findings, there is a connection between applying manure and the key elements of cumin essential oil beneath the water. Manure and water stress have a considerable impact on the components of essential oils. With manure treatment and three irrigations, the largest concentrations of cumin, aldehyde, and -cymene and the lowest concentrations of -pinene, -terpinene, and -pinene was attained [88].

5. HEALTH BENEFITS OF ESSENTIAL OILS

5.1. Important Roles in Hormonal Balance

Hormone essential oils can help you balance your estrogen, progesterone, cortisol, thyroid, and testosterone levels [89, 90]. Some essential oils, such as clary sage, geranium, and thyme (https://draxe.com/essential-oils/thyme-oil/.), assist in regulating estrogen and progesterone levels in your body, which can treat illnesses such as infertility and PCOS, as well as PMS and menopause symptoms [90, 91]. According to a 2017 study published in Neuro Endocrinology Letters, geranium and rose to have the ability to impact the salivary levels of estrogen in women [92]. This may be beneficial for people having menopausal symptoms caused by decreased estrogen secretion. Certain oils can also assist in boosting your mood and minimizing symptoms of depression by lowering cortisol levels [93] and increasing testosterone levels (https://draxe.com/essential-oils/essential-oils-for-hormones/) [93 - 95].

5.2. Increase Immunity and Fight Infections

Many essential oils include anti-inflammatory, antiviral, antibacterial, antiseptic, and antifungal qualities that aid in the immune system's function and the battle against infections. Terpenes, esters, phenolics, ethers, and ketones are chemical compounds present in oils that can fight invading microorganisms that can damage your health. Oregano, myrrh, ginger, lemon, eucalyptus, frankincense, peppermint (*Mentha piperita*), and cinnamon are some of the greatest essential oils for immunity [96, 97].

Essential oils have been demonstrated in studies to efficiently eliminate a variety of fungal, viral, and bacterial pathogens, including methicillin-resistant *Staphylococcus aureus*, *Helicobacter pylori*, and *Candida albicans* infections [98]. Because antibiotic resistance is becoming such a serious problem in modern medicine, using these oils as a kind of independent or combination therapy can aid in the fight against bacterial infections more safely and naturally [99]. Choose oregano oil with significant immune-boosting characteristics, as it has been shown in lab studies to have both antiviral and antibacterial properties. Carvacrol and thymol, two chemicals found in oregano oil, have antibacterial properties and can impede the creation and proliferation of many bacteria [100]. The immune-boosting properties of frankincense oil may include aiding in the destruction of harmful germs, viruses, and even cancer. Laboratory research, for example, discovered that frankincense oil has substantial immunostimulant action [101]. When studied in lab experiments and on animals, frankincense also exhibits anti-cancer, anti-inflammatory, and anti-tumor actions, notably aiding in the battle against cancer cells [102]. According to a 2012 study, AKBA, a chemical component found in frankincense, may kill cancer cells that have become resistant to chemotherapy ;https: //publik ation en.sulb.u nisaar land.de/ha ndle/20.500.1 1880/22895;jses sion id=A0A5 B03 2CBD 0B3B692E0 5AB7 6B12 A195) [103, 104].

5.3. Helps in the Improvement of Digestion

Another well-studied essential oil benefit is its ability to help and improve digestion. Some oils can aid with stomach discomfort, indigestion, diarrhea, stomach spasms, and even gastrointestinal diseases like IBS. Oils can also help with digestion by stimulating digestive enzymes, which make it simpler to break down and absorb the nutrients, fats, and protein you require. For example, ginger essential oil is believed to improve digestive health by alle*via*ting indigestion, constipation, and ulcers. Ginger oil increasesstomach emptying in persons with dyspepsia, according to a study published in the World Journal of Gastroenterology. Ginger oil is also used to treat flatulence, nausea, and abdominal pain. Peppermint is another essential oil that might help with digestion [105]. According to research, peppermint oil works quickly to relieve IBS symptoms. In a 4-week randomized, double-blind, placebo-controlled clinical trial, 72 IBS patients were randomly assigned to receive peppermint oil or a placebo. After four weeks, the peppermint group observed a 40% reduction in total IBS symptoms, compared to a 24% reduction in symptoms reported by the placebo group. The treatment group showed a 19.6 percent reduction in symptoms after only 24 hours of taking peppermint oil [106]. Fennel, lemongrass, marjoram, black pepper, and juniper berries are some more essential oils that may aid digestion.

5.4. Promotes Energy Towards Higher Levels

Did you know that using essential oils can increase your energy and even help you perform better in sports? Some oils have energizing properties and may even boost the amount of oxygen getting to your brain, leaving you feeling reenergized, sharp, and concentrated. According to research in the Journal of the International Society of Sports Nutrition, healthy male athletes who drank peppermint oil with water for 10 days experienced greater exercise performance, higher brain oxygen concentrations, and less weariness [107]. Other excellent essential oils for energy include rosemary, eucalyptus, grapefruit, lemon, and lemongrass.

5.5. Boost Cognitive Function

Essential oil advantages, which include neuroprotective effects and cognitive performance-boosting properties, have benefited many patients with neurodegenerative disorders including Alzheimer's and dementia. Researchers discovered that essential oils aid in naturally improving brain function and reducing inflammation because they include potent antioxidants that operate to block free radical scavenging, according to a scientific review that was published in Frontiers in Aging Neuroscience. Additionally, studies on essential oils have demonstrated that they enhance memory, focus, and learning. Both energizing and sedative essential oils have their uses. For example, peppermint oil can help with sustained focus over a longer length of time, while lavender oil can be helpful for persons who are dealing with challenging tasks or circumstances. They can also be helpful in calming agitation in dementia sufferers. This occurs as a result of their sedative and soothing properties [108, 109].

5.6. Reduce Anxiety and Emotional Stress

The power of essential oils to lessen tension and anxiety is perhaps one of their most well-known advantages. Some are sedative and produce feelings of calmness, tranquility, elevation, and relaxation. Lavender, Roman chamomile, bergamot, ylang, orange, rose, frankincense, and vetiver are among the greatest essential oils for reducing anxiety and tension. Inhaling rose water for four weeks dramatically reduced the condition and characteristics of anxiety in patients receiving hemodialysis treatment, according to a 2016 randomized controlled clinical research [110]. In a pilot study that was published in Complementary Therapies in Clinical Practice, it was discovered that using aromatherapy as a complementary therapy helped postpartum women experience less anxiety and despair. A treatment group of postpartum women who inhaled a concoction of rose and lavender oils was separated from the control group, which received no aromatherapy treatment, for a period ranging from zero to 18 months. Comparing the ladies utilizing aromatherapy to those in the control group after four weeks, the former had a significant reduction in anxiety and depressive symptoms [111]. Additionally, an 82-participant study from 2014 assessed the efficacy of aromatherapy for older patients with chronic pain and signs of anxiety and despair. Researchers discovered that the intervention group's levels of negative emotions, such as worry, stress, and depression, significantly decreased following four weeks of essential oil therapy [112]. These are only a few of the research that has demonstrated the ability to combat anxiety and relieve stress [113 - 115].

5.7. Reduce Pain and Aches

Aromatherapy significantly reduces pain when compared to placebo or control therapies, according to a comprehensive review and meta-analysis published in Pain Research and Treatment. Researchers looked at 12 studies on this subject and discovered that using essential oils to treat gynecological, obstetrical, and postoperative pain was particularly effective [116]. Many different oils can be used aromatically or topically to ease body aches and pains. One study that demonstrates this advantage of essential oils examined their effectiveness in treating neck discomfort. The control group used an unscented cream whereas the experimental group used a cream that contained the oils of marjoram, black pepper, lavender, and peppermint. Following a bath, the creams were administered directly to the sore area for 4 weeks. Researchers discovered that the experimental group demonstrated considerable improvement in the 10 mobility areas that were examined, as well as better pain tolerance in the neck [117]. Lavender, peppermint, eucalyptus, chamomile, rosemary, marjoram, thyme, frankincense, turmeric, ginger, and myrrh are among the greatest essential oils for reducing aches and pains.

5.8. Improve the Health of Your Skin and Hair

Using essential oils on your skin and in hair and beauty products is a natural and effective approach to maintaining your personal care routine without using products containing chemicals or hydrogenated oils. Essential oils can help to soothe irritated skin, diminish aging symptoms such as age spots, alleviate acne, protect your skin from sun damage, and thicken your hair. "At least 90 essential oils can be recognized as being indicated for dermatological usage, with at least 1,500 combinations," according to a review published in Evidence-Based Complementary and Alternative Medicine. The capacity of these oils to fight microorganisms that cause dermatological diseases is what gives them their skin advantages. Oils can also help with inflammatory skin problems such as dermatitis, eczema, and lupus, as well as improve the overall appearance of your skin and even aid in wound healing [118]. There have also been numerous studies that show essential oils to be beneficial for hair development. A 2015 study looked at the effects of rosemary oil on patients with androgenetic alopecia, or male or female pattern baldness. For a six-month treatment period, patients were randomly assigned to either rosemary oil or minoxidil (a drug routinely used to treat hair loss). At the six-month mark, researchers discovered that both groups had a considerable rise in hair count. They also found that scalp irritation was more common in the minoxidil group [119]. Lavender, Roman chamomile, frankincense, tea tree, geranium, myrrh, helichrysum, rosemary, and clary sage are among the greatest essential oils for skin and hair. The Use section of the following page includes blends that incorporate certain oils with particular carrier oils.

5.9. Decrease Toxicity

By supporting your body's and home's detoxification processes, essential oils may aid in reducing toxins. These days, many chemicals and environmental contaminants that can be harmful to human health are being inhaled and ingested by everyone. Some have minor diuretic properties, which boost urine production and enhance detoxification. Additionally, certain oils aid in digestion and encourage the removal of toxins that accumulate in the body [120]. Lemon, grapefruit, parsley, fennel, lemongrass, peppermint, and ginger oils are among those that support internal cleansing. By using detoxifying oils, you may assist your body to getrid of harmful toxins bypurifying the air in your house. In reality, essential oils can organically clean your home by removing hazardous bacteria and pollutants, unlike the majority of household cleaning products that are packed with chemicals. Grapefruit, orange, lemon, lemongrass, eucalyptus, cinnamon, peppermint, and tea tree oils are the greatest for lowering toxins in your home or place of employment.

5.10. Reduce Migraines and Headaches

Essential oils may be useful as natural headache and migraine remedies because they target the source of the problem rather than disguising it as medications do. Essential oils for headaches relieve pain, increase circulation, and reduce stress, which can be a contributing factor to headaches and migraines. In 2012, a placebo-controlled clinical experiment was done to assess the efficacy of breathing lavender oil for migraine headache therapy. Forty-seven migraine patients were separated into two groups: those who inhaled lavender oil for 15 minutes and those who utilized a colorful and odorless liquid. The researchers discovered a statistically significant difference between the controls and treated patients after asking the patients to record their headache severity and related symptoms every 30 minutes for a total of 2 hours. In the treatment group, 92 of the 129 headache bouts reacted completely or partially to lavender. 32 of 68 headache bouts in the control group responded to a placebo [121]. Other oils that can help relieve headache pain besides lavender include peppermint, which has a cooling impact and encourages blood flow, eucalyptus, which relieves sinus pressure by opening the nasal airways, and rosemary, which lowers inflammation, enhances circulation and has a relaxing effect [122 - 124].

5.11. Encourage Restful Sleep

Some essential oils have sedative characteristics that can aid those who have difficulty falling asleep or sleeping through the night. Because of its propensity to leave you feeling relaxed and tranquil, lavender oil is believed to be a great sleep aid. Roman chamomile, ylang, bergamot, and vetiver are some other oils that can be used to encourage deep sleep [115]. A comprehensive analysis published in 2014 by the University of Minnesota analyzed 15 quantitative studies, including 11 randomized controlled trials, on the effects of essential oils on sleep. The majority of the study findings imply that oils have a good effect on sleep deprivation and disturbance, according to the researchers. Lavender oil was the most commonly examined oil, and no adverse events were documented in any of the trials that were reviewed [125]. Another recent study, published in Nursing in Critical Care, looked at the impact of lavender oil on sleep quality in patients in the coronary critical care unit (ICU). Sixty patients took part in the study and were randomly assigned to either the intervention or control groups.

The intervention group inhaled lavender oil for 15 days, and the researchers discovered that they had considerably better sleep quality than the control group, which received no therapy. According to the researchers, lavender oil is a non-invasive, low-cost, and simple intervention for hospital patients who have difficulty sleeping and suffer from anxiety [126].

5.12. Relief from Inflammation

When applied to the skin, certain essential oils' potent anti-inflammatory characteristics help lessen skin irritation and inflammation. These oils can be used either alone or in combination with a carrier oil, straight on the skin. Examples of essential oils that can be used to reduce inflammation include:

- Both acne and skin irritation can be effectively treated with tea tree oil. Additionally, it can lessen inflammation-related redness.
- Peppermint essential oil has a lot of potential as a treatment for intestinal inflammation. Due to digestive issues, peppermint essential oil might lessen intestinal irritation.
- Rosemary and eucalyptus essential oils can help relieve sinus and throat discomfort caused by colds. These two oils can also help to cleanse clogged sinus passages and free up congested airways.
- The use of rosemary essential oil can significantly reduce irritation if you have dandruff or an itchy scalp.
- The power of thyme essential oil as an anti-inflammatory is well documented. When breathed, it has been found to lessen respiratory irritation.

5.13. The Advantages of Essential Oils for Pain Relief

Because the oils can be absorbed through the skin, aromatherapy can considerably relieve discomfort. The topical application of essential oils for pain relief is safe and effective [127]. The following are some essential oils that can be used to relieve pain:

- Ginger, frankincense, and myrrh essential oils can provide quick relief for arthritis pain in the muscles, joints, and tendons.
- Helichrysum oil can help mend damaged muscle tissue and relieve discomfort caused by disorders like fibromyalgia.
- Chamomile oil can instantly ease digestive tract pain as well as period cramps. Chamomile oil is also a great pain reliever for the lower back and muscles.
- When taken, peppermint essential oil can rapidly reduce the pain associated with gas. It can also be used to treat nausea and indigestion.
- Essential oils of lavender and rosemary have been demonstrated to significantly alleviate tension headaches and migraines. Inhaling these oils directly on the temples and either side of the nose provides immediate pain alleviation because these oils are received by the brain in seconds.

5.14. Skin Irritations Can Be Healed

Strong anti-inflammatory and antibacterial qualities can be found in several essential oils [128]. They are, therefore, a very powerful natural remedy for treating all types of skin irritations. These essential oils swiftly penetrate deeper layers of skin tissue when applied topically to the skin, promoting healing [129]. The following are some instances of how to treat skin irritation with essential oils. Get Rid of Skin Irritations:

- Tea tree essential oil kills the bacteria on the face that causes acne, which effectively reduces zits and blemishes. Additionally, it can lessen eczema and offer prompt relief from insect bites and sunburn.
- Apply lavender essential oil directly to the skin to hasten the healing of cuts. Lavender essential oil's antimicrobial qualities will expedite the healing process.
- Lemongrass essential oil is a powerful astringent for the face that effectively treats acne and greatly minimizes the appearance of big pores.
- Insect bites and eczema-related itchiness and irritation can be lessened by using basil essential oil.
- Rosemary essential oil acts as a mild anti-inflammatory and can help lessen skin irritation on the face and scalp.
- Apply carrot seed essential oil to the skin to treat sun damage. This successfully lessens sunburns.

5.15. Alternatives to Candles and Incense that are Less Dangerous

Aromatherapy is a safe and effective technique to make your house smell great. Candles and incense might cause a fire in your home. They are particularly hazardous if you have pets or young children. However, by employing an oil diffuser, you may drastically change the smell of your home without jeopardizing your valuable possessions. A little device that can be placed on any surface in your home is an oil diffuser. It functions as a small humidifier, emitting steam or acoustically generated water vapor into the room. Fill the tank halfway with water and add 10-15 drops of your preferred essential oil blend. The smell will take over your home as the water vapor "diffuses," allowing you to enjoy the advantages of aromatherapy while going about your routine.

CONCLUSION

The present article is about the beneficial use of essential oils in our day-to-day lives. We made an effort to link as frequently as we could to the more in-depth studies in which the benefits of essential oils are found. Understanding the many advantages of essential oils can help us to find fully safe, all-natural ways to treat our bodies and mind. Using aromatherapy to treat a wide range of illnesses has been used for ages. We can get an essential oil beginning kit here if we are unfamiliar with the idea of aromatherapy. Additionally, this oil diffuser is one of our favorites if we want to benefit from using one in our house.

REFERENCES

[1] Adorjan B, Buchbauer G. Biological properties of essential oils: An updated review. Flavour Fragrance J 2010; 25(6): 407-26. [http://dx.doi.org/10.1002/ffj.2024]

[2] Amorati R, Foti MC, Valgimigli L. Antioxidant activity of essential oils. J Agric Food Chem 2013; 61(46): 10835-47. [http://dx.doi.org/10.1021/jf403496k] [PMID: 24156356]

[3] Jahan SJAHAN, Chowdhury SF, Mitu SA, Shahriar MSHAHRIA, Bhuiyan MABH. Genomic DNA extraction methods: A comparative case study with gram–negative organisms. Banat's J Biotechnol 2015; VI(11): 61-8. [http://dx.doi.org/10.7904/2068-4738-VI(11)-61]

[4] Ouis N, Hariri A. Antioxidant and antibacterial activities of the essential oils of Ceratonia siliqua. Banat's J Biotechnol 2018; IX(17): 13-23. [http://dx.doi.org/10.7904/2068-4738-IX(17)-13]

[5] Baser KH, Buchbauer G. Handbook of essential oils: science, technology, and applications. CRC press 2009. [http://dx.doi.org/10.1201/9781420063165]

[6] Caissard JC, Joly C, Bergougnoux V, Hugueney P, Mauriat M, Baudino S. Secretion mechanisms of volatile organic compounds in specialized cells of aromatic plants. Recent Res Dev Cell Biol 2004; 2: 1-5.

[7] Antoń S, Kamińska M, Stpiczyńska M. Comparative structure of the osmophores in the flowers of Stanhopea graveolens Lindley and Cycnoches chlorochilon Klotzsch (Orchidaceae). Acta Agrobot 2012; 65(2): 11-22. [http://dx.doi.org/10.5586/aa.2012.054]

[8] Curry KJ, McDowell LM, Judd WS, Stern WL. Osmophores, floral features, and systematics of Stanhopea (Orchidaceae). Am J Bot 1991; 78(5): 610-23. [http://dx.doi.org/10.1002/j.1537-2197.1991.tb12585.x]

[9] Effmert U, Große J, Röse USR, Ehrig F, Kägi R, Piechulla B. Volatile composition, emission pattern, and localization of floral scent emission in *Mirabilis jalapa* (Nyctaginaceae). Am J Bot 2005; 92(1): 2-12.
[http://dx.doi.org/10.3732/ajb.92.1.2] [PMID: 21652378]

[10] Kay QON, Daoud HS, Stirton CH. Pigment distribution, light reflection and cell structure in petals. Bot J Linn Soc 1981; 83(1): 57-83.
[http://dx.doi.org/10.1111/j.1095-8339.1981.tb00129.x]

[11] Chen F, Tholl D, D'Auria JC, Farooq A, Pichersky E, Gershenzon J. Biosynthesis and emission of terpenoid volatiles from Arabidopsis flowers. Plant Cell 2003; 15(2): 481-94.
[http://dx.doi.org/10.1105/tpc.007989] [PMID: 12566586]

[12] Glover BJ, Perez-Rodriguez M, Martin C. Development of several epidermal cell types can be specified by the same MYB-related plant transcription factor. Development 1998; 125(17): 3497-508.
[http://dx.doi.org/10.1242/dev.125.17.3497] [PMID: 9693152]

[13] Weryszko-Chmielewska E, Chwil M. Ecological adaptations of the floral structures of Galanthus nivalis L. Acta Agrobot 2012; 63(2): 41-9.
[http://dx.doi.org/10.5586/aa.2010.031]

[14] Peter AJ, Shanower TG. Plant glandular trichomes. Resonance 1998; 3(3): 41-5.
[http://dx.doi.org/10.1007/BF02837613]

[15] Weryszko-Chmielewska E, Chernetskyy M. Structure of trichomes from the surface of leaves of some species of Kalanchoë Adans. Acta Biol Cracov Ser; Bot 2005; 47(2): 15-22.

[16] Osman AK. Trichome micromorphology of Egyptian Ballota (Lamiaceae) with emphasis on its systematic implication. Pak J Bot 2012; 44(1): 33-46.

[17] Wang G, Tian L, Aziz N, *et al.* Terpene biosynthesis in glandular trichomes of hop. Plant Physiol 2008; 148(3): 1254-66.
[http://dx.doi.org/10.1104/pp.108.125187] [PMID: 18775972]

[18] Boughton AJ, Hoover K, Felton GW. Methyl jasmonate application induces increased densities of glandular trichomes on tomato, Lycopersicon esculentum. J Chem Ecol 2005; 31(9): 2211-6.
[http://dx.doi.org/10.1007/s10886-005-6228-7] [PMID: 16132222]

[19] Carpenter KJ. Specialized structures in the leaf epidermis of basal angiosperms: morphology, distribution, and homology. Am J Bot 2006; 93(5): 665-81.
[http://dx.doi.org/10.3732/ajb.93.5.665] [PMID: 21642131]

[20] Turner GW, Gershenzon J, Croteau RB. Distribution of peltate glandular trichomes on developing leaves of peppermint. Plant Physiol 2000; 124(2): 655-64.
[http://dx.doi.org/10.1104/pp.124.2.655] [PMID: 11027715]

[21] Jasim RK. Isolation and molecular characterisation xylanase produced by sporolactobacilli. Banat's J Biotechnol 2016; VII(14): 30-7.
[http://dx.doi.org/10.7904/2068-4738-VII(14)-30]

[22] Bakari M, Yusuf HO. Utilization of locally available binders for densification of rice husk for biofuel production. Banat's J Biotechnol 2018; IX(18): 47-55.
[http://dx.doi.org/10.7904/2068-4738-IX(18)-47]

[23] Eed AM, Burgoyne AH. Tissue culture of Simmondsia chinensis (Link) Schneider. Banat's. J Biotechnol 2015; 6: 11.

[24] Nikolova I, Georgieva N. Effect of biological products on the population of aphids and chemical components in alfalfa. Banat's J Biotechnol 2018; IX(18): 38-46.
[http://dx.doi.org/10.7904/2068-4738-IX(18)-38]

[25] Rahimian Y, Akbari SM, Karami M, Fafghani M. Effect of different levels of Fenugreek powder supplementation on performance, Influenza, Sheep red blood cell, New Castle diseases anti-body titer

and intestinal microbial flora on Cobb 500 broiler chicks. Banat's J Biotechnol 2018; IX(18): 29-37. [http://dx.doi.org/10.7904/2068-4738-IX(18)-29]

[26] Saidi A, Eghbalnegad Y, Hajibarat Z. Study of genetic diversity in local rose varieties (Rosa spp.) using molecular markers. Banat's J Biotechnol 2017; VIII(16): 148-57. [http://dx.doi.org/10.7904/2068-4738-VIII(16)-148]

[27] Zerkaoui L, Benslimane M, Hamimed A. The purification performances of the lagooning process, case of the Beni Chougrane region in Mascara (Algerian N.W.). Banat's J Biotechnol 2018; IX(18): 20-8. [http://dx.doi.org/10.7904/2068-4738-IX(18)-20]

[28] Hariri A, Ouis N, Bouhadi D, Ould Yerou K. Evaluation of the quality of the date syrups enriched by cheese whey during the period of storage. Banat's J Biotechnol 2017; VIII(16): 75-82. [http://dx.doi.org/10.7904/2068-4738-VIII(16)-75]

[29] Bozhanska T. Botanical and morphological composition of artificial grassland of bird's–foot–trefoil (Lotus Corniculatus L.) treated with lumbrical and lumbrex. Banat's J Biotechnol 2018; IX(18): 12-9. [http://dx.doi.org/10.7904/2068-4738-IX(18)-12]

[30] Mahmoodi M, Afshari KP, Seyedabadi HR, Aboozari M. Sequence analysis of 12S rRNA and 16S rRNA mitochondrial genes in Iranian Afshari sheep. Banat's J Biotechnol 2018; IX(18): 5-11. [http://dx.doi.org/10.7904/2068-4738-IX(18)-5]

[31] Satimehin FP, Tiamiyu LO, Okayi RG. Proximate and phytochemical changes in hydrothermally processed rubber (Hevea brasiliensis) leaf meal. Banat's J Biotechnol 2017; VIII(16): 12-7. [http://dx.doi.org/10.7904/2068-4738-VIII(16)-12]

[32] Dlilali BDLILAL, Ahmed HAHMED, Zouaoui BZOUAOUI, Fatima SFATIMA, Karima OY. Kinetic of batch production of lactic acid from carob pods syrup. Banat's J Biotechnol 2017; VIII(15): 57-65. [http://dx.doi.org/10.7904/2068-4738-VIII(15)-57]

[33] Egu UN, Okonkwo JC. Effect of Gonadotrophin (Diclair®) on semen characteristics, hormonal profile and biochemical constituents of the seminal plasma of mature Balami rams. Banat's J Biotechnol 2017; VIII(15): 90-7. [http://dx.doi.org/10.7904/2068-4738-VIII(15)-90]

[34] Danilchuk YVD. Selective crystallization of maltose by isopropanol and acetone from glucose-maltose syrups. Banat's J Biotechnol 2016; VII(14): 120-5. [http://dx.doi.org/10.7904/2068-4738-VII(14)-120]

[35] Ojogu NA, Annune PA, Okayi GR. Toxicological effects of aqueous extract of piptadeniastrium africanum bark on clarias gariepinus juveniles. Banat's J Biotechnol 2017; VIII(15): 123-35. [http://dx.doi.org/10.7904/2068-4738-VIII(15)-123]

[36] Mallavarapu GR, Kulkarni RN, Baskaran K, Rao L, Ramesh S. Influence of plant growth stage on the essential oil content and composition in Davana (Artemisia pallens wall.). J Agric Food Chem 1999; 47(1): 254-8. [http://dx.doi.org/10.1021/jf980624c] [PMID: 10563881]

[37] Singh N, Luthra R, Sangwan R. Effect of leaf position and age on the essential oil quantity and quality in lemongrass (Cymbopogon flexuosus) 1. Planta Med 1989; 55(3): 254-6. [http://dx.doi.org/10.1055/s-2006-961997] [PMID: 17262411]

[38] Croteau R, Felton M, Karp F, Kjonaas R. Relationship of camphor biosynthesis to leaf development in sage (Sal*via* officinalis). Plant Physiol 1981; 67(4): 820-4. [http://dx.doi.org/10.1104/pp.67.4.820] [PMID: 16661761]

[39] Duriyaprapan S, Britten EJ. The effect of age and location of leaf on quantity and quality of Japanese mint oil production. J Exp Bot 1982; 33(4): 810-4. [http://dx.doi.org/10.1093/jxb/33.4.810]

[40] Chalchat JC, Garry RP, Lamy J. Influence of harvest time on yield and composition of Artemisia annua oil produced in France. J Essent Oil Res 1994; 6(3): 261-8.

[http://dx.doi.org/10.1080/10412905.1994.9698374]

[41] Sakata I. Seasonal variations in menthyl glucoside, menthol, menthone and related monoterpenes in developing Japanese peppermint [mentha arvensis var. piperascens]. J Agricult Chem Socie Japan 1980.

[42] Góra J, Lis A, Kula J, Staniszewska M, Wołoszyn A. Chemical composition variability of essential oils in the ontogenesis of some plants. Flavour Fragrance J 2002; 17(6): 445-51. [http://dx.doi.org/10.1002/ffj.1126]

[43] Maffei M, Codignola A. Photosynthesis, photorespiration and herbicide effect on terpene production in peppermint (Mentha piperita L.). J Essent Oil Res 1990; 2(6): 275-86. [http://dx.doi.org/10.1080/10412905.1990.9697886]

[44] Tajidin NE, Ahmad SH, Rosenani AB, Azimah H, Munirah M. Chemical composition and citral content in lemongrass (Cymbopogon citratus) essential oil at three maturity stages. Afr J Biotechnol 2012; 11(11): 2685-93. [http://dx.doi.org/10.5897/AJB11.2939]

[45] Weiss EA. Essential oil crops. Cab International 1997.

[46] Lattoo SK, Dhar RS, Dhar AK, Sharma PR, Agarwal SG. Dynamics of essential oil biosynthesis in relation to inflorescence and glandular ontogeny in *Salvia* sclarea. Flavour Fragrance J 2006; 21(5): 817-21. [http://dx.doi.org/10.1002/ffj.1733]

[47] Karousou R, Grammatikopoulos G, Lanaras T, Manetas Y, Kokkini S. Effects of enhanced UV-B radiation on Mentha spicata essential oils. Phytochemistry 1998; 49(8): 2273-7. [http://dx.doi.org/10.1016/S0031-9422(98)00385-9]

[48] Johnson CB, Kirby J, Naxakis G, Pearson S. Substantial UV-B-mediated induction of essential oils in sweet basil (Ocimum basilicum L.). Phytochemistry 1999; 51(4): 507-10. [http://dx.doi.org/10.1016/S0031-9422(98)00767-5]

[49] Ioannidis D, Bonner L, Johnson CB. UV-B is required for normal development of oil glands in Ocimum basilicum L. (sweet basil). Ann Bot 2002; 90(4): 453-60. [http://dx.doi.org/10.1093/aob/mcf212] [PMID: 12324268]

[50] Chang X, Alderson PG, Wright CJ. Enhanced UV-B radiation alters basil (Ocimum basilicum L.) growth and stimulates the synthesis of volatile oils. J Hortic For 2009; 12: 27-31.

[51] Maffei M, Scannerini S. UV-B effect on photomorphogenesis and essential oil composition in peppermint (Mentha piperita L.). J Essent Oil Res 2000; 12(5): 523-9. [http://dx.doi.org/10.1080/10412905.2000.9712150]

[52] Maffei M, Canova D, Bertea CM, Scannerini S. UV-A effects on photomorphogenesis and essential-oil composition in Mentha piperita. J Photochem Photobiol B 1999; 52(1-3): 105-10. [http://dx.doi.org/10.1016/S1011-1344(99)00110-4]

[53] Behn H, Albert A, Marx F, Noga G, Ulbrich A. Ultraviolet-B and photosynthetically active radiation interactively affect yield and pattern of monoterpenes in leaves of peppermint (Mentha x piperita L.). J Agric Food Chem 2010; 58(12): 7361-7. [http://dx.doi.org/10.1021/jf9046072] [PMID: 20481601]

[54] Vinutha M. Effect of sUV-B on Essential Oil from Aerial and Sub-Aerial Parts of Cymbopogonflexuosus (Nees Ex Steud) Wats. Int J Adv Res 2013; 1(7): 263-71.

[55] Sharafzadeh SH. Growth and secondary metabolites of basil, mint and thyme as affected by light. Int J Pharma Bio Sci 2012; 3(1): 43-6.

[56] Sangwan RS, Arora B, Sangwan NS. Spectral modulation of essential oil biogenesis in the scented geranium, Pelargonium graveolens L. J Herbs Spices Med Plants 2003; 10(1): 85-91. [http://dx.doi.org/10.1300/J044v10n01_10]

[57] Hälvä S, Craker LE, Simon JE, Charles DJ. Light levels, growth, and essential oil in dill (Anethum graveolens L.). J Herbs Spices Med Plants 1992; 1(1-2): 47-58. [http://dx.doi.org/10.1300/J044v01n01_06]

[58] Hälvä S, Craker LE, Simon JE, Charles DJ. Light quality, growth, and essential oil in dill (Anethum graveolens L.). J Herbs Spices Med Plants 1992; 1(1-2): 59-69. [http://dx.doi.org/10.1300/J044v01n01_07]

[59] Li YL. Effect of light level on the growth and essential oil production of two herbs:: sage (Sal*via* officinalis) and thyme (Thymus vulgaris). Masters Theses , University of Massachusetts Amherst 2014.

[60] Mattana RS, Vieira MAR, Marchese JA, Ming LC, Marques MOM. Shade level effects on yield and chemical composition of the leaf essential oil of Pothomorphe umbellata (L.) Miquel. Sci Agric 2010; 67(4): 414-8. [http://dx.doi.org/10.1590/S0103-90162010000400006]

[61] Farooqi AHA, Samgwan NS, Sangwan RS. Effect of different photoperiodic regimes on growth, flowering and essential oil in Mentha species. Plant Growth Regul 1999; 29(3): 181-7. [http://dx.doi.org/10.1023/A:1006248019007]

[62] Omobolanle Ade-Ademilua E, Oghenekome Obi H, Craker LE. Growth and essential oil yield of African Basil, Ocimum gratissimum, under light and water stress. Journal of Medicinally Active Plants 2013; 1(4): 143-9.

[63] Muhammad Z, Hussain F. Vegetative growth performance of five medicinal plants under NaCl salt stress. Pak J Bot 2010; 42(1): 303-16.

[64] Omer EA, Said-Al Ahl HA, Hendawy SF. Production, chemical composition and volatile oil of different basil species/varieties cultivated under Egyptian soil salinity conditions. Res J Agric Biol Sci 2008; 4(4): 293-300.

[65] Ghassemi-Golezani K, Zehtab-Salmasi S, Dastborhan S. Changes in essential oil content of dill (Anethum graveolens) organs under salinity stress. J Med Plants Res 2011; 5(14): 3142-5.

[66] Karray-Bouraoui N, Rabhi M, Neffati M, *et al.* Salt effect on yield and composition of shoot essential oil and trichome morphology and density on leaves of Mentha pulegium. Ind Crops Prod 2009; 30(3): 338-43. [http://dx.doi.org/10.1016/j.indcrop.2009.06.003]

[67] Khan MM, Hanif MA, Abraham AS. Variations in basil antioxidant contents in relation to deficit irrigation. J Med Plants Res 2012; 6(11): 2220-3.

[68] Scharff AM, Jakobsen I, Rosendahl L. The effect of symbiotic microorganisms on phytoalexin contents of soybean roots. J Plant Physiol 1997; 151(6): 716-23. [http://dx.doi.org/10.1016/S0176-1617(97)80069-7]

[69] Benhamou N. Elicitor-induced plant defence pathways. Trends Plant Sci 1996; 1(7): 233-40. [http://dx.doi.org/10.1016/S1360-1385(96)86901-0]

[70] Larose G, Chênevert R, Moutoglis P, Gagné S, Piché Y, Vierheilig H. Flavonoid levels in roots ofMedicago sativa are modulated by the developmental stage of the symbiosis and the root colonizing arbuscular mycorrhizal fungus. J Plant Physiol 2002; 159(12): 1329-39. [http://dx.doi.org/10.1078/0176-1617-00896]

[71] Kapoor R, Giri B, Mukerji KG. Improved growth and essential oil yield and quality in Foeniculum vulgare mill on mycorrhizal inoculation supplemented with P-fertilizer. Bioresour Technol 2004; 93(3): 307-11. [http://dx.doi.org/10.1016/j.biortech.2003.10.028] [PMID: 15062827]

[72] Kapoor R, Chaudhary V, Bhatnagar AK. Effects of arbuscular mycorrhiza and phosphorus application on artemisinin concentration in Artemisia annua L. Mycorrhiza 2007; 17(7): 581-7.

[http://dx.doi.org/10.1007/s00572-007-0135-4] [PMID: 17578608]

[73] Khaosaad T, Vierheilig H, Nell M, Zitterl-Eglseer K, Novak J. Arbuscular mycorrhiza alter the concentration of essential oils in oregano (Origanum sp., Lamiaceae). Mycorrhiza 2006; 16(6): 443-6. [http://dx.doi.org/10.1007/s00572-006-0062-9] [PMID: 16909287]

[74] Chaudhary V, Kapoor R, Bhatnagar AK. Effectiveness of two arbuscular mycorrhizal fungi on concentrations of essential oil and artemisinin in three accessions of Artemisia annua L. Appl Soil Ecol 2008; 40(1): 174-81. [http://dx.doi.org/10.1016/j.apsoil.2008.04.003]

[75] Singh K, Singh DV. Effect of rates and sources of nitrogen application on yield and nutrient uptake of Citronella Java (Cymbopogon winterianus Jowitt). Fert Res 1992; 33(3): 187-91. [http://dx.doi.org/10.1007/BF01050873]

[76] Samiullah VA, Afridi MM, Mohmmad F, Afaq SH. Nitroge n requirements of lemongrass for optimum performance in Uttar Pradesh. Indian perfumer 1988; 32: 225.

[77] Orlova LM. Principles of essential oil rose nutrient requirement sdetermination by leaf analysis. Trudy vsesoyuznogo nauchno issledovatel, skogo instituta efiromaslichnykhkul 1984; 16: 11.

[78] Malwatkar GM, Kokje BA, Kelkar GD. Seasonal variations in aldehyde content in oil: leaf yellowing and crinkling and leaf browning in java citronella (Cymbopogon winterianus Jowitt). Indian perfumer 1984.

[79] Nandi RP, Chatterjee SK. Improved cultivation and distillation methods, followed by citronella plantations of Darjeeling hills. Indian Perfumer 1991; 35(1): 24-9.

[80] Carrubba A, Scalenghe R. The scent of *Mare Nostrum* : medicinal and aromatic plants in Mediterranean soils. J Sci Food Agric 2012; 92(6): 1150-70. [http://dx.doi.org/10.1002/jsfa.5630] [PMID: 22419102]

[81] Misra A, Sharma S. Critical Zn concentration for essential oil yield and menthol concentration of Japanese mint. Fert Res 1991; 29(3): 261-5. [http://dx.doi.org/10.1007/BF01052394]

[82] Misra A, Srivastava NK, Srivastava AK. Influence of Zn stresses on growth and physiology in Khus-khus (Vetiveria zizanoides Nash.) and its essential sesquiterpene oil (s), in relation to roots diameter circumferential positions. J Ecol Nat Environ 2012; 4(2): 58-61.

[83] Sharma SN, Singh A, Tripathi RS. Response of palmarosa to nitrogen, phosphorus, potassium and zinc. Indian J Agron 1980; 25(4): 719-23.

[84] Nasiri Y, Zehtab-Salmasi S, Nasrullahzadeh S, Najafi N, Ghassemi-Golezani K. Effects of foliar application of micronutrients (Fe and Zn) on flower yield and essential oil of chamomile (Matricaria chamomilla L.). J Med Plants Res 2010; 4(17): 1733-7.

[85] Aziz EE, Gad N, Khaled SM. Effect of cobalt on growth and chemical composition of peppermint plant grown in newly reclaimed soil. Aust J Basic Appl Sci 2011; 5(11): 628-33.

[86] Shiyab S, Shatnawi M, Shibli R, Al-Zweiri M, Akash M, Aburijai T. Influence of developmental stage on yield and composition of Origanum syriacum L. oil by multivariate analysis. J Med Plants Res 2012; 6(15): 2985-94.

[87] Alizadeh A, Khoshkhui M, Javidnia K, Firuzi O, Tafazoli E, Khalighi A. Effects of fertilizer on yield, essential oil composition, total phenolic content and antioxidant activity in Satureja hortensis L.(Lamiaceae) cultivated in Iran. J Med Plants Res 2010; 4(1): 33-40.

[88] Ahmadian A, Tavassoli A, Amiri E. The interaction effect of water stress and manure on yield components, essential oil and chemical compositions of cumin (Cuminum cyminum). Afr J Agric Res 2011; 6(10): 2309-15.

[89] Kavlock RJ, Daston GP, DeRosa C, *et al.* Research needs for the risk assessment of health and environmental effects of endocrine disruptors: a report of the U.S. EPA-sponsored workshop. Environ

Health Perspect 1996; 104(Suppl 4): 715-40.
[http://dx.doi.org/10.1289/ehp.96104s4715] [PMID: 8880000]

[90] Zoeller RT, Brown TR, Doan LL, *et al.* Endocrine-disrupting chemicals and public health protection: A statement of principles from The Endocrine Society. Endocrinology 2012; 153(9): 4097-110. [http://dx.doi.org/10.1210/en.2012-1422] [PMID: 22733974]

[91] Tanos T, Rojo LJ, Echeverria P, Brisken C. ER and PR signaling nodes during mammary gland development. Breast Cancer Res 2012; 14(4): 210. [http://dx.doi.org/10.1186/bcr3166] [PMID: 22809143]

[92] Shinohara K, Doi H, Kumagai C, Sawano E, Tarumi W. Effects of essential oil exposure on salivary estrogen concentration in perimenopausal women. Neuroendocrinol Lett 2017; 37(8): 567-72. [PMID: 28326753]

[93] Kim IH, Kim C, Seong K, Hur MH, Lim HM, Lee MS. Essential oil inhalation on blood pressure and salivary cortisol levels in prehypertensive and hypertensive subjects. Evid Based Complement Alternat Med 2012; 2012: 1-9. [http://dx.doi.org/10.1155/2012/984203] [PMID: 23259002]

[94] Diamanti-Kandarakis E, Bourguignon JP, Giudice LC, *et al.* Endocrine-disrupting chemicals: an Endocrine Society scientific statement. Endocr Rev 2009; 30(4): 293-342. [http://dx.doi.org/10.1210/er.2009-0002] [PMID: 19502515]

[95] Diaz A, Luque L, Badar Z, Kornic S, Danon M. Prepubertal gynecomastia and chronic lavender exposure: Report of three cases. J Pediatr Endocrinol Metab 2016; 29(1): 103-7. [http://dx.doi.org/10.1515/jpem-2015-0248] [PMID: 26353172]

[96] Burt S. Essential oils: their antibacterial properties and potential applications in foods—a review. Int J Food Microbiol 2004; 94(3): 223-53. [http://dx.doi.org/10.1016/j.ijfoodmicro.2004.03.022] [PMID: 15246235]

[97] Deyno S, Mtewa AG, Abebe A, *et al.* Essential oils as topical anti-infective agents: A systematic review and meta-analysis. Complement Ther Med 2019; 47: 102224. [http://dx.doi.org/10.1016/j.ctim.2019.102224] [PMID: 31780027]

[98] Kuriyama H, Watanabe S, Nakaya T, *et al.* Immunological and psychological benefits of aromatherapy massage. Evid Based Complement Alternat Med 2005; 2(2): 179-84. [http://dx.doi.org/10.1093/ecam/neh087] [PMID: 15937558]

[99] Yap PSX, Yiap BC, Ping HC, Lim SHE. Essential oils, a new horizon in combating bacterial antibiotic resistance. Open Microbiol J 2014; 8(1): 6-14. [http://dx.doi.org/10.2174/1874285801408010006] [PMID: 24627729]

[100] Swamy MK, Akhtar MS, Sinniah UR. Antimicrobial properties of plant essential oils against human pathogens and their mode of action: An updated review. Evid-based Compl Alterna Med 2016; 2016: 3012462. [http://dx.doi.org/10.1155/2016/3012462]

[101] Mikhaeil BR, Maatooq GT, Badria FA, Amer MMA. Chemistry and immunomodulatory activity of frankincense oil. Z Naturforsch C J Biosci 2003; 58(3-4): 230-8. [http://dx.doi.org/10.1515/znc-2003-3-416] [PMID: 12710734]

[102] Chen Y, Zhou C, Ge Z, *et al.* Composition and potential anticancer activities of essential oils obtained from myrrh and frankincense. Oncol Lett 2013; 6(4): 1140-6. [http://dx.doi.org/10.3892/ol.2013.1520] [PMID: 24137478]

[103] Miguel MG. Antioxidant and anti-inflammatory activities of essential oils: a short review. Molecules 2010; 15(12): 9252-87. [http://dx.doi.org/10.3390/molecules15129252] [PMID: 21160452]

[104] Valdivieso-Ugarte M, Gomez-Llorente C, Plaza-Díaz J, Gil Á. Antimicrobial, antioxidant, and immunomodulatory properties of essential oils: A systematic review. Nutrients 2019; 11(11): 2786.

[http://dx.doi.org/10.3390/nu11112786] [PMID: 31731683]

[105] Hu ML, Rayner CK, Wu KL, *et al.* Effect of ginger on gastric motility and symptoms of functional dyspepsia. World J Gastroenterol 2011; 17(1): 105-10. [http://dx.doi.org/10.3748/wjg.v17.i1.105] [PMID: 21218090]

[106] Cash BD, Epstein MS, Shah SM. A novel delivery system of peppermint oil is an effective therapy for irritable bowel syndrome symptoms. Dig Dis Sci 2016; 61(2): 560-71. [http://dx.doi.org/10.1007/s10620-015-3858-7] [PMID: 26319955]

[107] Meamarbashi A, Rajabi A. The effects of peppermint on exercise performance. J Int Soc Sports Nutr 2013; 10(1): 15. [http://dx.doi.org/10.1186/1550-2783-10-15] [PMID: 23517650]

[108] Ayaz M, Sadiq A, Junaid M, Ullah F, Subhan F, Ahmed J. Neuroprotective and anti-aging potentials of essential oils from aromatic and medicinal plants. Front Aging Neurosci 2017; 9: 168. [http://dx.doi.org/10.3389/fnagi.2017.00168] [PMID: 28611658]

[109] Wang ZJ, Heinbockel T. Essential oils and their constituents targeting the gabaergic system and sodium channels as treatment of neurological diseases. Molecules 2018; 23(5): 1061. [http://dx.doi.org/10.3390/molecules23051061] [PMID: 29724056]

[110] Barati F, Nasiri A, Akbari N, Sharifzadeh G. The effect of aromatherapy on anxiety in patients. Nephrourol Mon 2016; 8(5): e38347. [http://dx.doi.org/10.5812/numonthly.38347] [PMID: 27878109]

[111] Conrad P, Adams C. The effects of clinical aromatherapy for anxiety and depression in the high risk postpartum woman – A pilot study. Complement Ther Clin Pract 2012; 18(3): 164-8. [http://dx.doi.org/10.1016/j.ctcp.2012.05.002] [PMID: 22789792]

[112] Tang SK, Tse MYM. Aromatherapy: does it help to relieve pain, depression, anxiety, and stress in community-dwelling older persons? BioMed Res Int 2014; 2014: 1-12. [http://dx.doi.org/10.1155/2014/430195] [PMID: 25114901]

[113] Haskins JT. Generalized anxiety disorder. Epidemiology, impact of comorbidity, and natural history. Postgrad Med 1999; 106(6): 3-9. [PMID: 19667498]

[114] Kasper S, Müller WE, Volz HP, Möller HJ, Koch E, Dienel A. Silexan in anxiety disorders: Clinical data and pharmacological background. World J Biol Psychiatry 2018; 19(6): 412-20. [http://dx.doi.org/10.1080/15622975.2017.1331046] [PMID: 28511598]

[115] Bano Z, Ejaz M, Ahmad I. Assessment of prevalence of Anxiety in adult population and development of anxiety scale: A study of 819 patients with anxiety disorder. Pak J Med Sci 2021; 37(2): 472-6. [http://dx.doi.org/10.12669/pjms.37.2.2158] [PMID: 33679934]

[116] Lakhan SE, Sheafer H, Tepper D. The effectiveness of aromatherapy in reducing pain: a systematic review and meta-analysis. Pain Res Treat 2016; 2016: 8158693. [http://dx.doi.org/10.1155/2016/8158693]

[117] Ou MC, Lee YF, Li CC, Wu SK. The effectiveness of essential oils for patients with neck pain: a randomized controlled study. J Altern Complement Med 2014; 20(10): 771-9. [http://dx.doi.org/10.1089/acm.2013.0453] [PMID: 25192562]

[118] Orchard A, van Vuuren S. Commercial essential oils as potential antimicrobials to treat skin diseases. SEvid-Based Complemen Alternat Med2017; 2017: 4517971. [http://dx.doi.org/10.1155/2017/4517971]

[119] Panahi Y, Taghizadeh M, Marzony ET, Sahebkar A. Rosemary oil vs minoxidil 2% for the treatment of androgenetic alopecia: a randomized comparative trial. Skinmed 2015; 13(1): 15-21. [PMID: 25842469]

[120] Guan YS, He Q. Plants consumption and liver health. Evid Based Complement Alternat Med 2015;

2015: 1-10.
[http://dx.doi.org/10.1155/2015/824185] [PMID: 26221179]

[121] Sasannejad P, Saeedi M, Shoeibi A, Gorji A, Abbasi M, Foroughipour M. Lavender essential oil in the treatment of migraine headache: a placebo-controlled clinical trial. Eur Neurol 2012; 67(5): 288-91. [http://dx.doi.org/10.1159/000335249] [PMID: 22517298]

[122] Apaydin EA, Maher AR, Shanman R, *et al.* A systematic review of St. John's wort for major depressive disorder. Syst Rev 2016; 5(1): 148. [http://dx.doi.org/10.1186/s13643-016-0325-2] [PMID: 27589952]

[123] Cipriani A, Furukawa TA, Salanti G, *et al.* Comparative efficacy and acceptability of 21 antidepressant drugs for the acute treatment of adults with major depressive disorder: a systematic review and network meta-analysis. Lancet 2018; 391(10128): 1357-66. [http://dx.doi.org/10.1016/S0140-6736(17)32802-7] [PMID: 29477251]

[124] Sánchez-Vidaña DI, Po KKT, Fung TKH, *et al.* Lavender essential oil ameliorates depression-like behavior and increases neurogenesis and dendritic complexity in rats. Neurosci Lett 2019; 701: 180-92. [http://dx.doi.org/10.1016/j.neulet.2019.02.042] [PMID: 30825591]

[125] Lillehei AS, Halcon LL. A systematic review of the effect of inhaled essential oils on sleep. J Altern Complement Med 2014; 20(6): 441-51. [http://dx.doi.org/10.1089/acm.2013.0311] [PMID: 24720812]

[126] Karadag E, Samancioglu S, Ozden D, Bakir E. Effects of aromatherapy on sleep quality and anxiety of patients. Nurs Crit Care 2017; 22(2): 105-12. [http://dx.doi.org/10.1111/nicc.12198] [PMID: 26211735]

[127] Cino K. Aromatherapy hand massage for older adults with chronic pain living in long-term care. J Holist Nurs 2014; 32(4): 304-13. [http://dx.doi.org/10.1177/0898010114528378] [PMID: 24733781]

[128] Kalemba D, Kunicka A. Antibacterial and antifungal properties of essential oils. Curr Med Chem 2003; 10(10): 813-29. [http://dx.doi.org/10.2174/0929867033457719] [PMID: 12678685]

[129] Lis-Balchin M. Essential oils and 'aromatherapy': their modern role in healing. J R Soc Health 1997; 117(5): 324-9. [http://dx.doi.org/10.1177/146642409711700511] [PMID: 9519666]

CHAPTER 5

Essential Oils Toxicity and Conflicts

Archana Shukla[1,*], **Angel Kushwaha**[2], **Suman Sanju**[3], **Priyanka Spring**[3], **Ashwani Kumar**[4], **Pragati Misra**[5] and **Pradeep Kumar Shukla**[1]

[1] *Department of Biological Sciences, Faculty of Science, Sam Higginbottom University of Agriculture, Technology and Sciences, Prayagraj, Uttar Pradesh, India*

[2] *Department of Molecular and Cellular Engineering, Jacob Institute of Biotechnology and Bioengineering, Sam Higginbottom University of Agriculture, Technology and Sciences, Prayagraj, Uttar Pradesh, India*

[3] *Department of Botany, Abhilashi PG Institute of Science, Mandi, Himanchal Pradesh University, Himanchal Pradesh, India*

[4] *Department of Entomology, Naini Agricultural Institute, Sam Higginbottom University of Agriculture, Technology and Sciences, Prayagraj, Uttar Pradesh, India*

[5] *Centre for Tissue Culture Technology, Jacob Institute of Biotechnology and Bioengineering Sam Higginbottom University of Agriculture Technology and Sciences, Prayagraj Uttar Pradesh, India*

Abstract: The importance of medicinal plants in enhancing people's lives all around the world is undeniable. The primary metabolites of therapeutic plants are essential oils, which are widely used in a variety of businesses since their biological qualities were first identified in mythology. The biological effects of essential oils include insecticidal, antiviral, antibacterial, and antioxidant activities. These distinctive qualities raise their attraction and favourability in several international businesses. They are crucial as scent providers in the cosmetics business and have been employed as food preservatives in the food sector. Surprisingly, some components of essential oils are used in medicine since research has shown that some plant-based essential oils may be able to prevent, delay, or even reverse the growth of cancerous cells, the current focus is on investigating aromatherapy's potential in terms of Essential Oils biological qualities. This chapter's goal is to present a short and in-depth examination of Essential Oils' cytotoxicity, activity, therapeutic and pharmacological potential, and common misunderstandings regarding these issues.

Keywords: Biological properties, Cytotoxicity, Dermal absorption, EO, Misconception, Pharmacological potential, Therapeutic, Treatogenicity.

* **Corresponding author Archana Shukla:** Department of Biological Sciences, Faculty of Science, Sam Higginbottom University of Agriculture, Technology and Sciences, Prayagraj, Uttar Pradesh, India;
E-mail: archana.shukla@shiats.edu.in

Pradeep Kumar Shukla, Ajeet Kumar Srivastav, Deepti Chopra, Shikha Agnihotry, Pragati Misra and Jyoti Singh (Eds.)

1. INTRODUCTION

Essential Oils (EOs) are natural compounds having pharmacological, cosmetic, agrochemical, and nutritional uses that have an extensive history in the pharmaceutical sciences [1]. Aromatherapy and phytotherapy make considerable use of EOs, with some of them acting as anti-anxiety medications [2]. Phytotherapy is the "art and science" of utilizing medicinal plants to cure, prevent, or even threaten illness. Aromatherapy is the sanative use of EOs and is considered a subcategory of phytotherapy. These objects have long been in use and are acknowledged by both traditional and modern medical systems. Although medicinal plants are commonly used to treat central nervous system disorders, preclinical and clinical research is sometimes limited [3].

J. B. Dumas (1800-1844), a renowned French scientist who began his career as a pharmacist, is credited for evaluating stearoptenes and being the first to do systematic research on EOs. His first EO article appeared in Liebig's Annalen der Pharmacie. Turpentine oil appears to be linked to nearly every key discovery in the history of EOs. Turpentine oil was the first EO to be mass-produced in the USA (United States of America) Naturally, there were legitimate reasons for this, such as enormous expanses of pine trees, notably in North and South Carolina, Georgia, and Alabama, and the massive and ever-increasing need for oil, both locally and internationally [4].

Terpenoids are the principal ingredients of EOs, which are lipophilic secondary metabolites obtained from plants. Numerous studies have shown that EOs are neurotoxic, and they paralyze insects before killing them, Such property allows us to consider EO components as natural pesticides. One of the best studied effects of EOs is suppression of acetylcholinesterase (AChE). Nevertheless, EOs only have a minor inhibitory effect on AChE. The positive allosteric regulation of GABA (gamma-aminobutyric acid) receptors is another hypothesized mechanism of action for EOs, which respond to the neurotransmitter (GABArs). Numerous studies show that EOs increases the GABA effect on mammalian receptors. On the other hand, no information is available on the binding of EO components to insect GABArs. EOs also displays an impact on the octopaminergic systems of insects. Recent information indicates that EOs exhibit the ability to elevate the levels of calcium and cyclic adenosine monophosphate (cAMP) in nerve cells. In addition, other EO compounds compete with octopamine for the attention of the receptor. Electrophysiological research on the *Periplaneta americana* has demonstrated parallels in the activities of EO constituents and octopamine. According to this, EOs may have the ability to influence neuronal activity *via* octopamine receptors. EO constituents are ideal intrants for bio-insecticides application due to the vast array of potential targets in the insect nervous system [5].

Bergapten (BPs) or furocoumarin, also known as 5-methoxy psoralen (5-MOP), is a kind of psoralen found in grapefruit juice, citrus EOs, and bergamot EOs [6, 7]. Numerous medicinal plants contain this furanocoumarin derivative, notably belonging to the Rutaceae and Umbelliferae families, such as plum, coriander, parsley, and cardamom [8, 9]. Many research efforts have been carried out to look at the biological consequences of furanocoumarins obtained from using herbal and citrus extracts, including the fact that they serve as antimicrobial, antioxidant, anti-inflammatory agents, necrotic, and antitumor agents [10].The combination of BP's anti-inflammatory and pro-resolution qualities suggests it could be salutary for treating chronic inflammatory illnesses [11]. It has also been demonstrated to have analgesic and anticoagulant characteristics, hepatoprotective quality, and anticonvulsant effects [12 - 14] Additionally, numerous investigations showed that BP inhibits topoisomerase 1, cyclooxygenase (COX), and 5-lipoxygenase (5-LOX) [13, 15] Fig. (**1**).

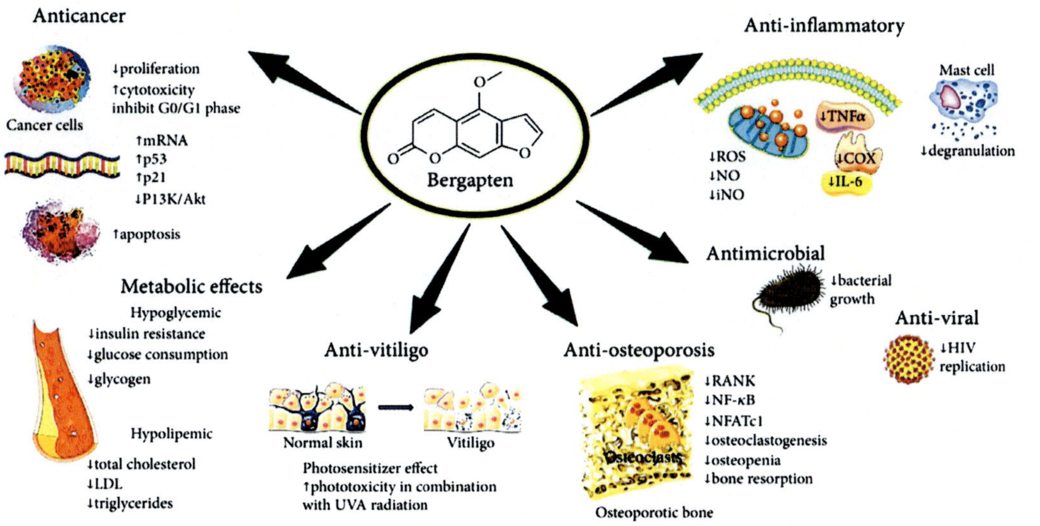

Fig. (1). Representative scheme regarding pharmacological activities and molecular mechanisms of bergapten. ↑: increased; ↓: decreased; mRNA: messenger ribonucleic acid; LDL: low-density lipoprotein; ROS: reactive oxygen species; NO: nitric oxide; iNO: inducible nitric oxide; RANK: receptor activator of nuclear factor-κB; P13k/Akt: phosphoinositide-3-kinase–protein kinase B/Akt; NF-κB: nuclear factor kappa light chain enhancer of activated B cells; NFATc1: nuclear factor-activated T cells c1; TNF-α: tumor necrosis alpha; COX: cyclooxygenase; IL-6: interleukin-6; HIV: human immunodeficiency virus [16].

2. TOXICITY MYTHS ABOUT EOS

Terpenoids, the major ingredients of EOs, are natural, complex compounds obtained from numerous plant organs [17] People have profited from EOs and the unique components that make them up for many centuries. A detailed overview of the historical features of the use of EOs was recently presented [18, 19] Currently, more than 3000 known varieties of EOs are in use. Farmers traditionally use EOs to safeguard the grain that is being stowed. EOs are commonly used to repel insects, particularly mosquitoes [19, 20] The active components in quasi-deterrent products intended for children are EOs derived from lemon and eucalyptus. Furthermore, a number of research show that EOs act on insects as neurotoxic substances in addition to acting as insect repellents [21 - 26].

Environmental issues and food safety worries have gotten a lot of attention lately. The use of antimicrobial compounds in chicken diets has been declining due to the emergence of antimicrobial germs and a decline in consumer acceptance of these feed additives [27]. Therefore, there is a definite need for secure substitute feed additives in the chicken business. Prebiotics, acidifiers, and probiotic microflora have all been researched as potential diet options to replace the use of non-antibiotic growth promoters, including plant-based commercial additions such as aromatic phytoextracts and EOs. According to [28] the swine and poultry sectors have given EOs higher priority. Numerous scientific studies have shown how beneficial EOs are for the growth and health of broilers and other meat-eating animals [29 - 32]. EOs tend to have a larger effect on Gram-positive bacteria over Gram-negative bacteria, owing to differences in the composition of the two types of bacteria's cell walls [33 - 36]. There are no generally accepted criteria for Gram sensitivity.The tested EOs did not appear to cause DNA damage to HEL (12469 human embryonic lung cells) and were not seems to be cytotoxic by the National Cancer Institute's standards. EOs can be regarded as safe for people at relatively low doses and may offer an alternative method to combat microbial contamination. In general, reliable *in vitro* tests are required before recommending the use of EOs for different environmental disinfection procedures [37].

In Ghana and other West African countries, lime fruits and their juice are frequently used in traditional medicine. The juice has been used to treat diabetes, malaria, and other illnesses when combined with neem leaf extract. It serves as an effective deodorant and is also used to enhance the flavor and mask the odor of local alcoholic beverages (Akpeteshie). In the area, lime juice combined with other plant extracts has shown to be a successful treatment for boils. A typical treatment for gonorrhea and other associated disorders is the bark extract. The plant's roots are consumed in Nigeria to relieve headaches and used as a vermifuge, leaves are applied topically to treat eye issues and colds [38]. However, the quest for medicinal and aromatic plants and their phytoconstituents as treatments for a variety of ailments has captured the attention of researchers. Though its precise origin is uncertain, *C. aurantifolia* (also known as lime) is believed to have originated in Southeast Asia or Indonesia before spreading to the Mediterranean region and northern Africa about the year 1000 CE [39].

The American Food and Drug Administration (FDA) states that lime essential oil (EO) is generally recognized as safe (GRAS) and utilized as a flavor enhancer and food component. The perniciousness of lime EO when taken frequently as a prescription medicine or dietary supplement, however, has not been the subject of published investigations. According to [40], it is uncertain if lime EOs used in food or pharmaceuticals are harmful. "Every substance is a poison; there is none that is not a poison," added Paracelsus, the founder of toxicology, "the proper dosage distinguishes a poison from a remedy." Furthermore, nothing is known regarding the harmful effects of Ghanaian lime EO, Since unripe oil has been successful in treating many regional disorders, it is imperative to look into the perniciousness of lime EO from unripe fruits. The majority of EOs, including lime Eos, has not been premeditated at high concentrations internally, even if some of the EOs is considered GRAS [41 - 43].

The possible toxicity and carcinogenicity of EOs depends on how much is consumed and for how long, much like conventionally safe EOs. Natural detoxifying systems in individuals may be able to withstand sporadic low-dose consumption of such possibly carcinogenic compounds without any issues, according to human experience with "traditional" medicines like calamus. The Human Exposure/Rodent Potency Index (HERP) was created to compare the chemicals contained in food, drink, and other items that are carcinogenic in rats to the expected human exposure. It uses data from research done on animals and in labs, including the Ames test. A "TD50" (total dosage) number was used to demonstrate this [44]. The long history of human exposure to naturally occurring chemicals has yet to be properly examined. There is a disparity in the evidence and acuity of possible human carcinogenic hazards from chemical exposures since such testing at the maximum tolerated dose (MTD) frequently might result in persistent cell death and consequent cell regeneration [45].

3. EOS' ORAL TOXICITY, BOTH SHORT-TERM (ACUTE) AND LONG-TERM (CHRONIC)

The criteria of toxicity were assessed using essential oil of *L. organoids*. According to the acute toxicity test results, Wistar rats were given *L. organoids* oil and had normal physiology and behavior in all treatment groups. The lack of evidence of organ damage in the histopathology examinations implies that the *L. organoids* oil had no adverse effects. The *L. organoids* oil application exhibited an inappreciable impact as equated to the control group since the hematological values were within the reference range. Histopathology of the heart, liver, and kidneys showed insignificant dose-dependent variations in the histology between the treated groups and the control. The results concluded that the oral administration of *L. organoid* oil for 2 weeks, at the concentrations used in this study were not hazardous [47, 46].

In the study on the long-term toxicity of *L. organoids*, it was discovered that the average corpuscular volume (MCV), a measure of erythrocyte size, had drastically reduced [46, 47]. The amount of hemoglobin in erythrocytes as measured by mean corpuscular hemoglobin (MCH) decreased as well. These results, which are below those for the control animals and above the reference range for Wistar rats, might indicate an erythropoiesis disruption [48, 49]. Levels of Aspartate Aminotransferase (AST), Alanine Transaminase (ALT), Urea, and Creatinine in the blood did not alter after 2 or 4 weeks of *L. organoids* oil administration. This advocates that consuming *L. organoids* oil did not exhibit any negative impact on these rats. The histology analyses of the kidney, heart, and liver did not cover any evident anomalies (Fig. **2**). Since AST and ALT are considered sensitive indicators of hepatotoxicity and liver damage, and within the reference, range can offer a qualitative evaluation to confirm the damage degree of hepatocytes, the result indicated that no damages in the liver were noticed following treatment with *L. organoids* oil [50]. There were no differences in the features of the feces, urine, or eye color of any of the rats in the control and test groups, indicating that this oil cannot be hepatotoxic when consumed at the observed doses [51].

During an acute toxicity study, Ocimum oil demonstrated a dose-dependent tranquilizing effect on mice and rats; however, in subchronic trials, this effect vanished after one week of daily application [51]. These results suggest that Ocimum oil may have calmative and central nervous system (CNS) depressing effects. EOs from *Lavandula angustifolia* has been found to have similar effects [52]. Calculations revealed that Ocimum oil had LD_{50} values of 0.27g/kg, and 0.43g/kg, and LD_{100} values of 0.59g/kg and 0.74g/kg in mice and rats, respectively, when supplied with intraperitoneal injection. Orally given Ocimum oil was shown to have LD_{50} and LD_{100} values of 1.41 and 2.50 g/kg in mice and 2.29 and 4.07 g/kg in rats, respectively. Despite studies categorizing EOs with comparable LD_{50} values as the least toxic to rats, these numbers designate that the oil exhibits potential hazards according to Lorke's classification [53, 54]. The primary constituent of Ocimum oil, thymol, which has an LD50 of 3.75–5.67 g/kg body weight, is most likely to be on the basis of potential hazards [55]. The Ocimum oil at the recommended amounts produced noticeable languor in the animals as well as dose-dependent gross behavioral impairments with increasing dosage and treatment times. Relaxation, sedation, sleep time, as well as impulsive exploratory and stereotaxic activity, all decreased in a dose-related manner. Previous research into the oil's anti-diarrheal effects revealed that it can decrease gastrointestinal (GIT) motility, possibly *via* stabilizing GIT parasympathetic impulses [56].

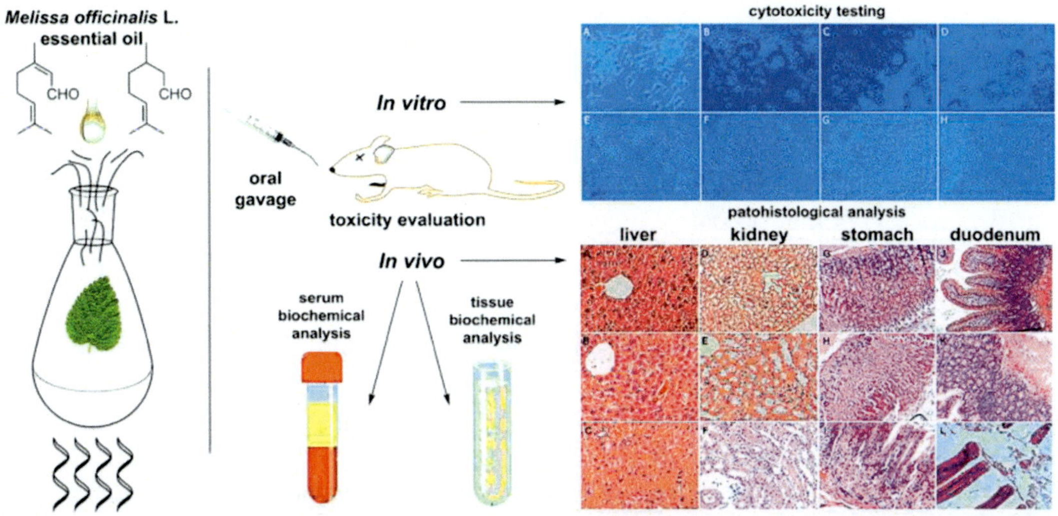

Fig. (2). Oral feeding of *M. officinalis* EO's LD50 (2.57 g/ kg-1) in BALB/c (An albino, laboratory-bred strain mouse) resulted in significant behavioral changes in the mice, liver and kidney functions and also resulted in a reduction in antioxidant capacities in the liver and kidneys and an increase in the rate of lipid peroxidation, indicating that the EO is only potentially toxic [62].

The widely held assumption that all herbal treatments and associated formulations manufactured from natural sources are solely advantageous and entirely safe to use may have detrimental effects on the general public's health [57]. Physicochemical processes including extraction method, hydro distillation, pressing, *etc.* are used to create extracts, the most popular kind of plant preparation. *Melissa officinalis* (Lemon balm), a plant species, is widely distributed throughout Europe due to its soothing, antispasmodic, intestinal, antimicrobial, and antiviral, qualities [58]. There is inadequate data to back up the assertion that *M. Officinalis* has a wide variety of other advantageous properties besides the above-mentioned uses. These comprise the capacity to cure severe gastric, cardiovascular, CNS, and tumor conditions. On occasion, it is even touted as a natural cure-all [58]. It is widely known that psychiatric patients struggling with anxiety, depression, and insomnia utilize dry extracts of *M. officinalis* or other herbal treatments that comprise this taxon and other species [59]. It is uncertain what *M. Officinalis* extract doses work best to provide the whole intended effect while still being safer to use. *M. officinalis* has been listed in the FDA and GRAS, signifying it is safe when taken orally for up to 30 days at dosages normally found in food, according to [58]. Theoretically, it should not be taken by minors, thyroid disease sufferers, pregnant, or breastfeeding women, or when mixed with sedatives .The majority of European Union (EU) members commercially market it as drops, capsules, pills, *etc* [60]. Lemon balm can be supplementary to meals in small amounts, according to the Council of Europe, which recognizes M. officinalis folium as a naturally occurring flavor agent for food in category N_2 [58].

3.1. Dermal Absorption and Detoxification

Aromatherapy with EO has been associated with an improvement in cognitive performance in dementia patients. Active EO constituents must penetrate the skin, pass the blood-brain barrier (BBB), and reach the circulation in order to have a systemic effect [61] (Fig. **3**).

The two layers of skin are the dermis, which is highly vascularized, and the epidermis, which is non-vascular, epidermis' top layer, the stratum corneum, serves as an absorption barrier. Most drugs' rate of cutaneous absorption is controlled by diffusion *via* the stratum corneum. Penetration may increase if chemicals have the potential to damage or partially destroy the stratum corneum. The majority of EOs' natural terpenes have historically been used in transdermal medicine administration methods to promote skin penetration [63]. Terpenes are very small compounds having only three hydrogens, oxygen, and carbon atoms. It has been proposed that terpenes change the stratum corneum's intercellular lipid structure [64].

The most important properties of EOs for skin absorption are explicit molecular shapes, molecule size/surface area, flexibility (type of bonding), connectivity index of the third order, and valence connectivity index of zero order. Molecular flexibility is represented by molecular unsaturation since bond rotation is limited and only one molecular conformation is allowed in the sp2 hybridization state [65]. While valence indices convey details on heteroatoms, high-order molecular connection indices provide data on the size-reliant degree of carbon branching [66]. The zero-order valence index ($0\ \chi$ v), although being a connectivity index, overlooks the molecule's divergent structure and gives information on its heteroatoms, as opposed to higher-order valence indices, which give information on the molecular volume and surface area. As the length and number of branches of the hydrocarbon chains increase, the compounds containing heteroatoms have decreased values of the ($0\ \chi$ v) index in contrast to the values of their hydrocarbon equivalent compounds. Terpenes and terpenoids may be distinguished by a valence index of zero order. The flavonoid groups, ester functional groups, non-aromatic ring, nitrogen, and hydrogen bond acceptors are a few examples of descriptors that are important in the cutaneous permeability hypothesis [61], (Fig. **3**).

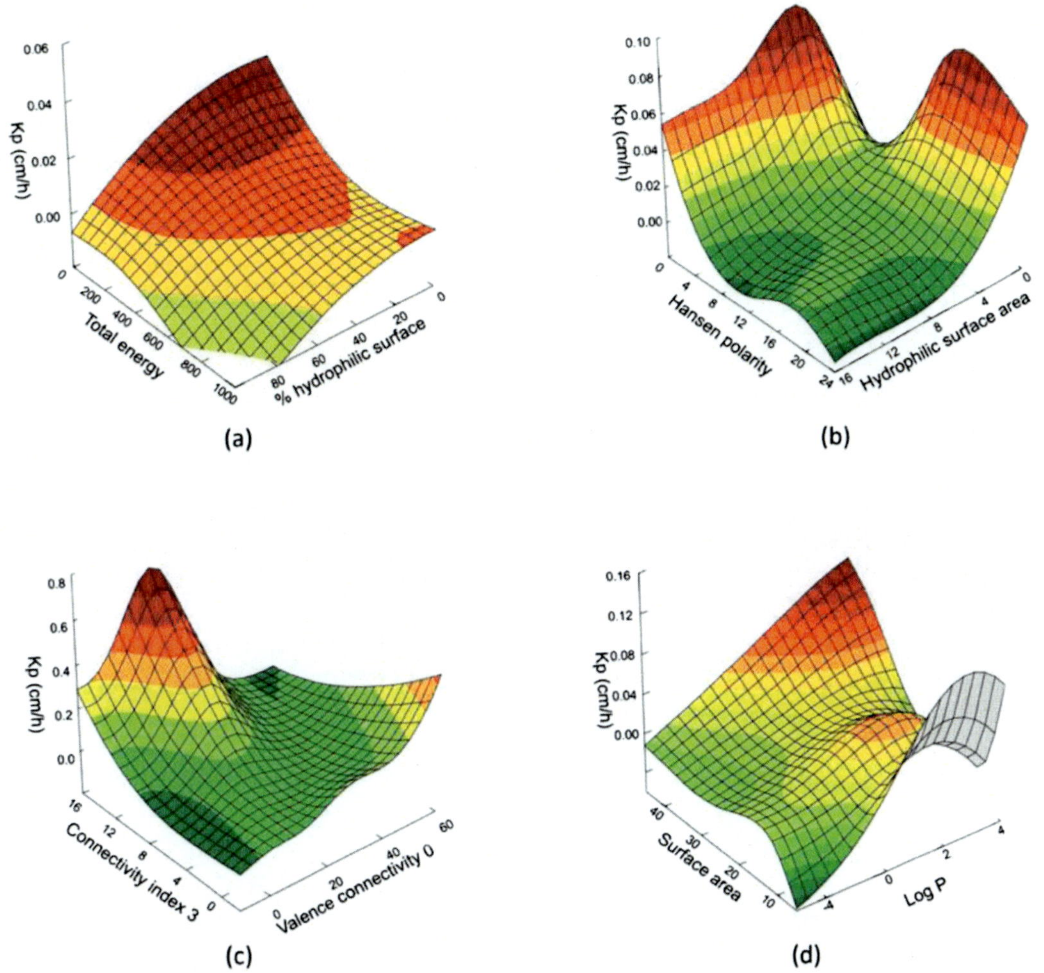

Fig. (3). Response graph of Kp (skin penetration constant) versus selected molecular descriptors [67].

Since cutaneous malignancies are growing more prevalent, many treatment approaches are needed. Even though surgical methods endure the cornerstone of care, efficient tactics are still mandatory to lessen morbidity and mortality. Complementary treatments and the creation of effective chemotherapeutic medications are necessary for the treatment of skin cancer. One such method is to use natural substances' propensity to be operative in cancer treatment and chemoprevention, particularly those originating from floras [68].

3.1.1. EOs and EO Components' Chemo-preventive Efficacy on Tumorigenesis

Cancer has appeared to be the world's most worrisome disease during the past several decades [69]. It is a complex condition that leads to abnormal cells' unchecked invasion and proliferation, which causes tumors to grow (National Cancer Institute, 2013). The study of natural plant products as a feasible source of novel chemical species as anticancer medicines is one of the topics of exploration that is getting plenty of interest. Many plant compounds, classified as diuretics, phenolics, coumarins, flavonoids, and other phytochemicals, have shown incredibly promising anticancer effects in both *in vitro* and *in vivo* studies.

According to reports, over a thousand plants have power full anticancer properties [70]. Camptothecin, podophyllotoxin, lepachol, irinotecan, ellipticine, vincristine, vinblastine, colchicine, etoposide, taxol, and paclitaxel are traditional examples of plant-predicated chemical constituents that are used in various cancer therapies [71]. Pharmaceuticals derived from plants are anticipated to have fewer negative consequences than manufactured drugs. Amongst plant-predicated compounds, EOs from fragrant plants exhibit anticancer properties [72, 73]. Moreover, it has been demonstrated that EOs recuperate the eminence of life for cancer patients by reducing their degree of agony (National Cancer Institute 2013). Skin cancer can be stopped, prevented, or even reversed by several numbers of phytochemicals. Turmeric EO (TEO) pointedly delayed and prevented the expansion of cutaneous papillomas in mice given DMBA (7,12-dimethyl benzene anthracene) and croton oil treatments. TEO's ability to inhibit cytochrome P450 (an enzyme that plays a pivotal role in the detoxification of xenobiotics) was shown in *in vitro* tests [74] (Fig. **4**). By significantly lowering skin papilloma frequency, multiplicity, and TPA (tetradecanoylphorbol acetate) persuaded ornithine decarboxylase (ODC) activity in CD-1 mice after topical administration and pretreatment with the oil, sandalwood oil's chemopreventive properties have been proven [75, 76]. EOs are intricate combinations of compounds that may include alcohols, ethers, aldehydes, esters, ketones, triterpenes, sesquiterpenes, and alcohol [1] majority of these chemical components in EOs are monoterpenes, sesquiterpenes, and their oxygenated derivatives [77, 78], which evaluated the cytotoxic impact of EOs and their main constituents are citral, geraniol, D-limonene, humulene, myrcene, and thymol.

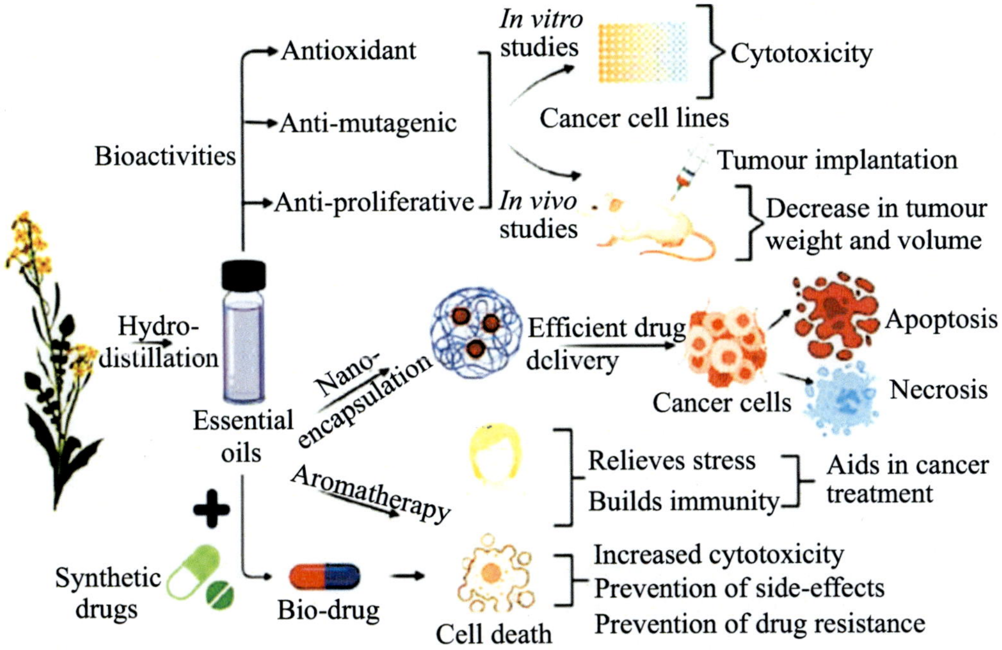

Fig. (4). The potential involvement of EOs as anticancer agents in the treatment of cancer, drug delivery systems, and immune system stimulation [69].

3.1.2. Skin-damaging Consequences of EOs and EO Components

The prevalence of allergic reactions to EOs has grown in the field of dermatology due to the rising usage of EOs application to the skin. The negative effects of EOs include phototoxicity, allergy symptoms, and local inflammation (*e.g.*, turpentine, bergamot oil, and limonene). The quantity, chemical makeup, physical-chemical characteristics, exposure technique, and dosage of EOs and their active components all have a significant impact on their toxicity. Due to EOs' lipid solubility, which makes them easily absorbed through intact skin, the respiratory system, or the gastrointestinal tract, they may be harmful to the entire body. When applied to a substantial region of the skin or wounded skin, excessive use of highly concentrated oils might lead to considerable systemic absorption and upturn the risk of pensive adverse effects, such as convulsions [80]. EOs, which are well-known sensitizers, are implicated in cases of contact dermatitis and allergies, according to previous reports. Among the oils that are light sensitizers include cyminum oil, dill, rosewood oil, lime oil, Ylang, ylang, and eucalyptus oil. Sensitization is probably caused by the EO components D and R- limonene, licareol, citronella, cinnamic alcohol, and Psoralea. There is evidence that some sensitizers interact with different substances. For instance, cinnamaldehyde combined with proteins shows immunomodulatory properties. Citronella's main parameters that cause photosensitization are the exposure area and the drug dosage. Citrus oil is photosensitive (*e.g.*, Citrus bergamia, pomelo, lemon, citrus limon, citrus reticulata, and wild orange). Due to their ultraviolet (UV) sensitivity, these oils cause skin irritation and darkening when exposed to sunshine. For the safe use of EOs, clinical research on skin exposure patterns is required [81, 82], (Fig. **5**).

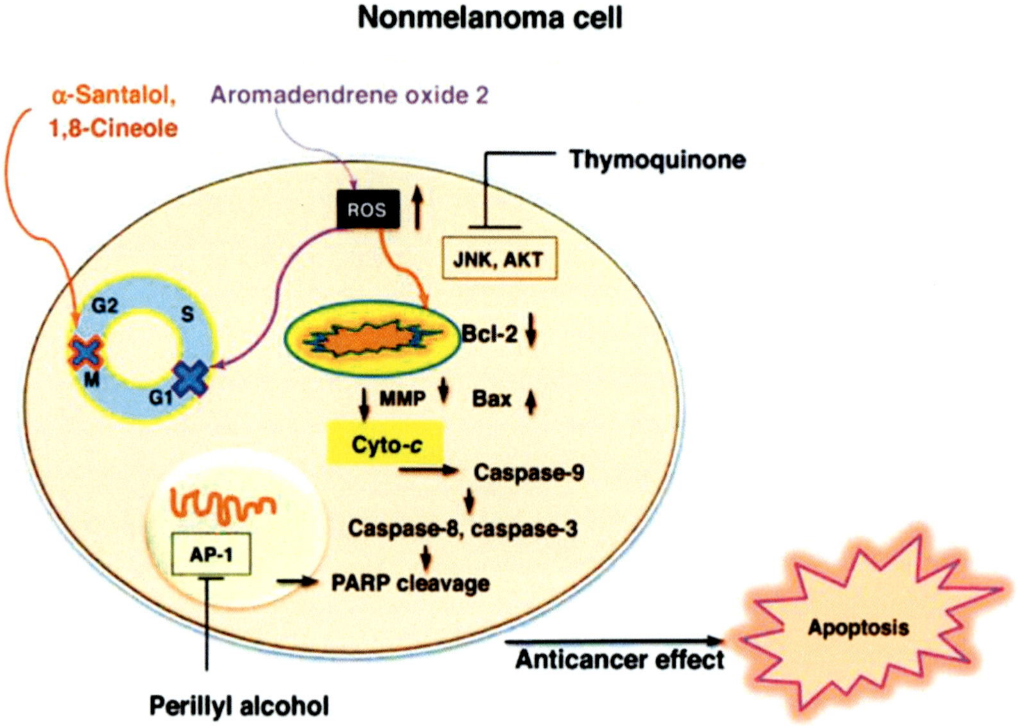

Fig. (5). An illustration of the anti-nonmelanoma action of several EO constituents. Each EO component interacts with a different cellular target, leading to apoptosis, which results in cell death. Colored arrows show the influence that specific EO components have on various cell cycle stages that results in cell cycle arrest, such as the arrest of the G2/M phase by -santalol and 1,8-cineole. G1 phase arrest is brought on by aromadendrene oxide 2, which raises intracellular reactive oxygen species (ROS). The transcription factor activator protein (AP)-1 is inhibited by perillyl alcohol. Thymoquinone prevents the phosphorylation of JNK and Akt pathways [79].

3.2. Inhalation: Absorption and Detoxification

Olfactory aromatherapy, which has been demonstrated to enhance physical and emotional well-being as well as promote serenity, relaxation, and regeneration, was made possible by the inhalation of EOs. Smells that are enjoyable and bring back memories of past odors are intertwined with the decompression of tension. EOs should never be used instead of medical treatment; they are a supplement to it [83]. Inhalation is the most popular technique and the one that is most usually associated with aromatherapy. Patients breathe in smoke from burning oil or water-vaporized oils. The body absorbs the oils through the lungs and nasal mucosa, wherein they reach the bloodstream and influence the patient's cognitive performance. One should smell and inhale the vapors of EO solutions using special equipment that guides the vapor stream into the nostrils and the mouth cavity [84].

Inhaling EOs is a simple, useful, and safe method. A vapor balm, nasal inhaler, light diffusion method, air spray (room deodorizer), or direct inhalation can all be used to apply EOs. Aromatherapy, on the other hand, works wonders by reducing stress, improving mood, regaining equilibrium and well-being, soothing minor aches and pains, and boosting the circulatory, respiratory, and immune systems. Serious illnesses are not, however, treated by it [85]. Aromatherapy benefits immunological, respiratory, and circulatory health as well as relaxation, stress reduction, mood enhancement, balance, well-being, and relief from minor discomfort. According to research [86] when two drops of lavender EO are breathed within half an hour, anxiety is greatly reduced. Additionally, it improves interrupted sleep, sleep duration, sleep quality, sleep latency, and anxiety in those who experience it. Additionally, lavender oil alone was less effective than lavender plus bergamot oil in promoting relaxation, promoting sleep, and lowering tension and anxiety [87]. According to the physiological view, the potential of various odors to directly and organically interact and alter the autonomic or CNS, which affects mood and behavior [88]. Exercise increased people's feelings of well-being, reduced tiredness, and improved their mood. Aroma has a significant emotional impact on exercisers and can increase exercise satisfaction and persistence [89]. The brain's glucose stage receptors are tricked by the aromas of *Vanilla planifolia* and *Citrus reticulata,* which reduces the perception of being “low energy.” To improve a person's mental health and fitness, bergamot EO aromatherapy might be a useful complementary treatment. Additionally, aromatherapy may be used precisely in nursing homes and mental health settings. It has been demonstrated that aromatherapy may reduce dementia-related agitation as well as symptoms linked to stress and tension [90]. Lemon balm aromatherapy EO is a safe and effective therapy to cure clinically relevant anxiety in people with severe dementia, and it also has additional advantages for important quality-of-life indicators [91].

EOs are recognized to relieve and refresh individuals, inhaling and applying them topically are the basic ways of aromatherapy for addressing mental and physical balance [92]. The nasal nerves that connect to the brain are stimulated by these EOs, which then have an effect. These oils exhibit acclaimed antiviral and antimicrobial properties, and numerous other studies and folklore practitioners have suggested they may be useful in treating a variety of ailments, including Alzheimer's [93], cardiovascular disease [94] cancer [95] and pregnancy labor pain, among others [96]. After breathing lavender oil, patients who have undergone bypass grafting have less discomfort. Most patients regarded the perfume of lavender EO to be pleasant, even though the fact that using it to ease anxiety before having an esophagogastroduodenoscopy or colonoscopy did not function [97]. Deep breathing exercises and lavender aromatherapy have a considerable calming impact on preoperative patient anxiety. Nausea is among the most typical postoperative side effects. According to studies, the degree of nausea can be reduced by the same amount by inhaling peppermint EOs at 10% and 30% concentrations. EOs display antibiotic and anti-inflammatory qualities that may aid in the treatment of respiratory tract infections, colds, flu, nasal congestion, and fever [98]. In conjunction with other conventional treatments, aromatherapy with rose hydrosol can help preterm neonates with hypoxia attacks and pulse oximetry [99].

3.2.1. Detoxification

The study of plant EO's antibacterial properties mostly concentrated on how they inhibited bacterial growth, certain mold development traits, and the buildup of toxin-producing mycotoxins. Some EOs include specific compounds that may positively impact the amount of mycotoxins generated by some fungi. The trials showed that when ochratoxin (OTA) awareness reached one thousand or thousand mg/kg, *Aframomum daniellii* (African cardamom) EO'sshould dissolve it, with estimates of decay being 90 -95% or 100%, respectively [100]. Cinnamon oil emulsion droplets may offer a defense against FB1/AFB1 persuading oxidative stress, cytotoxicity, and reproductive/generative damage in male rats. Mycotoxins can be diminished by plant EOs, opening up new opportunities to lessen the harm they do to both humans and animals. Nevertheless, certain issues still exist. First, further research is required to improve the extraction process since different EO extraction techniques have varying impacts on how mycotoxins degrade. Additionally, the process by which plants EOsdegrade mycotoxins has not been explored, particularly in terms of whether or not the breakdown products are still dangerous [101]. Consumption of Allium species foods, associated with epidemiological studies, showed a lower risk of cancer [102].

3.3. Dermatitis and Sensitization

Contact dermatitis (CD), referred to as dermatitis attributable to outside irritants or allergens, is the most typical occupational skin ailment and is commonly connected with cutaneous contacts at the workplace [103]. Deodorants can result in scent contact dermatitis and frequently bring on the initial signs of fragrance allergy. Occlusion, moieties, hair follicles, and irritation from shaving increase their persistence and skin penetration. The exposure changes depending on the smell, concentration, and application regularity. Deodorants are used by 90 percent of women, 87 percent of men, and 31.5 percent of female teenagers. Scent contents for spray and roll-ons are 3 percent and 5 percent, accordingly [104, 105].The primary purposes of fragrances, which are used in cosmetics and home items, are to produce aromas that are aesthetically acceptable or to cover up offensive ones. They can be created in labs or they might be natural, like EO's [106].

Fragrances are found in absorbent hygiene items including sanitary pads, pantyliners, and tampons (Dipentene, licareol, citronellal, geranyl, 7-hydroxycitronellal, hexyl cinnamaldehyde, and benzyl salicylate) have scent content more than 10 g/g [107]. *M. Pereira* can be found in over-the-counter diaper products. When used on moist occluded regions, these products have a significant risk of sensitization [108]. EOs are fragrant chemicals that are frequently obtained from plants but very seldom from animals. Some might also be created synthetically with petrolatum and coal. Evaporation, soaking, solvent, and carbon dioxide separation, and enfleurage are a few extraction techniques. A large portion of them is hydrocarbons, such as Dipentene, licareol, citronellal, geranyl, 7-hydroxycitronellal, and hexyl cinnamaldehyde, as well as other organic substances like aromatic hydrocarbons, aliphatics alicyclic compounds, and heterocyclics [109].

Topical traditional Chinese medicine makes use of EOs and fragrances such as camphor, Cinnamomum oil, olive oil, chamomile oil, citrus oil, Lavandula oil, cajeput oil, wintergreen oil, mastic, myrrh, bone setter's herbs, and menthol. Tiger Balm red N® has been linked to cases of contact dermatitis in patients who evince allergies to cinnamyl alcohol, fragrance mix (FM), *Cananga odorata*, and *M. Pereira* oil [110]. Chronic poisoning symptoms might appear after repeated low-dose exposure to Sabina EO. The use of plant EOs in livestock farming is still relatively new. Future methods of livestock farming may substitute plant EOs for medications to improve intestinal health, reduce feed mildew, and accelerate animal growth. The diverse applications of plant EOs in animal production necessitate further study [111].

Primary sensitization and subsequent allergic response are required for allergic contact dermatitis (ACD), a delayed type IV hypersensitivity condition. People with a weakened natural skin barrier, such as those with atopic dermatitis, often known as "eczema," and those who frequently come into contact with allergens are more likely to develop ACD. Aromatherapists and masseuses regularly employ EOs in their work [112]. An allergic reaction normally occurs 2-3 days after being exposed to the allergen. The production of cytokines by CD4+ T cells, which recognize an antigen on the surface of the skin, activates the immune system. The most prevalent CD symptoms include skin redness, itchy sores, and dry, scaly skin. These symptoms can appear and affect anywhere on the body, however, they typically appear on the hands and face. Atopic dermatitis history patients are more prone to exposure to sensitive chemicals due to increased sensitivity and allergic response. The direct application of oils, the use of products for personal hygiene infused with EOs, or the dispersion of oils are the causes of airborne CD [113].

The Pre-Emptive Avoidance Strategy research and the Danish Contact Dermatitis Group (2012–2016) examined and contrasted major allergens regularly found in adolescents were nickel (Ni), cobalt (Co), neomycin, Myroxylonpereirae, FM I, FM II, methylisothiazolinone (MCI)/methylchloroisothiazolinone, methanol, and lanolin. One study found that all ages with suspected ACD received similar percentages of affirmative responses, accenting the need for patch testing [114]. Four people were reported to have experienced allergic contact cheilitis (lip inflammation) after coming into contact with the peppermint oil included in lip balm, according to a case study both the patient's lips and the surrounding skin are inflamed [115].Peppermint EOs are used in food, personal care products, aesthetics, and pharmaceuticals because of their flavoring and scenting abilities. Peppermint oil contains more than 30 recognized chemicals, including large quantities of menthone (30%), menthol (35–60%), menthyl acetate, pulegone, limonene, and eucalyptol. In people with eczema or conditions of the oral mucosa, it has been demonstrated to cause ACD [116].

3.4. Photosensitization and Phototoxicity of EOs

When some of the chemical components in EOs absorb light, altering their molecular structure and leading to negative effects including skin allergy. This condition is known as photosensitization. Psoralens, commonly referred to as furanocoumarins, are a class of phototoxic compounds that can elicit phototoxic reactions, which manifest as erythema and blister formation, after having an initial photosensitizing effect [117] which are mostly present in citrus, marigold, and parsley EOs. Phototoxicity is caused by the most common chemicals, bergapten and psoralen [118 - 120]. To treat vitiligo, furanocoumarins are used sparingly and in therapeutic doses. After the first formation of erythema, a distinctive coloring happens. Other simpler coumarin derivatives, such as hydrangine, herniarin, and 6,7-dihydroxy coumarin, have the function of sunscreen because they absorb UV rays between 280 and 315 nm. Citrus oils, particularly those prepared by distillation, including bergapten (BP) oil, have been demonstrated to have phototoxic or photosensitizing activity. When the skin is exposed to sunlight after the application of Eau de Cologne (a kind of fragrance), the skin turns red (photodermatitis pigmentary). Some Apiaceae (angel, parsley) family oils, especially those from Giant hogweed (*Heracleum mantegazzianum*), can have light irritation effects [121, 122].

Several experimental models, including lab animals, green algae, fungi, and cultured human skin systems, have been used in studies to examine the phototoxic potential of furanocoumarins [123]. The phototoxic effects of BP oil on guinea pig skin exposed to monochromatic UV light were examined [124]. To demonstrate the photosensitizing effects of BP oil, the group of sunburnt cells (SBCs) in the interfollicular epidermis was significantly enhanced when the skin was exposed to UVA radiation, and BP oil, but not after UVA alone. In a different experiment, the photoaddition of BP to DNA resulted in a phototoxic reaction, which was then followed by an improvement in the pigmentation of human skin, shielding the epidermal cell DNA from further damage [125]. The phototoxic potential of oxypeucedanin, an active ingredient in EOs belonging to the Rutaceae family, is just one-fourth of the BP oil. It is possible to cure skin diseases, including vitiligo and psoriasis, by utilizing BP oils in conjunction with UVA radiation. The principal components of *Brosimum gaudichaudii's* crude extract, psoralen, and BP, which are frequently used in vitiligo photochemotherapy, were investigated for their electrochemical activity [126]. The research showed that BP, but not psoralen, exhibits electro-activity related to electron transfer pathways that may change the DNA of epidermal cells, therefore, decreasing skin regeneration and inflammation.

Volatile oils' phototoxic qualities are related to their constituents, the majority of which share similarities with the constituents of other species but in varying proportions. Eucalyptol and -pinene have been found as the major components of myrtle EO [127 - 130]. The main ingredients of myrtle leaf oil were found to include linalool, citronellal-pinene, and myrtenyl acetate [131]. Citrus plants' phototoxic activity is mostly caused by the plentiful selinene, pinene, limonene, sabinene, and myrcene that are present in citrus plants [132].

3.5. Commonest Allergenic EOs and Components

Among the 20 thousand herbal remedies thought to be available in the US, research suggests that ginkgo and garlic are beneficial. This scientific information is occasionally undermined by poor technique, erroneous end measurements, conflicting findings, and a lack of thorough examination of the effectiveness of medicinal herbs [133]. Although present in variable concentrations and formulations, the medicinal plants employed in various topical and beauty treatments have unknown therapeutic qualities [134]. The majority of herbal remedies also come with a broad list OF side effects, being allergic contact dermatitis the most common. In addition, it is important to evaluate the possibility of irritating CD, contact urticaria, photosensitization, phototoxic reactions, airborne dermatitis, drug interactions, and poisoning [134 - 137]. Aloe, calendula, jasmine, propolis, tea tree oil, and marigold are all frequently utilized by different industries but are also known to cause allergies and irritants [134,138,139]. Women were thought to be more prone than men to have unpleasant cutaneous reactions while using topical herbal medications, with 6.22% of users reporting such reactions, according to a study from the University of Ferrara in Italy. The possibility of unfavorable reactions to herbal remedies depends on several factors, including age, skin integrity, application method, and oil content. EOs is an illustration of a plant employed in the industry; these oils have repeatedly been connected to ACD and photosensitization when applied topically, in addition to perfumes and cosmetics [135, 140, 141]. The Faculty of Dermatology at the University of Gottingen in Germany did a retrospective study and found that 638 (4.06%) of the 15,683 patients tested with at least one EO responded favorably. Patch testing findings for ylang-ylang oil were the most commonly positive among the studied EOs, followed by those for lemongrass, jasmine, pure rosewood, and clove oil [142] The psoralens, which include 5-methoxy psoralen, BP, bergamottin, 4,5,8-trimethylpsoralen (TMP), and methoxsalen are known for their capacity to produce photosensitization, is thought to be the reason for the photosensitizing effect experienced with EOs [136, 143] .EOs have been related to ACD in several occupational groups, although it is difficult to pinpoint the precise sensitizing component because of the diverse composition and concentrations of the oil [141] .Additionally, the complex interactions between the constituents of EOs frequently have what is known as a “quenching effect,” which lessens the sensitization potential of a single constituent when added to EOs concoctions [140] Several herbal treatments, predominantly Chinese herbal balms, have been discovered to regularly include corticosteroids without prescription in addition to the numerous risks that come with taking them [136].A significant quantity of corticosteroids was added to 24% of the samples in a thorough analysis of the ingredients in Chinese herbal remedies [144] The two most typical adulterants are dexamethasone and clobetasol propionate [135]. Using skin-lightening cosmetics, cases of mercury exposure and poisoning have also happened. Unfortunately, US patients may still get mercury and mercury salts on the global market even if their use in cosmetic products is prohibited in the US [145].

Generally, consuming many typical EOs might make you feel nauseous or give you diarrhea while also burning your tongue and throat. An extreme dosage may be followed by lethargy, ataxia, coma, agitation, and spasms [146]. EO substances included in foods like cinnamon may cause contact gingivitis, lesions that resemble lichen planus, or a bullous stomachache. Furthermore, foods that have fragrance allergens, like terpenes in citrus oil, can cause allergic dermatitis through skin contact. Irritation of the gastrointestinal mucosa is the main disadvantage of using EOs orally as it is generally more susceptible to damage than the skin. Because the irritation is concentration-reliant, EOs must be thoroughly disseminated or dissolved in the opposite vehicle prior to consumption. It is advocated to consume EOs as capsules, alcoholic beverages, or a lipophilic medium like vegetable oil while observing that compounds with high viscosity, including vegetable oils, have been reported to cause gastrointestinal absorption delays. The European Commission reported 29 allergen components in EOs arc tcrpcncs, limonene, estragole, phenylacetaldehyde, methyl octanoate, citronellol, geraniol, benzyl alcohol, neral, and geranial, as well as isomethyl octanoate, methyl eugenol, and hydroxy citronellal [147].

3.6. Abortifacient and Teratogenic Oils

During the female reproductive cycle, the uterus, ovaries, breast, and hormone levels all go through a series of incredibly complex changes. Several molecular mechanisms, metabolic circuits, and enzymes regulate and control the blood levels of reproductive hormones. During the reproductive cycle, these endogenous hormones modulate implantation preparation and milk production [148, 149]. Some expectant mothers opt to treat pregnancy-related symptoms (stomach pain, uneasiness, vomiting, indigestion, *etc.*) with herbal supplements, or EOs rather than with conventional drugs out of concern that doing so may harm the unborn child [150, 151]. Some plants are beneficial during pregnancy, delivery, and the postnatal period, and many can improve female reproductive function [152, 153]. Many oils have the GRAS classification, just as how EOs are frequently safe. However, it is highly controversial whether or not women should use herbs and EOs while pregnant. It's crucial to remember that the therapeutic and medicinal uses of EOs are influenced by their unique composition and the possible risk of a single or combination. Some plant EOs have a wide range of compositions and are extremely changeable, which can lead to a variety of EO chemotypes, some of which may be harmful to the development of the baby in pregnant women. It is widely acknowledged that emmenagogic plants EOs are dangerous or detrimental during pregnancy since they can cause miscarriage and menstrual bleeding. However, it's not always the case. It's possible that the oils don't operate in the same way as the whole plant. These oils can unquestionably promote menstruation; however, no indication utilizing them in aromatherapy quantities will result in abortion. For instance, the whole rue, tansy, pennyroyal, and savin plants can result in miscarriage and their oils were classified as abortifacient oils [154]. These oils haven't yet resulted in fetal death or had any noticeable effects on an isolated human uterus' uterine muscles [155 - 157].

Spanish sage (*Salvia lavandulifolia*) is a Labiatae species found in Spain and other countries in the Mediterranean region. It can grow in the wild or in cultivation [158, 159]. There are several subspecies of Spanish sage identified [160].The plant's pleasant aroma is derived from EOs extracted from leaves and flowers [158, 161]. *Salvia lavandulifolia* leaves have been used for a long time in traditional folk medicine and as a spice in Spain as a choleretic, antibacterial, abrasive, cicatrizing, and diabetic remedy [162]. Their anti-spasmodic was established in isolated organs [163, 164]. Additionally, the factory works in the cosmetics industry [158, 159, 165, 166]. Savin (*Juniperus sabina*) and *Plectranthus fruticosus* (Labiatae) are two additional EOs that contain quite high quantities (50%) of the terpenoid compound sabinyl acetate [167 - 169]. Savin is commonly thought to have an abortifacient effect [170 - 175] and it was suggested that the major ingredient Sabinal acetate was the cause of this activity. In a study done in identical experimental conditions, it was discovered that the *Plectranthus fruticosus* EOs also had some abortifacient properties, that were also blamed for embryotoxicity, which led to lesions including severe eye damage, including anophthalmia and mono-or bilateral microphthalmia., which were again probably brought on by the presence of Sabinal acetate [176, 177].

3.7. Genotoxicity of EOs

The majorities of EOs is safe and have no adverse side effects when used appropriately [178]. The most important aspect of safety is the EO dosage. EOs have shown little toxicity and effective anticancer properties in both *in vitro* and animal studies [179, 180]. While, it has also been shown that several have detrimental effects on the body when used in large doses [181]. It is demonstrated that, only at higher concentrations, the EOs exhibit a cytotoxic effect on HEL cells in an *in vitro* environment. A 24-hour treatment with a particular EO lowered the viability of HEL cells, however, the effect was concentration-dependent. It may be due to differences in cell sensitivity because the cytotoxic impact of EOs was seen in a diversity of cell lines, including the human hepatocarcinoma cell line (HepG2), human keratinocytes (HaCaT), and human melanoma cell line (HMB-2). In accordance with the standards set by the National Cancer Institute [182] only organic compounds having an EC50 (20 g/mL) are regarded as cytotoxic. Turmeric EO (TEO) has to go through more extensive testing for its efficiency and safety as a result of the growing demand for its purported therapeutic applications. According to a computer model of toxicity, many TEO components are safe to consume [183] The primary component of TEO, turmerone, was discovered by GC/MS, and its bioavailability was determined to be 13%. The research was done to investigate the safety of TEO at various doses for 13 weeks, assessing acute, subchronic, and genotoxicity [184, 185]. TEO, which varies from oleoresin in its composition, has not had its toxicity properly evaluated, according to a study of the literature. 13 weeks of TEO administration, there were no discernible differences between the treated groups and the control group in terms of general behavior, body weight, and food and water intake of rats. Oral administration of TEO did not affect the growth and physiology of rats at a dose of 5g/kg. [186].

One of the most subtle indicators to evaluate the toxicity of medications in both people and animals is the hematopoietic system [187]. Any liver damage leads to increased ALT and AST values. Furthermore, it is believed that the presence of ALT in the serum serves as a warning signal for liver and cell damage [187, 188]. Since increases in creatinine indicate clear damage to the functional nephrons, they are regarded as a trustworthy marker for renal function [187, 189]. In mice treated with TEO, ALT, and AST, urea, creatinine, serum bilirubin, and total protein levels did not alter substantially from those of untreated mice. These results advocate that TEO exhibits no adverse effect on renal and liver function. The current analysis also examined serum electrolytes and cholesterol levels, LDL/VLDL (low-density lipoprotein/very low-density lipoprotein), proving that TEO did not affect the rats' lipid and carbohydrate metabolism. When the treated group of rats' organs were inspected under a microscope, the TEO's safety was established. Because terpenoids are present, TEO is believed to have significant antioxidant activity and has been demonstrated to have chemo-preventive effects [184, 190]. TEO is reportedly able to stop human oral submucosa fibrosis [191]. Additionally, significant anti-arthritic, anti-inflammatory, and anti-nociceptive benefits are reported [184, 192, 193]. It has been shown that TEO enhances curcumin (BCM-95) bioavailability in humans and clinical studies are being done to determine the safety and effectiveness of using BCM-95 to treat oral premalignant lesions and cervical cancer [194, 195]. These outcomes conclude that TEO has an enormous therapeutic potential that has not yet been properly appreciated.

3.8. Neurotoxicity of EOs

People have used aromatherapy and other EOs to accomplish their calming and uplifting effects for millennia [196]. Clinical research suggests that EOs like lavender, EO (LEO), and coriander when breathed or administered topically, impact the brain and central nervous system. In complementary and alternative medicine (CAM), aromatherapy employs plant EOs to influence the patient's state of mind or physical well-being [3, 93]. Since EOs has a substantial impact on neurotransmitter pathways, notably the serotonin system, it has also recently been proposed that they may have antidepressant benefits [197]. There has been limited research conducted on the pharmacological consequences of EOs to comprehend the molecular mechanisms behind the CNS impacts of a variety of neurological and psychiatric conditions, such as Parkinson's disease, epilepsy, and early damage. By modifying the N-methyl-D-aspartate (NMDA) receptors, LEO may have calming effects [198 - 206].

Alzheimer's disease (AD), which has emerged as one of the most common neurodegenerative disorders, is characterized by slow cognitive decline and memory loss [207]. The abnormal synthesis of amyloid peptide (AP), which is created proteolytically from the processing of amyloid precursor protein (APP), and the hyperphosphorylation of Tau protein are critical aspects of AD pathogenesis [208]. Conferring to the amyloid cascade theory, the A1-42 peptide, the principal component of intracellular and extracellular aggregates, is the primary catalyst for the neurodegeneration seen in AD. In particular, the intracellular accumulation and aggregation of A1-42 oligomers affect cell survival, synapse function, and brain network activity [209]. Molecular damage regulated by A1-42 oligomers, *viz.* Caspase-3 activation, a key enzyme in apoptosis, and an upsurge in intracellular reactive oxygen species concentration (ROS) can be controlled by LEO, as well as coriander at a concentration of 10 g/mL. These findings support prior *in vivo* studies showing that LEO protects against AD neurodegeneration and that coriander EO possesses antioxidant and antiapoptotic characteristics, which have the potential to provide neuroprotection [210, 211]. In this competition, coriander EO exhibited *in vitro* antioxidant activity due to its ability to absorb and neutralize hydrogen peroxide (H2O2), which was associated with its chemical constituents, such as monoterpene hydrocarbons [212]. The 2,2-diphenyl-1-picrylhydrazyl radical was stabilized by linalool in the same research, suggesting that it may have antiradical characteristics [212]. Furthermore, additional chemical constituents of lavender and coriander EOs may have unique positive benefits or cooperate with linalool to offset A1-42's neurotoxic effects. Although cells treated with A1-42 oligomers alone or in combination with lavender, coriander, and linalool showed a similar improvement in cell viability, it is conceivable that the processes behind this advantageous outcome may vary or be more pronounced for one constituent in comparison to the others. It is challenging, however, to extrapolate from the results of the current study that linalool contributes to the positive effects of lavender and coriander EOs [213]. Due to their ability to inhibit AChE, EOs are well-known for having antioxidant properties [214, 215]. It is well known that using EOs such as chamomile, lavender, and rosemary during aromatherapy might help AD patients behave less agitatedly. EOs mostly consists of terpenes and terpenoids, which are terpenes' oxygenated derivatives. AChE has been demonstrated to be inhibited *in vitro* by a few monoterpenoids found in the EOs of, thyme, Spanish sage, and lavender [216 - 218]. The positive effects of taking EOs therapeutically have been witnessed in several investigations, including clinical trials with AD demented persons.

Another explanation for other EOs' anti-agitational actions is that it has been demonstrated that they change brain neurotransmitters. For instance, it has been shown that ylang-ylang (*Cananga odorata*) EO had calming effects on male rats by reducing dopamine levels in the striatum and increasing serotonin levels in the brain [219]. Unexpectedly, linalool is one of the main constituents of EO. The antidepressant-like actions of the EO extracted from *Eugenia uniflora* in animal models including the modulatory and adrenal systems [220]. It has been demonstrated that the herbal sedative *M.officinalis* (lemon balm) EO has a depressing effect on neurotransmission [221]. Similar findings with anxiolytics that are mediated by 5-HT1 receptors are shown with bitter orange EO [222]. These results lend credence to the idea that EOs' calming effects on the neurological system involve the neurobiological system. The elements of EO decrease the action of acetylcholinesterase (AChE), which is the key enzyme in neural circuits and neurological connections in insects and humans as well, shown to be less active when exposed to EOs [223 - 225]. AChE can be a specific target for recently discovered insecticides (harmless for non-target vertebrates) as insect AChE varies from mammalian AChE by a single residue, identified as the insect-specific cysteine residue [226, 227 - 230] EOs are considered a possible source of pesticides due to their capacity to change the AChE activity of insects [231 - 235] Chamomile (*Chamaemelum nobile*), *Eriocephalus punctulatus, Ormenis multicaulis, Santolina chamaecyparissus, Cyclotrichium niveum*, Thymus praecox subspecies. caucasicus, Echinacea purpurea, Echinacea pallida, and Sal are among the plants whose EOs have been shown to inhibit AChE [231 - 235]. 48 of the 73 chemicals examined have anti-AChE activity. The investigation's main focus, however, was on isolated AChE from certain mammal species and the electric eel (Electrophorus electricus). The AChE was evaluated on 28 compounds, and 23 of them inhibited the enzyme. The three most potent compounds were 11, eucalyptol, cis-ocimene, and nloticini, phellandrene, -limonene, carvacrol, -menthol, and –menthone [230, 236 - 241]. The bulk of the EO constituents demonstrated anti-AChE activity in mM doses. Only one specific study provided evidence that the carvacrol component of EOs inhibits AChE in μM concentration [239] (Fig. **6**).

3.9. Possible Hazards of Novel EOs and Plant Extracts

Plant-based volatile oils (VOs) called Aetherolea, which are falsely referred to as “EOs,” are used in aromatherapy or phytotherapy to alle*via*te sickness. Various plant parts, including flowers, leaves, roots, bark, seeds, *etc*, are used to create EOs [243]. The over 3000 different EOs that are currently recognized are composed of a composite blend of both volatile and non-volatile compounds, including hydrocarbons, quinones, amines, aldehydes, acids, esters, alcohols, ketones, epoxides, and sulfides [244]. VOs, which are byproducts of plant secondary metabolism, are released by specialized cells. VOs are stored as combustible aroma liquids in secretory channels or sacks inside the plant or outside the plant (in glandular brushes or papillae) [245]. EOs have long been used in the food, feed, cosmetic, and pharmaceutical industries due to their antiviral, antibacterial, and antiparasitic properties [1, 243, 246, 247]. The EOs generated from *Eucalyptus globules* (Myrtaceae family) also possess a contact-killing effect against larvae of *Aedes albopictus* and can repel three different species of adult mosquitoes [248, 249].

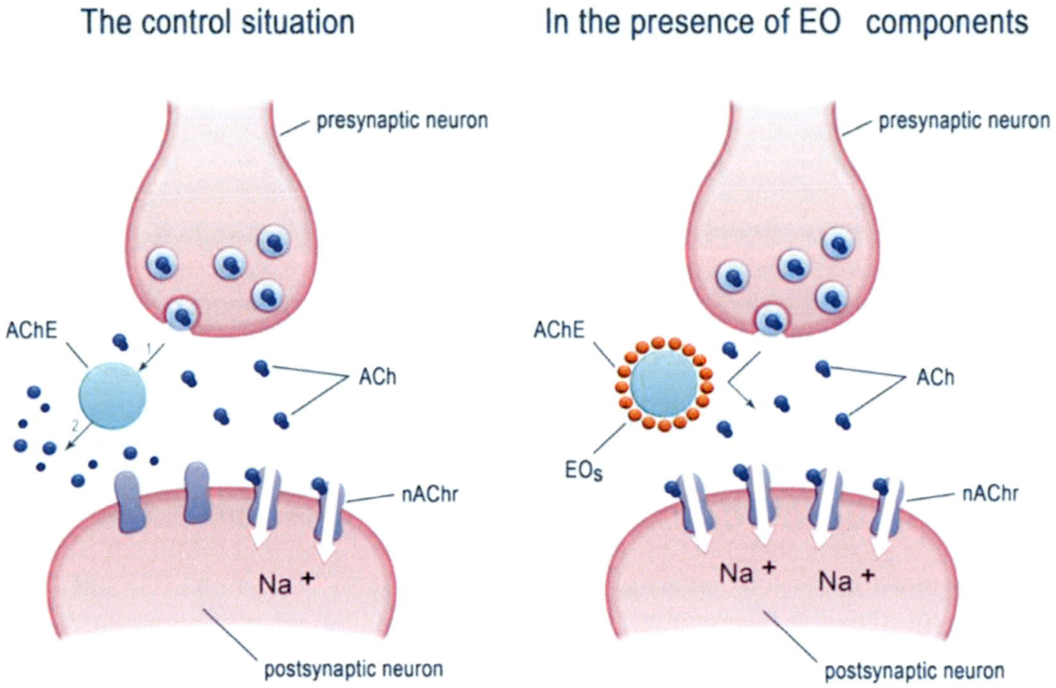

Fig. (6). The EO components inhibit the acetylcholinesterase (AChE) activity. ACh—acetylcholinesterase, nAChr—nicotinic acetylcholine receptors, EOs—essential oil components [242].

High-quality VOs are required for usage in medical applications. Unfortunately, many synthetic or imitation oils don't function as effectively as they ought to or might be harmful to your health. Therefore, it is crucial to look into the sources and producers of volatile oil in great detail. Volatile oils should only be used topically or breathed when pregnant (aromatherapy lamps, partial shower [250]. During pregnancy, it is strictly banned to consume any EOs, aniseed, coriander, fennel, hyssop, basil, juniper, nutmeg, or Spanish lavender. The same principle holds for Thuja and sage oils that have negative effects on the CNS [251]. included highly reactive oxygenated monoterpene ketones, methanol, pinocamphone, thymol, citronellal, pulegone, sabinyl, turpentine, eucalyptus, tansy, fennel, savin, hyssop, pennyroyal, rosemary, sage, thuja, and wormwood EOs were all strong convulsants. These claims' epileptogenic characteristics have been extensively documented and investigated in animal models [252].

4. SAFE EOS AND THEIR TOXICITY

Similar to general concerns regarding EO toxicity, an EO's potential toxicity or carcinogenicity relies on how much is eaten and for how long. Studies and human experience with "traditional" herbs like Calamus demonstrate that human beings' natural detoxification systems are capable of handling the occasional low-dose usage of such possibly carcinogenic compounds without any problems [253].

4.1. Clary Sage

The Lamiaceae family includes *Salvia sclarea* Linn., sometimes referred to as clary sage. The large, hairy, purple-hued green leaves of the perennial shrub Clary sage are the main source of its EOs. It differs from *Salvia officinalis* or common sage as it has a larger leaf size and becomes blue-white in the late summer. Its main components are geranyl, linalool, linalyl acetate, germacrene D, and alpha-terpineol (Price 1993). Linalyl acetate and linalool are recognized as the primary constituents of clary sage oil, while the chemical makeup of clary sage is modified by a variety of ecological, geographical, and environmental circumstances. When a woman is menstruating, giving birth, or going through menopause, clary sage oil is utilized in aromatherapy. Modern clinical studies have validated the effectiveness of Clary sage oil as a pain reliever, antidepressant, and stress reducer in primary dysmenorrhea. Clary sage displays antioxidant, antibacterial, cytotoxic, and anti-inflammatory properties. Additionally, Clary sage oil is well-known safe oil with no side effects. Future research must include a sizable clinical investigation to assess the oral effectiveness of clary sage oil for female illnesses [254].

4.2. Rosemary

Rosemary (*Rosmarinus officinalis* Linn.), belongs to the Lamiaceae family, can reach a height of 90 cm, and has tiny, pale blue blooms in the late spring or early summer. There are three types of it (silver, gold, and green stripe); the green variant is used for its therapeutic qualities. This plant is abundant in volatile oil, resins, tannic acid, and bitter principles. The active ingredients are cineol, unique camphor akin to that found in myrtle bornyl acetate esters. cineol, pinene, and camphene [255]. The literature evaluation confirms that rosemary EO has the potential to be employed as a secure alternative therapy strategy for mood disorders associated with stress [256].

4.3. Lavender

One of the most popular plants in the world is lavender, a member of the Lamiaceae family. Europe, the Middle East, Asia, and North Africa are the main areas where lavender is grown [257]. The genus *Lavandula*comprises over 40 distinct species, hundreds of varieties, and hybrids [258].The most widely cultivated species are *L. latifolia, L. stoechas*, and their hybrids. A lavender plant with narrow leaves, *L. angustifolia*, is frequently used medicinally. In addition to its antimicrobial properties, lavender EO possesses specific biological activity [259]. Even though adequate evidence to acclaim lavender for the short-term therapy of a number of neurological disorders is available, long-term trials and observational studies are essential to determine the safety of long-term usage as well as the overall efficiency in the milieu of treating and managing various conditions. The information at hand points to lavender therapy being generally risk-free short-term treatment. There have been occasional instances of negative outcomes following lavender application [260].

5. SAFETY WARNINGS IN AROMA THERAPY INDUSTRY

Plant EOs is a unique product that may be both beneficial and lethal. A plant's EOs' kind, quantity, receptor, and action time are all closely related to how safe they are. The acute toxicity of *Artemisia annua* and *Artemisia scoparia* by oralpercutaneousinhalation and skin irritation is minimal in mice, quail, bees, Trichogramma, beetles, and red crucian carp. Sabina EO can be used in various concentrations to decrease animal growth and food consumption. High dosages of Sabina EO can have teratogenic effects and alter sperm [249]. The most common negative effects of EOs (particularly containing phenols and aldehydes) can lead to eyes, mucous membrane, and skin problems.. Additionally, it has been asserted that certain EOs, such as Citrus bergamia, which contains furocoumarins, are phototoxic. Contact sensitization is more likely to occur as a consequence of monoterpene oxidation, which usually happens as a result of poor storage conditions [261]. Some substances that might trigger allergic reactions include menthol, hydroxycitronellal, isoeugenol, benzyl salicylate, cinnamaldehyde, coumarin, geraniol, anisyl alcohol, benzyl cinnamaldehyde, citronellal, eugenol, benzyl benzoate, limonene [84].

It is important to do the sensitivity test to avoid allergic reactions. Small quantities of oil blend in a particular carrier should be applied to a place with a potential for high sensitivity and permeability, and any possible reactions should be watched for 24 to 48 hours. If reddening, irritation, or swellings are seen, the tested oils should not be utilized. Note that EOs should not be used directly undiluted because they might have strong, occasionally unpleasant effects. For safety reasons, it's essential to choose the proper oil-solvent ratio (*e.g.*, water or a massage carrier). It is essential to keep on the recommended dosage because exceeding it might be dangerous and worsen adverse effects [85].

CONCLUSION

EOs derived from plants are more dangerous than people realize. Given the increased occurrence of serious skin reactions to topically applied herbal remedies and the lack of scientific data indicating that such natural components are more effective than synthetic ones, the incentives for seeking these products may be misguided. Another source of concern is the difficulty in identifying the active component and, as a result, standardization. This issue might be caused by a genetic, environmental, or harvesting-related plant feature, or it could be caused by differing manufacturing procedures or chemical interactions in the goods. However, the increase in negative responses might be attributed to the lack of standards and controls for plant-based commodities, as well as their rising popularity.

Natural furocoumarin is mostly derived from citrus EOs, including bergamot, and has demonstrated a range of biological effects with potential medicinal applications. In research employing cell lines and animal models, anti-inflammatory, anti-cancer, anti-microbial, hypolipemic, phototoxic, and photochemotherapy properties have been shown. In several of these studies, the mechanisms of action have been attempted to be clarified, and it has been shown that BP can be able to change several signaling pathways, such as nuclear factor(NF), kB, JNK, or PI3K/Akt. The limited clinical trials that have employed this furanocoumarin, meanwhile, have mostly been used to treat non-alcohol fatty liver, control the serum lipid profile, and cure skin disorders. However, there haven't yet been any clinical investigations on its potential anticancer properties. Vitiligo and psoriasis have both been effectively treated with BP and UVA radiation. When BP and UVA radiation was supplied combined rather than separately, a greater therapeutic effect was seen. Additionally, it has been demonstrated in several studies that BP, a crucial aspect of bergamot essence, lowers the levels of glucose and LDL cholesterol. More clinical trials with a large number of participants are needed to establish dosage and treatment guidelines and determine whether the benefits shown in preclinical investigations are transferable to clinical practice.A detailed examination of the hematological, biochemical and histological effects of *L. organoids* oil in animals revealed no apparent changes in an organ or physiological function. These findings imply that L. organoids oil might be effective as a veterinary antimicrobial. Further research on this medicinal plant is required for animal phytotherapy.

REFERENCES

[1] Bakkali F, Averbeck S, Averbeck D, Idaomar M. Biological effects of essential oils – A review. Food Chem Toxicol 2008; 46(2): 446-75.
[http://dx.doi.org/10.1016/j.fct.2007.09.106] [PMID: 17996351]

[2] Setzer William N. Essential oils and anxiolytic aromatherapy. Nat Prod Commun 2009; 4(9): 1934578X0900400928.
[http://dx.doi.org/10.1177/1934578X0900400928]

[3] Wheatley D. Medicinal plants for insomnia: A review of their pharmacology, efficacy and tolerability. J Psychopharmacol 2005; 19(4): 414-21.
[http://dx.doi.org/10.1177/0269881105053309] [PMID: 15982998]

[4] Gray R, Bonner J. An inhibitor of plant growth from the leaves of Encelia farinosa. Am J Bot 1948; 35(1): 52-7.
[http://dx.doi.org/10.1002/j.1537-2197.1948.tb05187.x] [PMID: 18909960]

[5] Jankowska M, Rogalska J, Wyszkowska J, Stankiewicz M. Molecular targets for components of essential oils in the insect nervous system- a review. Molecules 2017; 23(1): 34.
[http://dx.doi.org/10.3390/molecules23010034] [PMID: 29295521]

[6] Bauri AK, Foro S, Nhu Do QN. Crystal structure of bergapten: A photomutagenic and photobiologically active furanocoumarin. Acta Crystallogr E Crystallogr Commun 2016; 72(8): 1194-6.
[http://dx.doi.org/10.1107/S2056989016011221] [PMID: 27536412]

[7] Sicari V. Optimization of the supercritical carbon dioxide separation of bergapten from bergamot essential oil. J AOAC Int 2018; 101(1): 293-7.
[http://dx.doi.org/10.5740/jaoacint.17-0190] [PMID: 28762330]

[8] Liao M, Song G, Cheng X, Diao X, Sun Y, Zhang L. Simultaneous determination of six coumarins in rat plasma and metabolites identification of bergapten *in vitro* and *in vivo*. J Agric Food Chem 2018; 66(18): 4602-13.
[http://dx.doi.org/10.1021/acs.jafc.7b05637] [PMID: 29663811]

[9] Singh G, Singh A, Singh P, Bhatti R. Bergapten ameliorates vincristine-induced peripheral neuropathy by inhibition of inflammatory cytokines and NFκB signaling. ACS Chem Neurosci 2019; 10(6): 3008-17.
[http://dx.doi.org/10.1021/acschemneuro.9b00206] [PMID: 31064179]

[10] Mirzaei SA, Gholamian Dehkordi N, Ghamghami M, Amiri AH, Dalir Abdolahinia E, Elahian F. ABC-transporter blockage mediated by xanthotoxin and bergapten is the major pathway for chemosensitization of multidrug-resistant cancer cells. Toxicol Appl Pharmacol 2017; 337: 22-9.
[http://dx.doi.org/10.1016/j.taap.2017.10.018] [PMID: 29079042]

[11] Yang Y, Zheng K, Mei W, *et al.* Anti-inflammatory and proresolution activities of bergapten isolated from the roots of *Ficus hirta* in an *in vivo* zebrafish model. Biochem Biophys Res Commun 2018; 496(2): 763-9.
[http://dx.doi.org/10.1016/j.bbrc.2018.01.071] [PMID: 29337062]

[12] Łuszczki JJ, Andres-Mach M, Gleńsk M, Skalicka-Woźniak K. Anticonvulsant effects of four linear furanocoumarins, bergapten, imperatorin, oxypeucedanin, and xanthotoxin, in the mouse maximal electroshock-induced seizure model: A comparative study. Pharmacol Rep 2010; 62(6): 1231-6.
[http://dx.doi.org/10.1016/S1734-1140(10)70387-X] [PMID: 21273683]

[13] Azietaku T. Simultaneous determination of bergapten, imperatorin, notopterol, and isoimperatorin in rat plasma by high performance liquid chromatography with fluorescence detection and its application to pharmacokinetic and excretion study after oral administration of Notopterygium incisum extract. Int J Anal Chem 2016.

[14] Yu X-a, Azietaku JT, Li J, *et al.* The pharmacokinetics, bioavailability and excretion of bergapten after

oral and intravenous administration in rats using high performance liquid chromatography with fluorescence detection. Chem Central J 2016; 10(1): 016-212.
[http://dx.doi.org/10.1186/s13065-016-0212-x]

[15] Pattanayak SP, Bose P, Sunita P, Siddique MUM, Lapenna A. Bergapten inhibits liver carcinogenesis by modulating LXR/PI3K/Akt and IDOL/LDLR pathways. Biomed Pharmacother 2018; 108: 297-308.
[http://dx.doi.org/10.1016/j.biopha.2018.08.145] [PMID: 30227322]

[16] Quetglas-Llabrés MM, Quispe C, Herrera-Bravo J, *et al.* Pharmacological Properties of Bergapten: Mechanistic and Therapeutic Aspects. Oxid Med Cell Longev 2022; 2022: 1-10.
[http://dx.doi.org/10.1155/2022/8615242] [PMID: 35509838]

[17] Bassolé IHN, Juliani HR. Essential oils in combination and their antimicrobial properties. Molecules 2012; 17(4): 3989-4006.
[http://dx.doi.org/10.3390/molecules17043989] [PMID: 22469594]

[18] Pavela R. History, presence and perspective of using plant extracts as commercial botanical insecticides and farm products for protection against insects - a review. Plant Prot Sci 2016; 52(4): 229-41.
[http://dx.doi.org/10.17221/31/2016-PPS]

[19] Pavela R, Benelli G. Ethnobotanical knowledge on botanical repellents employed in the African region against mosquito vectors – A review. Exp Parasitol 2016; 167: 103-8.
[http://dx.doi.org/10.1016/j.exppara.2016.05.010] [PMID: 27260568]

[20] Mihajilov-Krstev T, Jovanović B, Jović J, *et al.* Antimicrobial, antioxidative, and insect repellent effects of Artemisia absinthium essential oil. Planta Med 2014; 80(18): 1698-705.
[http://dx.doi.org/10.1055/s-0034-1383182] [PMID: 25317772]

[21] Price DN, Berry MS. Neurophysiological effects of naturally occurring defensive compounds on the freshwater snail Planorbis corneus: Comparison with effects in insects. J Chem Ecol 2008; 34(8): 994-1004.
[http://dx.doi.org/10.1007/s10886-008-9511-6] [PMID: 18597145]

[22] Liu Z, Zhao N, Liu C, Zhou L, Du S. Identification of insecticidal constituents of the essential oil of Curcuma wenyujin rhizomes active against Liposcelis bostrychophila Badonnel. Molecules 2012; 17(10): 12049-60.
[http://dx.doi.org/10.3390/molecules171012049] [PMID: 23085655]

[23] Liu X, Zhou L, Liu Z, Du S. Identification of insecticidal constituents of the essential oil of Acorus calamus rhizomes against Liposcelis bostrychophila Badonnel. Molecules 2013; 18(5): 5684-96.
[http://dx.doi.org/10.3390/molecules18055684] [PMID: 23676474]

[24] Du SS, Yang K, Wang CF, *et al.* Chemical constituents and activities of the essential oil from Myristica fragrans against cigarette beetle Lasioderma serricorne. Chem Biodivers 2014; 11(9): 1449-56.
[http://dx.doi.org/10.1002/cbdv.201400137] [PMID: 25238085]

[25] Wang Y, You CX, Wang CF, *et al.* Chemical constituents and insecticidal activities of the essential oil from Amomum tsaoko against two stored-product insects. J Oleo Sci 2014; 63(10): 1019-26.
[http://dx.doi.org/10.5650/jos.ess14087] [PMID: 25213443]

[26] Zhang WJ, Yang K, You CX, *et al.* Bioactivity of essential oil from Artemisia stolonifera (Maxim.) Komar. and its main compounds against two stored-product insects. J Oleo Sci 2015; 64(3): 299-307.
[http://dx.doi.org/10.5650/jos.ess14187] [PMID: 25757434]

[27] Bozkurt M, Alçiçek A, Çabuk M, Küçükyilmaz K, Çatli AU. Effect of an herbal essential oil mixture on growth, laying traits, and egg hatching characteristics of broiler breeders. Poult Sci 2009; 88(11): 2368-74.
[http://dx.doi.org/10.3382/ps.2009-00048] [PMID: 19834088]

[28] Zeng Z, Zhang S, Wang H, Piao X. Essential oil and aromatic plants as feed additives in non-ruminant nutrition: A review. J Anim Sci Biotechnol 2015; 6(1): 7. [http://dx.doi.org/10.1186/s40104-015-0004-5] [PMID: 25774291]

[29] Botsoglou N, Florou-Paneri P, Botsoglou E, *et al.* The effect of feeding rosemary, oregano, saffron and a-tocopheryl acetate on hen performance and oxidative stability of eggs. S Afr J Anim Sci 2005; 35: 143-51.

[30] Falaki M, Shams Sharagh M, Dastar B, Hashemi SR, Sadeghi Mahoonak AR. Growth performance, carcass characteristics and intestinal microflora of broiler chickens fed diets containing carumcopticum essential oil. Poult Sci J 2016; 4: 37-46.

[31] Khaksar V, Krimpen M, Hashemipour H, Pilevar M. Effects of thyme essential oil on performance, some blood parameters and ileal microflora of Japanese quail. J Poult Sci 2012; 49(2): 106-10. [http://dx.doi.org/10.2141/jpsa.011089]

[32] Ghazanfari S, Moradi MA, Bardzardi MM. Intestinal morphology and microbiology of broiler chicken fed diets containig myrtle (Myrtus communis) essential oil supplementation. Iran J Appl Anim Sci 2014; 4: 549-54.

[33] Ratledge C, Wilkinson SG. An overview of microbial lipids in Microbial Lipids. Academic Press 1988; Vol. 1: pp. 3-22.

[34] Lambert RJW, Skandamis PN, Coote PJ, Nychas GJE. A study of the minimum inhibitory concentration and mode of action of oregano essential oil, thymol and carvacrol. J Appl Microbiol 2001; 91(3): 453-62. [http://dx.doi.org/10.1046/j.1365-2672.2001.01428.x] [PMID: 11556910]

[35] Mith H, Duré R, Delcenserie V, Zhiri A, Daube G, Clinquart A. Antimicrobial activities of commercial essential oils and their components against food borne pathogens and food spoilage bacteria. Food Sci Nutr 2014; 2(4): 403-16. [http://dx.doi.org/10.1002/fsn3.116] [PMID: 25473498]

[36] Fournomiti M, Kimbaris A, Mantzourani I, *et al.* Antimicrobial activity of essential oils of cultivated oregano (Origanum vulgare), sage (Salvia officinalis), and thyme (Thymus vulgaris) against clinical isolates of Escherichia coli, Klebsiella oxytoca, and Klebsiella pneumoniae. Microb Ecol Health Dis 2015; 26: 23289-95. [PMID: 25881620]

[37] Puškárová A, Bučková M, Kraková L, Pangallo D, Kozics K. The antibacterial and antifungal activity of six essential oils and their cyto/genotoxicity to human HEL 12469 cells. Sci Rep 2017; 7(1): 8211. [http://dx.doi.org/10.1038/s41598-017-08673-9] [PMID: 28811611]

[38] Ivine FR. Woody Plants of Ghana. Oxford University Press 1961.

[39] Narang N, Jiraungkoorskul W. Anticancer activity of key lime, Citrus aurantifolia. Pharmacogn Rev 2016; 10: 118-22.

[40] Christina B, Monice F. Safety Assessment of Citrus-derived Ingredients as Used in Cosmetics Cosmetic Ingredient Review. Washington, DC 2013.

[41] Trautmann N. The dose makes the poison or does it? Bioscience 2005.

[42] Frank P, Ottoboni MA. The Dose Makes the Poison: A Plain-Language Guide Toxicology. 3rd ed., New York: John Wiley & Sons, Inc. 2011. [http://dx.doi.org/10.1002/9780470918449]

[43] Wellness Mama Risks and Uses of Essential Oils, what you need to know about safety Wellness Mama. 2017. Available from:https://wellnessmama.com/26519/essential-oilsrisks/

[44] Cuba R. Toxicity myths essential oils and their carcinogenic potential. Int J Aromather 2001; 11(2): 76-83. [http://dx.doi.org/10.1016/S0962-4562(01)80021-7]

[45] Ames BN, Magaw R, Gold LS. Ranking possible carcinogenic hazards. Science 1987; 236(4799): 271-80.
[http://dx.doi.org/10.1126/science.3563506] [PMID: 3563506]

[46] Andrade V. Antimicrobial activity and acute and chronic toxicity of the essential oil of Lippiaoriganoides. Pesqui Vet Bras 2014; 34: 1153-61.
[http://dx.doi.org/10.1590/S0100-736X2014001200002]

[47] Fontenelle ROS, Morais SM, Brito EHS, *et al.* Chemical composition, toxicological aspects and antifungal activity of essential oil from Lippia sidoides Cham. J Antimicrob Chemother 2007; 59(5): 934-40.
[http://dx.doi.org/10.1093/jac/dkm066] [PMID: 17376793]

[48] Dantas JA, Ambiel CR, Cuman RKN, Baroni S, Bersani A, Ciomar A. Valores de referência de algunsparâmetrosfisiológicos de ratos do Biotério Central da UniversidadeEstadual de Maringá, Estado do Paraná. Acta Scient Health Sci 2006; 28: 165-7.

[49] Castello-Branco ACS, Diniz MFFM, Almeida RN, *et al.* Biochemical and hematological parameters of Wistar rat and Swiss mice in the Professor Thomas George Animal Laboratory. Revta Bras. Ciênc Saúde (Porto Alegre) 2011; 15: 209-14.

[50] Martin DW, Mayes PA, Rodwell YW, Harper S. Review of Biochemistry. California: Lange Medical 1981.

[51] Orafidiya LO, Agbani EO, Iwalewa EO, Adelusola KA, Oyedapo OO. Studies on the acute and sub-chronic toxicity of the essential oil of Ocimum gratissimum L. leaf. Phytomedicine 2004; 11(1): 71-6.
[http://dx.doi.org/10.1078/0944-7113-00317] [PMID: 14971724]

[52] Guillemain J, Rousseau A, Delaveau P. [Neurodepressive effects of the essential oil of Lavandula angustifolia Mill]. Ann Pharm Fr 1989; 47(6): 337-43.
[PMID: 2488249]

[53] Von Skramlik E. Über die Giftigkeit und Verträglichkeit von ätherischen Ölen. Pharmazie 1959; 14: 435-45.

[54] Lorke D. A new approach to practical acute toxicity testing. Arch Toxicol 1983; 54(4): 275-87.
[http://dx.doi.org/10.1007/BF01234480] [PMID: 6667118]

[55] Opdyke DLJ. Monographs of fragrance raw materials. Food Cosmet Toxicol 1974; 12(5-6): 703-4.
[http://dx.doi.org/10.1016/0015-6264(74)90242-9] [PMID: 4452542]

[56] Orafidiya OO, Elujoba AA, Iwalewa EO, Okeke IN. Evaluation of anti-diarrhoeal properties of Ocimumgratissimum volatile oil and its activity against enteroaggregative Escherichia coli. Pharm Pharmacol Lett 2000; 10: 9-1.

[57] Radulović NS, Jovanović I, Ilić IR, Randjelović PJ, Stojanović NM, Miltojević AB. Methyl and isopropyl N-methylanthranilates attenuate diclofenac- and ethanol-induced gastric lesions in rats. Life Sci 2013; 93(22): 840-6.
[http://dx.doi.org/10.1016/j.lfs.2013.10.002] [PMID: 24135460]

[58] Ulbricht C, Brendler T, Gruenwald J, *et al.* Lemon balm (Melissa officinalis L.): An evidence-based systematic review by the Natural Standard Research Collaboration. J Herb Pharmacother 2005; 5(4): 71-114.
[http://dx.doi.org/10.1080/J157v05n04_08] [PMID: 16635970]

[59] Stojanović NM, Samardžić L, Randjelović PJ, Radulović NS. Prevalence of self-medication practice with herbal products among non-psychotic psychiatric patients from southeastern Serbia: A cross-sectional study. Saudi Pharm J 2017; 25(6): 884-90.
[http://dx.doi.org/10.1016/j.jsps.2017.02.002] [PMID: 28951674]

[60] Barnes J, Anderson L, Phillipson JD. Herbal Medicines. A guide for healthcare professionals. 2nd ed.., London, Chicago, USA: Pharmaceutical Press 2002.

[61] Agatonovic-Kustrin S, Chloe KYC, Gegechkori V, Morton DW. Models for skin and brain penetration of major components from essential oils used in aromatherapy for dementia patients. J Biomol Struct Dyn 2019.
[PMID: 31204906]

[62] Stojanović NM, Randjelović PJ, Mladenović MZ, *et al.* Toxic essential oils, part VI: Acute oral toxicity of lemon balm (Melissa officinalis L.) essential oil in BALB/c mice. Food Chem Toxicol 2019; 133: 110794.
[http://dx.doi.org/10.1016/j.fct.2019.110794] [PMID: 31473339]

[63] Herman A, Herman AP. Essential oils and their constituents as skin penetration enhancer for transdermal drug delivery: A review. J Pharm Pharmacol 2015; 67(4): 473-85.
[http://dx.doi.org/10.1111/jphp.12334] [PMID: 25557808]

[64] Godwin DA, Michniak BB. Influence of drug lipophilicity on terpenes as transdermal penetration enhancers. Drug Dev Ind Pharm 1999; 25(8): 905-15.
[http://dx.doi.org/10.1081/DDC-100102251] [PMID: 10434134]

[65] Hückel E. QuantentheoretischeBeitrggezumBenzolproblem. I. Die Elekfronenkonfigurafion des Benzols und verwandferVerbindungen. Z Phys 1931; 70: 204-86.

[66] Contrera J, MacLaughlin P, Hall L, Kier L. QSAR modeling of carcinogenic risk using discriminant analysis and topological molecular descriptors. Curr Drug Discov Technol 2005; 2(2): 55-67.
[http://dx.doi.org/10.2174/1570163054064684] [PMID: 16472230]

[67] Agatonovic-Kustrin S, Chloe KYC, Gegechkori V, Morton DW. Models for skin and brain penetration of major components from essential oils used in aromatherapy for dementia patients. J Biomol Struct Dyn 2019.
[PMID: 31204906]

[68] Jung Park E, Pezzuto JM. Botanicals in cancer chemoprevention. Cancer Metastasis Rev 2002; 21(3/4): 231-55.
[http://dx.doi.org/10.1023/A:1021254725842] [PMID: 12549763]

[69] Sharma M, Grewal K, Jandrotia R, Batish DR, Singh HP, Kohli RK. Essential oils as anticancer agents: Potential role in malignancies, drug delivery mechanisms, and immune system enhancement. Biomed Pharmacother 2022; 146: 112514.
[http://dx.doi.org/10.1016/j.biopha.2021.112514] [PMID: 34963087]

[70] Mukherjee PK. Exploring botanicals in Indian system of medicine-regulatory perspectives. Clin Res Regul Aff 2003; 20(3): 249-64.
[http://dx.doi.org/10.1081/CRP-120023840]

[71] Cragg GM, Newman DJ. Plants as a source of anti-cancer agents. J Ethnopharmacol 2005; 100(1-2): 72-9.
[http://dx.doi.org/10.1016/j.jep.2005.05.011] [PMID: 16009521]

[72] Yu JQ, Lei JC, Zhang XQ, *et al.* Anticancer, antioxidant and antimicrobial activities of the essential oil of Lycopus lucidus Turcz. var. hirtus Regel. Food Chem 2011; 126(4): 1593-8.
[http://dx.doi.org/10.1016/j.foodchem.2010.12.027] [PMID: 25213932]

[73] Mitoshi M, Kuriyama I, Nakayama H, *et al.* Effects of essential oils from herbal plants and citrus fruits on DNA polymerase inhibitory, cancer cell growth inhibitory, antiallergic, and antioxidant activities. J Agric Food Chem 2012; 60(45): 11343-50.
[http://dx.doi.org/10.1021/jf303377f] [PMID: 23088772]

[74] Liju VB, Jeena K, Kuttan R. Chemopreventive activity of turmeric essential oil and possible mechanisms of action. Asian Pac J Cancer Prev 2014; 15(16): 6575-80.
[http://dx.doi.org/10.7314/APJCP.2014.15.16.6575] [PMID: 25169490]

[75] Dwivedi C, Abu-Ghazaleh A. Chemopreventive effects of sandalwood oil on skin papillomas in mice. Eur J Cancer Prev 1997; 6(4): 399-401.

[http://dx.doi.org/10.1097/00008469-199708000-00013] [PMID: 9370104]

[76] Dwivedi C, Zhang Y. Sandalwood oil prevents skin tumour development in CD1 mice. Eur J Cancer Prev 1999; 8(5): 449-56. [http://dx.doi.org/10.1097/00008469-199910000-00011] [PMID: 10548401]

[77] Carson C. Melaleuca alternifolia (tea tree) oil: A review of antimicrobial and other medicinal properties. Clin Microbiol Rev 2006; 19: 50-62.

[78] Gautam N, Mantha AK, Mittal S. Essential oils and their constituents as anticancer agents: A mechanistic view. BioMed Res Int 2014; 2014: 1-23. [http://dx.doi.org/10.1155/2014/154106] [PMID: 25003106]

[79] Pavithra PS, Mehta A, Verma RS. Essential oils: from prevention to treatment of skin cancer. Drug Discov Today 2019; 24(2): 644-55. [http://dx.doi.org/10.1016/j.drudis.2018.11.020] [PMID: 30508640]

[80] Bilia AR, Guccione C, Isacchi B, Righeschi C, Firenzuoli F, Bergonzi MC. Essential oils loaded in nanosystems: A developing strategy for a successful therapeutic approach. Evid Based Complement Alternat Med 2014; 2014: 1-14. [http://dx.doi.org/10.1155/2014/651593] [PMID: 24971152]

[81] Lis-Balchin M, Ed. Aromatherapy Science: A Guide for Healthcare Professionals. Pharmaceutical press 2006.

[82] Vangipuram R, Mask-Bull L, Kim SJ. Cutaneous implications of essential oils. World Journal of Dermatology 2017; 6(2): 27-31. [http://dx.doi.org/10.5314/wjd.v6.i2.27]

[83] Ali B, Al-Wabel NA, Shams S, Ahamad A, Khan SA, Anwar F. Essential oils used in aromatherapy: A systemic review. Asian Pac J Trop Biomed 2015; 5(8): 601-11. [http://dx.doi.org/10.1016/j.apjtb.2015.05.007]

[84] Michalak Monika. Aromatherapy and methods of applying essential oils. Arch Physiother Glob Res 2019; 22(2): 25-31.

[85] Schneider R, Singer N, Singer T. Medical aromatherapy revisited – basic mechanisms, critique, and new development. Hum Psychopharmacol Clin Exp 2018; 2018: e2683. [http://dx.doi.org/10.1002/hup.2683]

[86] Handayani S, Haryanto J, Makhfuddi M. Aromatherapy as the intervention of anxiety: systematic review. The 9th International Nursing Conference: Nurses at The Forefront in Transforming Care, Science, and Research. 07-08 April 2018, Surabaya, pp: 595-602.

[87] Lee I. Effects of inhalation of relaxing essential oils on electroencephalogram activity. International Journal of New Technology and Research 2016; 2: 37-45.

[88] Herz RS. Aromatherapy facts and fictions: A scientific analysis of olfactory effects on mood, physiology and behavior. Int J Neurosci 2009; 119(2): 263-90. [http://dx.doi.org/10.1080/00207450802333953] [PMID: 19125379]

[89] Kwon S, Ahn J, Jeon H. Can aromatherapy make people feel better through exercise? Int J Environ Res Public Health 2020; 17(12): 4559. [http://dx.doi.org/10.3390/ijerph17124559] [PMID: 32599887]

[90] Han X, Gibson J, Eggett DL, Parker TL. Bergamot (Citrus bergamia) essential oil inhalation improves positive feelings in the waiting room of a mental health treatment center: A pilot study. Phytother Res 2017; 31(5): 812-6. [http://dx.doi.org/10.1002/ptr.5806] [PMID: 28337799]

[91] Ballard CG, O'Brien JT, Reichelt K, Perry EK. Aromatherapy as a safe and effective treatment for the management of agitation in severe dementia: the results of a double-blind, placebo-controlled trial with Melissa. J Clin Psychiatry 2002; 63(7): 553-8.

[http://dx.doi.org/10.4088/JCP.v63n0703] [PMID: 12143909]

[92] Perry N, Perry E. Aromatherapy in the management of psychiatric disorders: clinical and neuropharmacological perspectives. CNS Drugs 2006; 20(4): 257-80. [http://dx.doi.org/10.2165/00023210-200620040-00001] [PMID: 16599645]

[93] Jimbo D, Kimura Y, Taniguchi M, Inoue M, Urakami K. Effect of aromatherapy on patients with Alzheimer's disease. Psychogeriatrics 2009; 9(4): 173-9. [http://dx.doi.org/10.1111/j.1479-8301.2009.00299.x] [PMID: 20377818]

[94] Shiina Y, Funabashi N, Lee K, *et al.* Relaxation effects of lavender aromatherapy improve coronary flow velocity reserve in healthy men evaluated by transthoracic Doppler echocardiography. Int J Cardiol 2008; 129(2): 193-7. [http://dx.doi.org/10.1016/j.ijcard.2007.06.064] [PMID: 17689755]

[95] Lin SSC, Lu TM, Chao PC, *et al. in vivo* cytokine modulatory effects of cinnamaldehyde, the major constituent of leaf essential oil from Cinnamomum osmophloeum Kaneh. Phytother Res 2011; 25(10): 1511-8. [http://dx.doi.org/10.1002/ptr.3419] [PMID: 21394803]

[96] Smith CA, Collins CT, Crowther CA. Aromatherapy for pain management in labour. Cochrane Libr 2011; (7): CD009215. [http://dx.doi.org/10.1002/14651858.CD009215] [PMID: 21735438]

[97] Seifi Z, Bikmoradi A, Bazrafshan MR, *et al.* The effect of inhalation aromatherapy with lavender essential oil on pain severity of patients after coronary artery bypass surgery: A single-blind randomised clinical trial. J Clin Diagn Res 2018; 12: LC01-5. [http://dx.doi.org/10.7860/JCDR/2018/34865.11721]

[98] Horváth G, Ács K. Essential oils in the treatment of respiratory tract diseases highlighting their role in bacterial infections and their anti inflammatory action: A review. Flavour Fragrance J 2015; 30(5): 331-41. [http://dx.doi.org/10.1002/ffj.3252] [PMID: 32313366]

[99] Aghagoli S, Salimi A, Salimi M, Ghazavi Z, Marofi M, Mohammadbeigi A. Aromatherapy with Rosa damascenes in apnea, bradycardia and SPO2 of preterm infants; a randomized clinical trial. Int J Pediatr 2016; 4: 1911-8.

[100] Aroyeun SO, Adegoke GO, Varga J, Teren J. Grading of fermented and dried cocoa beans using fungal contamination, ergosterol index and ochratoxin a production. Mycobiology 2009; 37(3): 215-7. [http://dx.doi.org/10.4489/MYCO.2009.37.3.215] [PMID: 23983536]

[101] Abdel-Wahhab MA, El-Nekeety AA, Hassan NS, Gibriel AAY, Abdel-Wahhab KG. Encapsulation of cinnamon essential oil in whey protein enhances the protective effect against single or combined sub-chronic toxicity of fumonisin B_1 and/or aflatoxin B_1 in rats. Environ Sci Pollut Res Int 2018; 25(29): 29144-61. [http://dx.doi.org/10.1007/s11356-018-2921-2] [PMID: 30112645]

[102] Bhalla Y, Gupta VK, Jaitak V. Anticancer activity of essential oils: A review. J Sci Food Agric 2013; 93(15): 3643-53. [http://dx.doi.org/10.1002/jsfa.6267] [PMID: 23765679]

[103] Brar KK. A review of contact dermatitis. Ann Allergy Asthma Immunol 2021; 126(1): 32-9. [http://dx.doi.org/10.1016/j.anai.2020.10.003] [PMID: 33091591]

[104] Heisterberg MV, Menné T, Andersen KE, *et al.* Deodorants are the leading cause of allergic contact dermatitis to fragrance ingredients. Contact Dermat 2011; 64(5): 258-64. [http://dx.doi.org/10.1111/j.1600-0536.2011.01889.x] [PMID: 21480912]

[105] Klaschka U. Contact allergens for armpits—Allergenic fragrances specified on deodorants. Int J Hyg Environ Health 2012; 215(6): 584-91. [http://dx.doi.org/10.1016/j.ijheh.2011.12.009] [PMID: 22261297]

[106] Pastor-Nieto MA, Gatica-Ortega ME. Ubiquity, Hazardous Effects, and Risk Assessment of Fragrances in Consumer Products. Curr Treat Options Allergy 2021; 8(1): 21-41. [http://dx.doi.org/10.1007/s40521-020-00275-7] [PMID: 33520600]

[107] Desmedt B, Marcelis Q, Zhilivoda D, Deconinck E. Sensitizing fragrances in absorbent hygiene products. Contact Dermat 2020; 82(5): 279-82. [http://dx.doi.org/10.1111/cod.13472] [PMID: 31951286]

[108] Scheinman PL. The foul side of fragrance-free products: What every clinician should know about managing patients with fragrance allergy. J Am Acad Dermatol 1999; 41(6): 1020-4. [http://dx.doi.org/10.1016/S0190-9622(99)70265-3] [PMID: 10570392]

[109] Trattner A, David M, Lazarov A. Occupational contact dermatitis due to essential oils. Contact Dermat 2008; 58(5): 282-4. [http://dx.doi.org/10.1111/j.1600-0536.2007.01275.x] [PMID: 18416758]

[110] Schliemann S, Geier J, Elsner P. Fragrances in topical over-the-counter medicaments - a loophole in EU legislation should be closed. Contact Dermat 2011; 65(6): 367-8. [http://dx.doi.org/10.1111/j.1600-0536.2011.01977.x] [PMID: 22077440]

[111] Cai J, Yan R, Shi J, *et al.* Antifungal and mycotoxin detoxification ability of essential oils: A review. Phytother Res 2021; 1-11. [http://dx.doi.org/10.1002/ptr.7281] [PMID: 34528300]

[112] Sindle A, Jacob SE, Martin K. Common allergens and considerations when performing pediatric patch testing. Dermatol Clin 2020; 38(3): 321-7. [http://dx.doi.org/10.1016/j.det.2020.02.003] [PMID: 32475510]

[113] Shah KM, Goldman SE, Agim NG. Airborne Contact Dermatitis Caused by Essential Oils in a Child. Dermatitis 2019; 30(1): 79-80. [http://dx.doi.org/10.1097/DER.0000000000000430] [PMID: 30570579]

[114] Tam I, Yu J. Pediatric contact dermatitis: what's new. Curr Opin Pediatr 2020; 32(4): 524-30. [http://dx.doi.org/10.1097/MOP.0000000000000919] [PMID: 32618793]

[115] Tran A, Pratt M, DeKoven J. Acute allergic contact dermatitis of the lips from peppermint oil in a lip balm. Dermatitis 2010; 21(2): 111-5. [http://dx.doi.org/10.2310/6620.2010.09040] [PMID: 20233551]

[116] Bourgeois P, Goossens A. Allergic contact cheilitis caused by menthol in toothpaste and throat medication: A case report. Contact Dermat 2016; 75(2): 113-5. [http://dx.doi.org/10.1111/cod.12571] [PMID: 27385520]

[117] Schilcher H. Effects and side-effects of essential oils. Essential oils and aromatic plants. Dordrecht: Springer 1985; pp. 217-31. [http://dx.doi.org/10.1007/978-94-009-5137-2_26]

[118] Averbeck D, Averbeck S, Dubertret L, Young AR, Morlière P. Genotoxicity of bergapten and bergamot oil in Saccharomyces cerevisiae. J Photochem Photobiol B 1990; 7(2-4): 209-29. [http://dx.doi.org/10.1016/1011-1344(90)85158-S] [PMID: 2128325]

[119] Kuttan R, Liju VB. Safety evaluation of essential oils. In: Hashemi SMB, Khaneghah AM, de Sant'Ana AS, Eds. Essential oils in Food Processing: Chemistry, Safety and Applications UK. 1st ed. West Sussex: John Wiley & Sons 2017; pp. 339-58. [http://dx.doi.org/10.1002/9781119149392.ch12]

[120] Vostinaru O, Heghes SC, Filip L. Safety profile of essential oils. Essential Oils-Bioactive Compounds, New Perspectives and Applications 2020; pp. 1-13.

[121] Frohne D, Pfander HJ. Giftpflanzen. Stuttgart: WissenschaftlicheVerlagsgesellschaft 1982; p. 4.

[122] Schilcher H. Essential Oils and Aromatic Plants. Dordrecht: Nijhof 1985.

[123] Stolk LML, Westerhof W, Cormane RH, Zwieten PAV. Serum and urine concentrations of 5-methoxypsoralen after oral administration. Br J Dermatol 1981; 105(4): 415-20. [http://dx.doi.org/10.1111/j.1365-2133.1981.tb00772.x] [PMID: 7295552]

[124] Yasui Y, Hirone T. Action spectrum for bergamot-oil phototoxicity measured by sunburn cell counting. J Dermatol 1994; 21(5): 319-22. [http://dx.doi.org/10.1111/j.1346-8138.1994.tb01746.x] [PMID: 8051317]

[125] Forlot P, Pevet P. Bergamot (*Citrus bergamia* Risso et Poiteau) essential oil: Biological properties, cosmetic and medical use. A review. J Essent Oil Res 2012; 24(2): 195-201. [http://dx.doi.org/10.1080/10412905.2012.659527]

[126] Alecrim MF, Lobón GS, D'Arc Machado R, *et al.* Electrochemical behavior of crude extract of Brosimumgaudchaudii and its major bioactives, psoralen and bergapten. Int J Electrochem Sci 2016; 11(11): 9519-28. [http://dx.doi.org/10.20964/2016.11.31]

[127] Flamini G, Cioni PL, Morelli I, Maccioni S, Baldini R. Phytochemical thpologies in some populations of Myrtus communis L. On caprione promontory (East Ligura, Italy). Food Chem 2004; 85(4): 599-604. [http://dx.doi.org/10.1016/j.foodchem.2003.08.005]

[128] Jamoussi B, Romdhane M, Abderraba A, Hassine BB, Gadri AEL. Effect of harvest time on the yield and composition of Tunisian myrtle oils. Flavour Fragrance J 2005; 20(3): 274-7. [http://dx.doi.org/10.1002/ffj.1453]

[129] Bouzabata Amel, Boussaha Faffani, Casanova Joseph, Tomi Félix. Composition and chemical variability of leaf oil of Myrtus communis from north-eastern Algeria. Nat Prod Commun 2010; 5(10): 1934578X1000501029. [http://dx.doi.org/10.1177/1934578X1000501029]

[130] Bouzabata A, Castola V, Bighelli A, Abed L, Casanova J, Tomi F. Chemical variability of Algerian Myrtus communis L. Chem Biodivers 2013; 10: 129-37.

[131] Yadegarinia D, Gachkar L, Rezaei MB, Taghizadeh M, Astaneh SA, Rasooli I. Biochemical activities of Iranian Mentha piperita L. and Myrtus communis L. essential oils. Phytochemistry 2006; 67(12): 1249-55. [http://dx.doi.org/10.1016/j.phytochem.2006.04.025] [PMID: 16777154]

[132] Razzaghi-Abyaneh M, Shams-Ghahfarokhi M, Rezaee MB, *et al.* Chemical composition and antiaflatoxigenic activity of Carum carvi L., Thymus vulgaris and Citrus aurantifolia essential oils. Food Control 2009; 20(11): 1018-24. [http://dx.doi.org/10.1016/j.foodcont.2008.12.007]

[133] Bent S. Herbal medicine in the United States: review of efficacy, safety, and regulation: grand rounds at University of California, San Francisco Medical Center. J Gen Intern Med 2008; 23(6): 854-9.

[134] Corazza M, Borghi A, Lauriola MM, *et al.* Use of topical herbal remedies and cosmetics: A questionnaire-based investigation in dermatology outpatients. J EurAcad Dermatol Venereol 2009; 23(11): 1298Y1303.

[135] Ernst E. Adverse effects of herbal drugs in dermatology. Br J Dermatol 2000; 143(5): 923Y929. [http://dx.doi.org/10.1046/j.1365-2133.2000.03822.x]

[136] Kiken DA, Cohen DE. Contact dermatitis to botanical extracts. Am J Contact Dermat 2002; 13(3): 148Y152.

[137] Corazza M, Borghi A, Gallo R, *et al.* Topical botanically derived products: Use, skin reactions, and usefulness of patch tests. A multicentre Italian study. . Contact Dermatitis 2014; 70(2): 90-7.

[138] Knight TE, Hausen BM. Melaleuca oil (tea tree oil) dermatitis. J Am Acad Dermatol 1994; 30(3): 423-7.

[139] Paulsen E. Contact sensitisation from Compositae-containing herbal remedies and cosmetics. Contact Dermatitis 2002; 47(4): 189-98.

[140] De Groot AC, Frosch PJ. Adverse reactions to fragrances: A clinical review. Contact Dermatitis 1997; 33336(2): 57-86. [http://dx.doi.org/10.1111/j.1600-0536.1997.tb00418.x]

[141] Bleasel N, Tate B, Rademaker M. Allergic contact dermatitis following exposure to essential oils. Australas J Dermatol 2002; 43(3): 211-3. [http://dx.doi.org/10.1046/j.1440-0960.2002.00598.x]

[142] Uter W, Schmidt E, Geier J, Lessmann H, Schnuch A, Frosch P. Contact allergy to essential oils: current patch test results (2000–2008) from the Information Network of Departments of Dermatology (IVDK) *. Contact Dermat 2010; 63(5): 277-83. [http://dx.doi.org/10.1111/j.1600-0536.2010.01768.x] [PMID: 20946456]

[143] Tisserand R, Young R. Essential Oil Safety: A Guide for Health Care Professionals. 2nd ed., Edinburgh, Scotland: Churchill Livingstone/ Elsevier 2014.

[144] Huang WF, Wen KC, Hsiao ML. Adulteration by synthetic therapeutic substances of traditional Chinese medicines in Taiwan. J Clin Pharmacol 1997; 37(4): 334-50.

[146] Price L, Price S. Essential oil science. In: Price L, Price S, Eds. Aromatherapy for health professionals. Elsevier 2007; pp. 43-61.

[147] Scientific Committee Members. Opinion on Fragrance allergens in cosmetic products. Scientific Committee on Consumer Safety 2012; 1459(11): 2-334. [http://dx.doi.org/10.2772/77628]

[148] Howes M-JR, Houghton PJ, Barlow DJ, Pocock VJ, Milligan SR. Assessment of estrogenic activity in some common essential oil constituents. J Pharm Pharmacol 2010; 54(11): 1521-8. [http://dx.doi.org/10.1211/002235702216] [PMID: 12495555]

[149] Ososki AL, Kennelly EJ. Phytoestrogens: A review of the present state of research. Phytother Res 2003; 17(8): 845-69. [http://dx.doi.org/10.1002/ptr.1364] [PMID: 13680814]

[150] Azaizeh H, Saad B, Cooper E, Said O. Traditional Arabic and Islamic medicine, a re-emerging health aid. Evidence-Based Complement. Evid Based Complement Alternat Med 2010; 7(4): 419-24. [http://dx.doi.org/10.1093/ecam/nen039] [PMID: 18955344]

[151] Al-Ramahi R, Jaradat N, Adawi D. Use of herbal medicines during pregnancy in a group of Palestinian women. J Ethnopharmacol 2013; 150(1): 79-84. [http://dx.doi.org/10.1016/j.jep.2013.07.041] [PMID: 23933314]

[152] Mbemya GT, Vieira LA, Canafistula FG, Pessoa ODL, Rodrigues APR. Reports on *in vivo* and *in vitro* contribution of medicinal plants to improve the female reproductive function. Reprodução Climatério 2017; 32(2): 109-19. [http://dx.doi.org/10.1016/j.recli.2016.11.002]

[153] Ali-Shtayeh MS, Jamous RM, Jamous RM. Plants used during pregnancy, childbirth, postpartum and infant healthcare in Palestine. Complement Ther Clin Pract 2015; 21(2): 84-93. [http://dx.doi.org/10.1016/j.ctcp.2015.03.004] [PMID: 25900613]

[154] aMacht DI. The action of so-called emmenagogue oils on the isolated uterine strip. J Pharm Exp Ther 1913; 4: 547-3.bSoares MC. Eucalyptol, an essential oil, reduces contractile activity in rat cardiac muscle. Braz J Med Biol Res 2005; 38: 453-61.

[155] Datnow MM. An experimental investigation concerning toxic abortion produced by chemical agents. J Obstet Gynaecol 1928; 35: 693-724.

[156] Kong Y, Lau C, Wat K, *et al.* Antifertility principle of Ruta graveolens. Planta Med 1989; 55(2): 176-8.

[http://dx.doi.org/10.1055/s-2006-961917] [PMID: 2748734]

[157] Soares MCMS, Damiani CEN, Moreira CM, Stefanon I, Vassallo DV. Eucalyptol, an essential oil, reduces contractile activity in rat cardiac muscle. Braz J Med Biol Res 2005; 38(3): 453-61. [http://dx.doi.org/10.1590/S0100-879X2005000300017] [PMID: 15761626]

[158] GavinaMugica De. L'huileessentielle de Sauged'Espagne (Salvia lavandulifoliaVahl). Parf Cosm Sav 1969; 12: 334-44.

[159] Marcos Sanz M E, Garcia Vallejo M C. Essential oils of Salvia lavandulifoliaVahl. Dev Food Sci 1988; 18: 147-60.

[160] Alziar G. Catalogue synonymique des Salvta L. (Lamiaceae). IV. BiocosmeMesogeen, Nice 1990; 7: 59.

[161] Tutin TG, Heywood VH, Burges NA, *et al.* Flora Europaea. Cambridge: Cambridge University Press 1972; Vol. 3: p. 189.

[162] Cafiigueral S, Iglesias J, Hamburger M, Hostettmann K. Phenolic constituents of Salvia lavandulifolia ssp. lavandulifolia. Pl' ita Med 1989; 55: 92.

[163] Cabo J, Crespo ME, Jimenez J, Navarro C, Peran E, Zarzuelo A. Sur I'huileessentielle de Salvia lavandulifoliaVahl. subsp. Oxyodon. PI. Med Phytother 1987; 21: 116-21.

[164] Crespo M, Jimenez J, Navarro C, Zarzuelo A. The essential oil of Salvia lavandulifolia subspecies Oxyodon. A study of its vegetative cycle. Planta Med 1986; 52(5): 367-9. [http://dx.doi.org/10.1055/s-2007-969187] [PMID: 17345342]

[165] Lawrence BM, Hogg JW, Terhune SJ. Essential oils and their constituents. J Chromatogr A 1970; 50: 59-65. [http://dx.doi.org/10.1016/S0021-9673(00)97916-0]

[166] Cordoba Rodriquez MA. €I AceiteEsencial de Salvia Espanola (Salvia lavandulifolia, Vahl.). Doctoral Thesis, Facultad de Farmacia, Universidad de Madrid 1983.

[167] Goryaev MI, Dzhalilov DR. Analysis of the essential oil of Cossack juniper. Trudy lnst. Khim. Nauk. Akad. Nauk Kazakh. SS R 1959; 4: 57-67.

[168] Rudloff EV. Gas-liquid chromatography of terpenes-Part IX. The volatile oil of the leaves of Juniperus sabina L. Can J Chem 1963; 41(11): 2876-81. [http://dx.doi.org/10.1139/v63-421]

[169] Fournier G, Paris M, Dumitresco S, Pages N, Boudene C. Contribution to the study of Plectranthusfruticosus leaf essential oil. Planta Med 1986; 52(6): 486-8. [http://dx.doi.org/10.1055/s-2007-969261] [PMID: 17345416]

[170] Papavassiliou MJ. Sur deux casd'intoxication par la sabine; la permeabiliteplacentaire a l'essence de sabine. SOC. Med Leg 1935; 15: 778-81.

[171] Revol L. L'essenceconstituet'elleI'uniqueprincipeactif des Juniperus de la section sabina? Bull Sci Pharmacol 1936; 43: 139-44.

[172] Patoir A, Patoir G, Bedrine H. Action toxique de I'essence de Sabine et de I'Armoise sur I'organisme. C. R. Seances. Soc Biol 1938; 127: 1325-6.

[173] Renaux J. Sur les effetsocytociques des essences de Rue et de Sabine. Acta Biol Belg 1941; 1: 334-5.

[174] Fourcade G. La Sabine des Pyrenees These Doct Etat. Toulouse: Pharmacie 1955.

[175] Pages N, Fournier G, Chamorro G, Salazar M, Paris M, Boudene C. Teratological evaluation of Juniperus sabina essential oil in mice. Planta Med 1989; 55(2): 144-6. [http://dx.doi.org/10.1055/s-2006-961908] [PMID: 2748731]

[176] Pages N, Salazar M, Chamorro G, *et al.* Teratological evaluation of Plectranthus fruticosus leaf essential oil. Planta Med 1988; 54(4): 296-8.

[http://dx.doi.org/10.1055/s-2006-962437] [PMID: 3222373]

[177] Pages N, Fournier G, Chamorro G, Salazar M. Teratogenic effects of *Plectranthus fruticosus* essential oil in mice. Phytother Res 1991; 5(2): 94-6. [http://dx.doi.org/10.1002/ptr.2650050213]

[178] Edris AE. Pharmaceutical and therapeutic Potentials of essential oils and their individual volatile constituents: A review. Phytother Res 2007; 21(4): 308-23. [http://dx.doi.org/10.1002/ptr.2072] [PMID: 17199238]

[179] Sertel S, Eichhorn T, Plinkert PK, Efferth T. Cytotoxicity of Thymus vulgaris essential oil towards human oral cavity squamous cell carcinoma. Anticancer Res 2011; 31(1): 81-7. [PMID: 21273584]

[180] Russo A, Formisano C, Rigano D, Cardile V, Arnold NA, Senatore F. Comparative phytochemical profile and antiproliferative activity on human melanoma cells of essential oils of three lebanese Salvia species. Ind Crops Prod 2016; 83: 492-9. [http://dx.doi.org/10.1016/j.indcrop.2015.12.080]

[181] Maistro EL, Mota SF, Lima EB, Bernardes BM, Goulart FC. Genotoxicity and mutagenicity of Rosmarinus officinalis (Labiatae) essential oil in mammalian cells *in vivo*. Genet Mol Res 2010; 9(4): 2120-9. [http://dx.doi.org/10.4238/vol9-4gmr857] [PMID: 21038297]

[182] Geran RI, Greenberg NH, Macdonald MM, Schumacher AM, Abbott BJ. Protocols for screening chemical agents and natural products against animal tumours and other biological systems. Cancer Chemother Rep 3 1972; 59-61.

[183] Balaji S, Chempakam B. Toxicity prediction of compounds from turmeric (Curcuma longa L). Food Chem Toxicol 2010; 48(10): 2951-9. [http://dx.doi.org/10.1016/j.fct.2010.07.032] [PMID: 20667459]

[184] Kuttan R, Liju VB, Jeena K. An evaluation of antioxidant, anti-inflammatory, and antinociceptive activities of essential oil from Curcuma longa. L. Indian J Pharmacol 2011; 43(5): 526-31. [http://dx.doi.org/10.4103/0253-7613.84961] [PMID: 22021994]

[185] Jayaprakasha GK, Rao LJ, Sakariah KK. Chemical composition of volatile oil from Cinnamomum zeylanicum buds. Z Naturforsch C J Biosci 2002; 57(11-12): 990-3. [http://dx.doi.org/10.1515/znc-2002-11-1206] [PMID: 12562082]

[186] Rahman MF, Siddiqui MK, Jamil K. Effects of Vepacide (Azadirachta indica) on asp artate and al anine aminotransferase profiles in a subchronic study with rats. Hum Exp Toxicol 2001; 20(5): 243-9. [http://dx.doi.org/10.1191/096032701678227730] [PMID: 11476156]

[187] Hilaly JE, Israili ZH, Lyoussi B. Acute and chronic toxicological studies of Ajuga iva in experimental animals. J Ethnopharmacol 2004; 91(1): 43-50. [http://dx.doi.org/10.1016/j.jep.2003.11.009] [PMID: 15036466]

[188] Lameire N, Vanbiesen W, Vanholder R. Acute renal failure. Lancet 2005; 365(9457): 417-30. [http://dx.doi.org/10.1016/S0140-6736(05)70238-5] [PMID: 15680458]

[189] Sertel S, Eichhorn T, Plinkert PK, Efferth T. Cytotoxicity of Thymus vulgaris essential oil towards human oral cavity squamous cell carcinoma. Anticancer Res 2011; 31(1): 81-7. [PMID: 21273584]

[190] Deepa Das A. Comparative study of the efficacy of curcumin and turmeric oil as chemopreventive agents in oral submucous fibrosis: A clinical and histopathological evaluation. JIAOMR 2010; 22: 88-92.

[191] Hastak K, Lubri N, Jakhi SD, *et al.* Effect of turmeric oil and turmeric oleoresin on cytogenetic damage in patients suffering from oral submucous fibrosis. Cancer Lett 1997; 116(2): 265-9. [http://dx.doi.org/10.1016/S0304-3835(97)00205-X] [PMID: 9215873]

[192] Lantz RC, Chen GJ, Solyom AM, Jolad SD, Timmermann BN. The effect of turmeric extracts on inflammatory mediator production. Phytomedicine 2005; 12(6-7): 445-52. [http://dx.doi.org/10.1016/j.phymed.2003.12.011] [PMID: 16008121]

[193] Funk JL, Frye JB, Oyarzo JN, Zhang H, Timmermann BN. Anti-arthritic effects and toxicity of the essential oils of turmeric (Curcuma longa L.). J Agric Food Chem 2010; 58(2): 842-9. [http://dx.doi.org/10.1021/jf9027206] [PMID: 20025215]

[194] Antony B, Merina B, Iyer VS, Judy N, Lennertz K, Joyal S. A pilot cross-over study to evaluate human oral bioavailability of BCM-95 ® CG (Biocurcumax ™), a novel bioenhanced preparation of curcumin. Indian J Pharm Sci 2008; 70(4): 445-9. [http://dx.doi.org/10.4103/0250-474X.44591] [PMID: 20046768]

[195] Anand P, Thomas SG, Kunnumakkara AB, *et al.* Biological activities of curcumin and its analogues (Congeners) made by man and Mother Nature. Biochem Pharmacol 2008; 76(11): 1590-611. [http://dx.doi.org/10.1016/j.bcp.2008.08.008] [PMID: 18775680]

[196] Dobetsberger C, Buchbauer G. Actions of essential oils on the central nervous system: An updated review. Flavour Fragrance J 2011; 26(5): 300-16. [http://dx.doi.org/10.1002/ffj.2045]

[197] Liu X, Li Y, Li H, *et al.* Identification of repellent and insecticidal constituents of the essential oil of Artemisia rupestris L. aerial parts against Liposcelis bostrychophila Badonnel. Molecules 2013; 18(9): 10733-46. [http://dx.doi.org/10.3390/molecules180910733] [PMID: 24005967]

[198] Bradley B F, Brown S L, Chu S, Lea R W. Effects of orally administered lavender essential oil on responses to anxietyprovoking film clips. Hum Psychopharmacol 2009; 24: 319-0.

[199] Faturi CB, Leite JR, Alves PB, Canton AC, Teixeira-Silva F. Anxiolytic-like effect of sweet orange aroma in Wistar rats. Prog Neuropsychopharmacol Biol Psychiatry 2010; 34(4): 605-9. [http://dx.doi.org/10.1016/j.pnpbp.2010.02.020] [PMID: 20211673]

[200] Tsang HWH, Ho TYC. A systematic review on the anxiolytic effects of aromatherapy on rodents under experimentally induced anxiety models. Rev Neurosci 2010; 21(2): 141-52. [http://dx.doi.org/10.1515/REVNEURO.2010.21.2.141] [PMID: 20614803]

[201] Kasper S, Gastpar M, Müller WE, *et al.* Silexan, an orally administered Lavandula oil preparation, is effective in the treatment of 'subsyndromal' anxiety disorder: A randomized, double-blind, placebo controlled trial. Int Clin Psychopharmacol 2010; 25(5): 277-87. [http://dx.doi.org/10.1097/YIC.0b013e32833b3242] [PMID: 20512042]

[202] Woelk H, Schläfke S. A multi-center, double-blind, randomised study of the Lavender oil preparation Silexan in comparison to Lorazepam for generalized anxiety disorder. Phytomedicine 2010; 17(2): 94-9. [http://dx.doi.org/10.1016/j.phymed.2009.10.006] [PMID: 19962288]

[203] Chioca LR, Pereira M, Baretta IP, *et al.* P.4.b.010 Anxiolytic-like effect of lavender and orange essential oil: participation of nitric oxide but not GABA-A benzodiazepine complex. Eur Neuropsychopharmacol 2011; 21: S538-8. [http://dx.doi.org/10.1016/S0924-977X(11)70875-6]

[204] Goes TC, Antunes FD, Alves PB, Teixeira-Silva F. Effect of sweet orange aroma on experimental anxiety in humans. J Altern Complement Med 2012; 18(8): 798-804. [http://dx.doi.org/10.1089/acm.2011.0551] [PMID: 22849536]

[205] Hritcu L, Cioanca O, Hancianu M. Effects of lavender oil inhalation on improving scopolamine-induced spatial memory impairment in laboratory rats. Phytomedicine 2012; 19(6): 529-34. [http://dx.doi.org/10.1016/j.phymed.2012.02.002] [PMID: 22402245]

[206] Schuwald AM, Nöldner M, Wilmes T, Klugbauer N, Leuner K, Müller WE. Lavender oil-potent anxiolytic properties *via* modulating voltage dependent calcium channels. PLoS One 2013; 8(4):

e59998.
[http://dx.doi.org/10.1371/journal.pone.0059998] [PMID: 23637742]

[207] Querfurth HW, LaFerla FM. Alzheimer's Disease. N Engl J Med 2010; 362(4): 329-44. [http://dx.doi.org/10.1056/NEJMra0909142] [PMID: 20107219]

[208] Selkoe DJ. Alzheimer's disease: genes, proteins, and therapy. Physiol Rev 2001; 81(2): 741-66. [http://dx.doi.org/10.1152/physrev.2001.81.2.741] [PMID: 11274343]

[209] Hardy JA, Higgins GA. Alzheimer's disease: the amyloid cascade hypothesis. Science 1992; 256(5054): 184-5. [http://dx.doi.org/10.1126/science.1566067] [PMID: 1566067]

[210] Xu P, Wang K, Lu C, *et al.* Protective effect of lavender oil on scopolamine induced cognitive deficits in mice and H_2O_2 induced cytotoxicity in PC12 cells. J Ethnopharmacol 2016; 193: 408-15. [http://dx.doi.org/10.1016/j.jep.2016.08.030] [PMID: 27558947]

[212] Samojlik I, Lakić N, Mimica-Dukić N, Đaković-Švajcer K, Božin B. Antioxidant and hepatoprotective potential of essential oils of coriander (Coriandrum sativum L.) and caraway (Carum carvi L.) (Apiaceae). J Agric Food Chem 2010; 58(15): 8848-53. [http://dx.doi.org/10.1021/jf101645n] [PMID: 20608729]

[215] Houghton PJ, Ren Y, Howes MJ. Acetylcholinesterase inhibitors from plants and fungi. Nat Prod Rep 2006; 23(2): 181-99. [http://dx.doi.org/10.1039/b508966m] [PMID: 16572227]

[217] Mukherjee PK, Kumar V, Mal M, Houghton PJ. Acetylcholinesterase inhibitors from plants. Phytomedicine 2007; 14(4): 289-300. [http://dx.doi.org/10.1016/j.phymed.2007.02.002] [PMID: 17346955]

[219] Zhang N, Zhang L, Feng L, Yao L. The anxiolytic effect of essential oil of Cananga odorata exposure on mice and determination of its major active constituents. Phytomedicine 2016; 23(14): 1727-34. [http://dx.doi.org/10.1016/j.phymed.2016.10.017] [PMID: 27912874]

[220] Victoria FN, de Siqueira Brahm A, Savegnago L, Lenardão EJ. Involvement of serotoninergic and adrenergic systems on the antidepressant-like effect of E. uniflora L. leaves essential oil and further analysis of its antioxidant activity. Neurosci Lett 2013; 544: 105-9. [http://dx.doi.org/10.1016/j.neulet.2013.03.054] [PMID: 23583586]

[221] Abuhamdah S, Huang L, Elliott MSJ, *et al.* Pharmacological profile of an essential oil derived from *Melissa officinalis* with anti-agitation properties: focus on ligand-gated channels. J Pharm Pharmacol 2010; 60(3): 377-84. [http://dx.doi.org/10.1211/jpp.60.3.0014] [PMID: 18284819]

[222] Costa CARA, Cury TC, Cassettari BO, Takahira RK, Flório JC, Costa M. Citrus aurantium L. essential oil exhibits anxiolytic-like activity mediated by 5-HT1A-receptors and reduces cholesterol after repeated oral treatment. BMC Complement Altern Med 2013; 13(1): 42. [http://dx.doi.org/10.1186/1472-6882-13-42] [PMID: 23432968]

[223] Ingkaninan K, Temkitthawon P, Chuenchom K, Yuyaem T, Thongnoi W. Screening for acetylcholinesterase inhibitory activity in plants used in Thai traditional rejuvenating and neurotonic remedies. J Ethnopharmacol 2003; 89(2-3): 261-4. [http://dx.doi.org/10.1016/j.jep.2003.08.008] [PMID: 14611889]

[224] Gnagey AL, Forte M, Rosenberry TL. Isolation and characterization of acetylcholinesterase from Drosophila. J Biol Chem 1987; 262(27): 13290-8. [http://dx.doi.org/10.1016/S0021-9258(18)45200-3] [PMID: 3115978]

[225] Bourguet D, Roig A, Toutant JP, Arpagaus M. Analysis of molecular forms and pharmacological properties of acetylcholinesterase in several mosquito species. Neurochem Int 1997; 31(1): 65-72. [http://dx.doi.org/10.1016/S0197-0186(96)00118-0] [PMID: 9185166]

[226] Kim JI, Jung CS, Koh YH, Lee SH. Molecular, biochemical and histochemical characterization of two

acetylcholinesterase cDNAs from the German cockroach *Blattella germanica*. Insect Mol Biol 2006; 15(4): 513-22.
[http://dx.doi.org/10.1111/j.1365-2583.2006.00666.x] [PMID: 16907838]

[227] Pezzementi L, Rowland M, Wolfe M, Tsigelny I. Inactivation of an invertebrate acetylcholinesterase by sulfhydryl reagents:The roles of two cysteines in the catalytic gorge of the enzyme. Invert Neurosci 2006; 6(2): 47-55.
[http://dx.doi.org/10.1007/s10158-006-0017-z] [PMID: 16586114]

[228] Pang YP, Singh SK, Gao Y, *et al.* Selective and irreversible inhibitors of aphid acetylcholinesterases: Steps toward human-safe insecticides. PLoS One 2009; 4(2): e4349.
[http://dx.doi.org/10.1371/journal.pone.0004349] [PMID: 19194505]

[229] Polsinelli GA, Singh SK, Mishra RK, *et al.* Insect-specific irreversible inhibitors of acetylcholinesterase in pests including the bed bug, the eastern yellowjacket, German and American cockroaches, and the confused flour beetle. Chem Biol Interact 2010; 187(1-3): 142-7.
[http://dx.doi.org/10.1016/j.cbi.2010.01.036] [PMID: 20109441]

[230] Pang YP, Brimijoin S, Ragsdale DW, Zhu KY, Suranyi R. Novel and viable acetylcholinesterase target site for developing effective and environmentally safe insecticides. Curr Drug Targets 2012; 13(4): 471-82.
[http://dx.doi.org/10.2174/138945012799499703] [PMID: 22280344]

[231] Perry NSL, Houghton PJ, Jenner P, Keith A, Perry EK. Salvia lavandulaefolia essential oil inhibits cholinesterase *in vivo*. Phytomedicine 2002; 9(1): 48-51.
[http://dx.doi.org/10.1078/0944-7113-00082] [PMID: 11926204]

[232] Orhan IE. Acetylcholinesterase inhibitory and antioxidant properties of Cyclotrichiumniveum, Thymus praecox subsp. caucasicus var. caucasicus, Echinacea purpurea and E. pallida. Food Chem Toxicol 2009; 47: 1304-10.
[http://dx.doi.org/10.1016/j.fct.2009.03.004] [PMID: 19285534]

[233] Tel G, Öztürk M, Duru ME, Harmandar M, Topçu G. Chemical composition of the essential oil and hexane extract of Salvia chionantha and their antioxidant and anticholinesterase activities. Food Chem Toxicol 2010; 48(11): 3189-93.
[http://dx.doi.org/10.1016/j.fct.2010.08.020] [PMID: 20732375]

[234] Erdogan Orhan I, Senol FS, Ozturk N, Celik SA, Pulur A, Kan Y. Phytochemical contents and enzyme inhibitory and antioxidant properties of Anethum graveolens L. (dill) samples cultivated under organic and conventional agricultural conditions. Food Chem Toxicol 2013; 59: 96-103.
[http://dx.doi.org/10.1016/j.fct.2013.05.053] [PMID: 23764360]

[235] Seo SM, Kim J, Kang J, *et al.* Fumigant toxicity and acetylcholinesterase inhibitory activity of 4 Asteraceae plant essential oils and their constituents against Japanese termite (Reticulitermes speratus Kolbe). Pestic Biochem Physiol 2014; 113: 55-61.
[http://dx.doi.org/10.1016/j.pestbp.2014.06.001] [PMID: 25052527]

[236] Park CG, Jang M, Yoon KA, Kim J. Insecticidal and acetylcholinesterase inhibitory activities of Lamiaceae plant essential oils and their major components against Drosophila suzukii (Diptera: Drosophilidae). Ind Crops Prod 2016; 89: 507-13.
[http://dx.doi.org/10.1016/j.indcrop.2016.06.008]

[237] Picollo MI, Toloza AC, Mougabure Cueto G, Zygadlo J, Zerba E. Anticholinesterase and pediculicidal activities of monoterpenoids. Fitoterapia 2008; 79(4): 271-8.
[http://dx.doi.org/10.1016/j.fitote.2008.01.005] [PMID: 18321657]

[238] Abdelgaleil SAM, Mohamed MIE, Badawy MEI, El-arami SAA. Fumigant and contact toxicities of monoterpenes to Sitophilus oryzae (L.) and Tribolium castaneum (Herbst) and their inhibitory effects on acetylcholinesterase activity. J Chem Ecol 2009; 35(5): 518-25.
[http://dx.doi.org/10.1007/s10886-009-9635-3] [PMID: 19412756]

[239] Anderson JA, Coats JR. Acetylcholinesterase inhibition by nootkatone and carvacrol in arthropods.

Pestic Biochem Physiol 2012; 102(2): 124-8.
[http://dx.doi.org/10.1016/j.pestbp.2011.12.002]

[240] Park IK. Fumigant toxicity of Oriental sweetgum (Liquidambar orientalis) and valerian (Valeriana wallichii) essential oils and their components, including their acetylcholinesterase inhibitory activity, against Japanese termites (Reticulitermes speratus). Molecules 2014; 19(8): 12547-58.
[http://dx.doi.org/10.3390/molecules190812547] [PMID: 25153870]

[241] Yeom HJ, Jung CS, Kang J, *et al.* Insecticidal and acetylcholine esterase inhibition activity of Asteraceae plant essential oils and their constituents against adults of the German cockroach (Blattella germanica). J Agric Food Chem 2015; 63(8): 2241-8.
[http://dx.doi.org/10.1021/jf505927n] [PMID: 25664467]

[242] Jankowska M, Rogalska J, Wyszkowska J, Stankiewicz M. Molecular targets for components of essential oils in the insect nervous system—A review. Molecules 2017; 23(1): 34.
[http://dx.doi.org/10.3390/molecules23010034] [PMID: 29295521]

[243] Aziz ZAA, Ahmad A, Setapar SHM, *et al.* Essential oils: Extraction techniques, pharmaceutical and therapeutic potential - a review. Curr Drug Metab 2018; 19(13): 1100-10.
[http://dx.doi.org/10.2174/1389200219666180723144850] [PMID: 30039757]

[244] Stevanovic ZD, Bosnjak-Neumuller J, Pajic-Lijakovic I, Raj J. Essential oils as feed additives-future perspectives. Molecules 2018.

[245] Grigoriu C, Varlas V, Călinescu G, *et al.* Phytotherapy in obstetrics – therapeutic indications, limits, and dangers. J Med Life 2021; 14(6): 748-55.
[http://dx.doi.org/10.25122/jml-2021-0353] [PMID: 35126743]

[246] Franz C, Baser KHC, Windisch W. Essential oils and aromatic plants in animal feeding – A European perspective. A review. Flavour Fragrance J 2010; 25(5): 327-40.
[http://dx.doi.org/10.1002/ffj.1967]

[247] Lanzerstorfer P, Sandner G, Pitsch J, Mascher B, Aumiller T, Weghuber J. Acute, reproductive, and developmental toxicity of essential oils assessed with alternative *in vitro* and *in vivo* systems. Arch Toxicol 2021; 95(2): 673-91.
[http://dx.doi.org/10.1007/s00204-020-02945-6] [PMID: 33159585]

[248] Amer A, Mehlhorn H. Repellency effect of forty-one essential oils against Aedes, Anopheles, and Culex mosquitoes. Parasitol Res 2006; 99(4): 478-90.
[http://dx.doi.org/10.1007/s00436-006-0184-1] [PMID: 16642384]

[249] Cai C, Ma R, Duan M, Deng Y, Liu T, Lu D. Effect of starch film containing thyme essential oil microcapsules on physicochemical activity of mango. Lebensm Wiss Technol 2020; 131: 109700.
[http://dx.doi.org/10.1016/j.lwt.2020.109700]

[250] Chen SF, Wang CH, Chan PT, *et al.* Labour pain control by aromatherapy: A meta-analysis of randomised controlled trials. Women Birth 2019; 32(4): 327-35.
[http://dx.doi.org/10.1016/j.wombi.2018.09.010] [PMID: 30344029]

[251] Bucur L, Ionus E, Moise G, Gird C, Schroder V. GC-MS analysis, and bioactive properties of Zingiberisrhizoma essential oil. Farmacia 2020; 68(2): 280-7.
[http://dx.doi.org/10.31925/farmacia.2020.2.13]

[252] Sharifi-Rad J, Sureda A, Tenore G, *et al.* Biological activities of essential oils: from plant chemoecology to traditional healing systems. Molecules 2017; 22(1): 70.
[http://dx.doi.org/10.3390/molecules22010070] [PMID: 28045446]

[253] Cuba R. Toxicity myths essential oils and their carcinogenic potential. International Journal of Aromatherapy 2001; 11(2): 76-83.
[http://dx.doi.org/10.1016/S0962-4562(01)80021-7]

[255] Price S. The aromatherapy workbook. London: Thorsons 1993.

[256] Svoboda KP, Deans SG. A study of the variability of Rosemary and Sage and their volatile oils on the British market: Their antioxidative properties. Flavour Fragrance J 1992; 7(2): 81-7. [http://dx.doi.org/10.1002/ffj.2730070207]

[257] Ghasemzadeh Rahbardar M, Hosseinzadeh H. Therapeutic effects of rosemary (*Rosmarinus officinalis* L.) and its active constituents on nervous system disorders. Iran J Basic Med Sci 2020; 23(9): 1100-12. [PMID: 32963731]

[259] Aprotosoaie AC, Gille E, Trifan A, Luca VS, Miron A. Essential oils of Lavandula genus: A systematic review of their chemistry. Phytochem Rev 2017; 16(4): 761-99. [http://dx.doi.org/10.1007/s11101-017-9517-1]

[260] Dzi̧eciol M. Comparison of phenolic acids and flavonoids contents in variouscultivars and parts of common lavender (Lavandula angustifolia) derived from Poland. Nat Prod Res 2017; 31: 2575-80. [http://dx.doi.org/10.1080/14786419.2017.1320792] [PMID: 28449600]

[261] Koulivand PH, Khaleghi Ghadiri M, Gorji A. Lavender and the nervous system. Evid Based Complement Alternat Med 2013; 2013: 1-10. [http://dx.doi.org/10.1155/2013/681304] [PMID: 23573142]

[262] Tisserand R, Balacs T. Essential oil safety: A guide for health professionals. Edinburgh: Churchill Livingstone 1995.

CHAPTER 6

Human Organs System and Essential Oils (EOs)

Sandeep Negi[1,*], **Ajeet Kumar Srivastav**[2,3] and **Lakshmi Bala**[2]

[1] *Photobiology Laboratory, Systems Toxicology and Health Risk Assessment Group CSIR-Indian Institute of Toxicology Research Vishvigyan Bhavan 31, P.O. Box No. 80, M.G. Marg Lucknow-226001, India*

[2] *Department of Biochemistry, Babu Banrasi Das University, Lucknow, India*

[3] *Redcliffe Hygiene Private Limited, Gurugram, India*

Abstract: Some patients prefer complementary and alternative medicine treatments because they are under the impression that these methods are safer than conventional medication because of their "natural" origins. EOs can be used in a bath, during a massage, as a spray, a paste, a gel, or *via* inhalation. People think that these oils get into the skin through the upper dermis. There are different ideas about how aromatherapy could help people. The components of EOs are essential for the treatment and prevention of cancer; the processes responsible for EOs' antimutagenic capabilities are numerous. These EOs boost immunity, improve blood circulation, protect from respiratory and skin diseases, and improve digestion. These are also helpful in relieving pain in joints and muscular regions. Their importance in boosting brain functioning helps in the treatment of various neurological problems. They have a significant impact on resolving human reproductive issues. They play a significant role in modern medicine and are increasingly used to treat a wide range of illnesses. Their value as a natural remedy of last resort is universally acknowledged. Their increasing application to the treatment of human health issues has paved the path for natural aromatherapy to find widespread acceptance among the general public.

Keywords: Aromatherapy, Anti-Cancer Activity, Antimutagenic, Anti-inflammatory Activity, Essential oils (EOs).

1. INTRODUCTION

Some patients prefer complementary and alternative medicine because they believe it is safer, less poisonous, and less likely to create side effects. After all, it is perceived as "natural." Essential oils can be applied topically, inhaled, blended into a paste or spray, added to a bath, or used in a variety of other ways. They are

* **Corresponding author Sandeep Negi:** Photobiology Laboratory, Systems Toxicology and Health Risk Assessment Group CSIR-Indian Institute of Toxicology Research Vishvigyan Bhavan 31, P.O. Box No. 80, M.G. Marg Lucknow-226001, India; E-mail: lakshmi266@gmail.com

Pradeep Kumar Shukla, Ajeet Kumar Srivastav, Deepti Chopra, Shikha Agnihotry, Pragati Misra and Jyoti Singh (Eds.)

thought to be absorbed into the skin through the dermis at the top layer [1] (Fig. **1**).

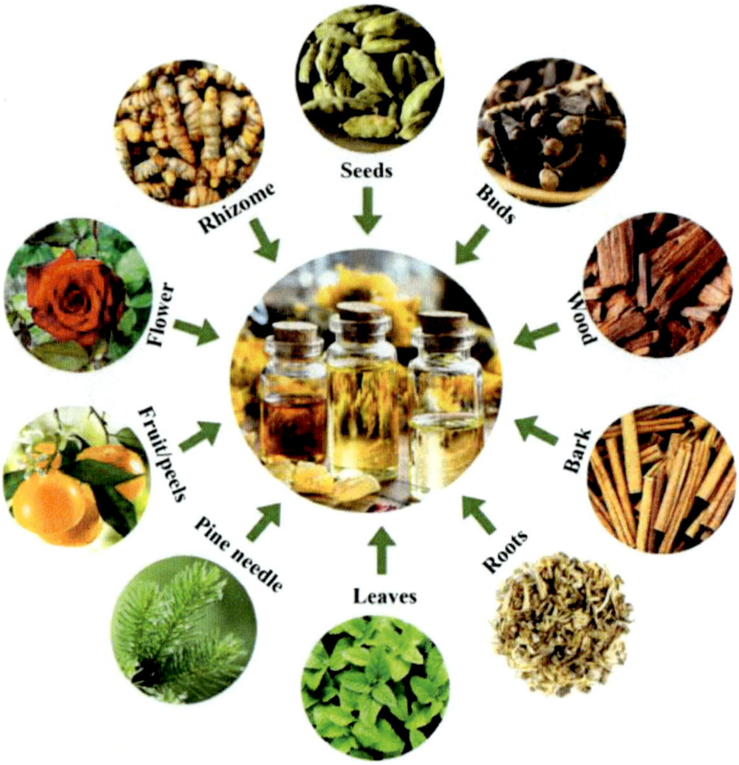

Fig. (1). Essential oils obtained from various plant components.

2. MECHANISMS OF ACTION OF NATURAL ESSENTIAL OILS

Several hypotheses explain how aromatherapy can produce therapeutic results, including systemic effects (working as a medicine or an enzyme), placebo effects, and general emotional or "reflective" effects that elicit happy emotions (Fig. **2**) [2].

Essential oils contain a variety of chemical components that have different medicinal properties. Essential oils can be derived from practically any part of the plant, including the leaves, flowers, wood, roots, vetivert, calamus, and sap of eucalyptus, peppermint, lavender, rose, juniper, and frankincense, to name a few. They often contain many naturally volatile organic compounds. These oils frequently contain a combination of numerous organic compounds having medicinal capabilities, which correspond to varying concentrations of each molecule in the oil. wound recovery. Ketone-rich oils have certain qualities, but alcohol-rich oils have properties that are antibacterial and anti-infectious [3].

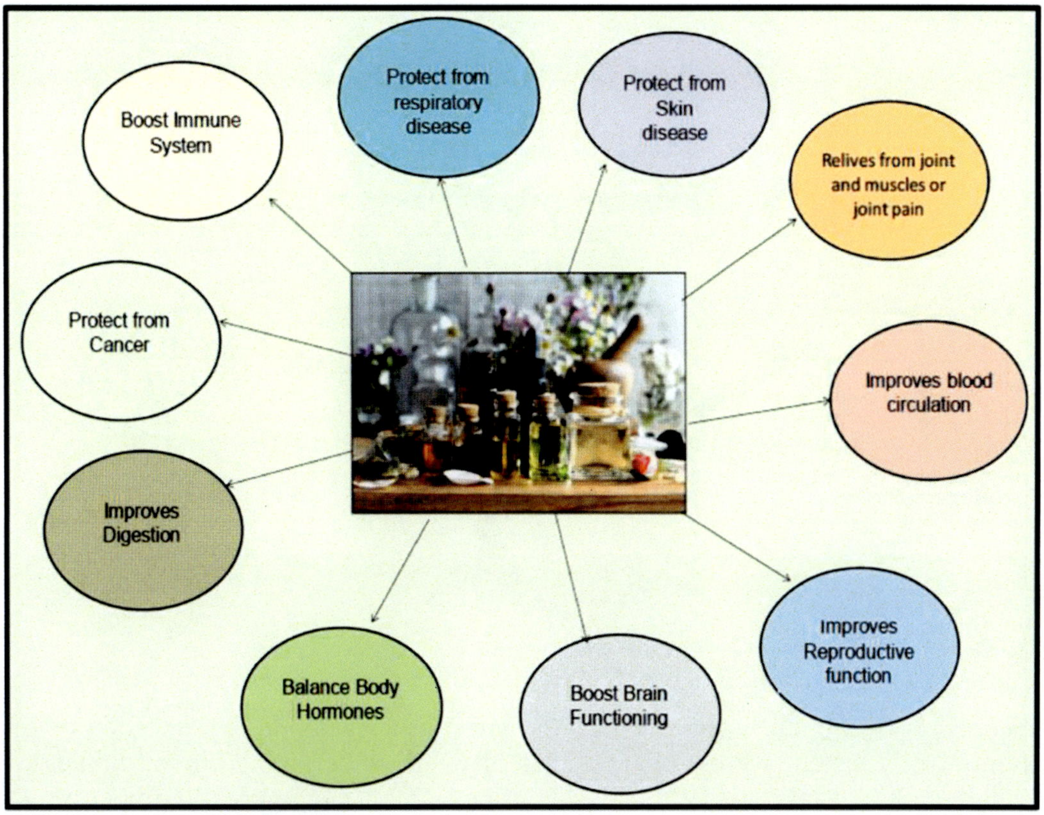

Fig. (2). Various uses of essential oils.

3. ANTI-CANCER ACTIVITY OF ESSENTIAL OILS (EOS)

EO constituents are crucial in the treatment and prevention of cancer. Because oxidation causes damage to various biological substances and, as a result, many diseases such as Parkinson's disease, Alzheimer's disease, liver disease, cancer, diabetes, arthritis, aging, AIDS inflammation, and atherosclerosis, antioxidant activity is one of the most researched topics in EOs [4]. Antioxidants have been used to treat a variety of ailments as they guard against oxidative damage [5]. To find natural antioxidants that are safe to use, researchers have been examining the antioxidant capabilities of several EOs. Numerous studies have demonstrated essential oils are the best natural providers of antioxidants [6]. In eukaryotes, hydrogen peroxide and superoxide anions combine to create hydroxyl radicals, which are particularly harmful to mitochondrial DNA. Damaged mitochondrial DNA hinders the formation of the electron transport protein, which exacerbates the buildup of reactive oxygen species (ROS) (Fig. **3**) [7]. Reactive phenoxy radicals are created when damaged mitochondrial membrane free radicals combine with EOs to stop further damage [8].

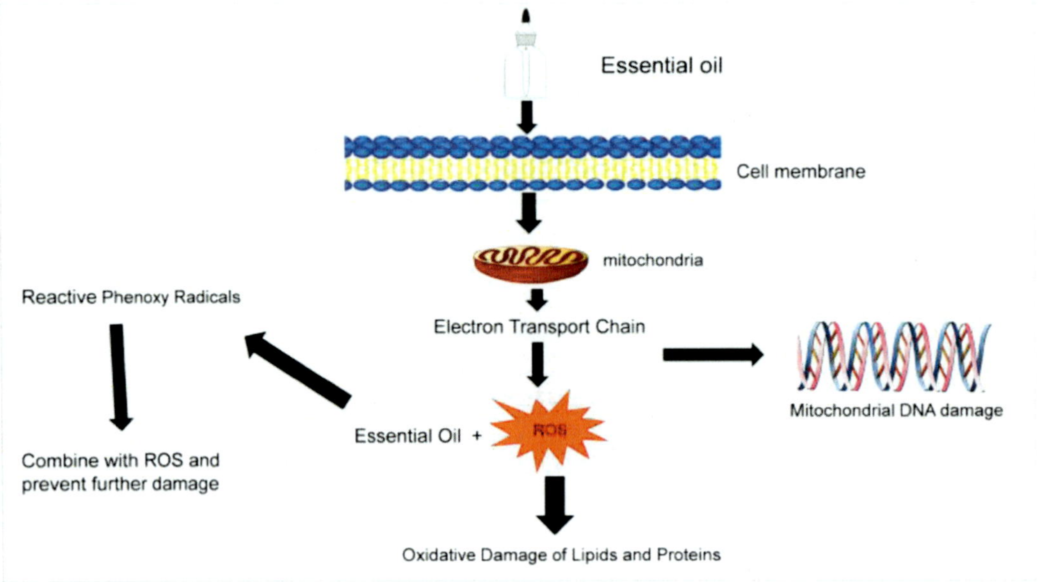

Fig. (3). Anti-cancer mechanism of essential oils.

According to one study, thyme had the strongest antioxidant properties of the essential oils tested, followed by a leaf of basil, eucalyptus, clove, cinnamon, basil, and chamomile oils [9]. The EOs of coriander, eucalyptus, juniper, cumin, and basil have been claimed to have antioxidant properties [10].

Due to the increased concentration of carvacrol [29.8%] and thymol [36.5%] in Thymus spathulifolius EOs, they also had antioxidant properties. Egyptian corn silk's high levels of thymol (20.5%) and carvacrol (58.1%) were shown to be responsible for the EOs' strong antioxidant action [11]. Essential oils of Salvia cryptantha and Salvia multicaulis were discovered to be more potent antioxidants than ascorbic acid or butylated hydroxytoluene (BHT) [12]. Furthermore, it was observed that the essential oils of Curcuma zedoaria are extremely powerful radical scavengers [13]. There are numerous EO aroma components, such as terpenes and terpenoids, that have been suggested to contribute to the antioxidant activity of EOs, including:- terpinene and terpinolene in tea tree (Melaleuca alternifolia); 1,8-cineole in Mentha aquatica L., Mentha longifolia L., and Mentha piperita L.; menthone and isomenth in Mentha longifolia and Mentha piperita; thymol, eugenol and linalool in black cumin, cinnamon bark and ginger; and thymol and eugenol in thyme and clove leaf [9]. The essential oils of Thymus caespititius, Thymus camphorates, and Thymus mastichina contained significant amounts of linalool and 1,8-cineole, which had antioxidant activity similar to that of -tocopherol. Strong antioxidant activity was discovered in the essential oil of lemon balm (*Melissa officinalis* L.), which contains neral/citral, citronellal, isomenthone, and menthone [14]. Additionally, reports about EOs' *in vivo* antioxidant activity also exist. When oregano oil was given to rabbits, lipid oxidation was postponed [15]. When the same oil was given to turkeys, a lipid oxidation reduction effect comparable to that of tocopheryl acetate was seen [16].The EOs of Achillea millefolium subsp. millefolium (Asteraceae) showed a hydroxyl radical-scavenging activity by reducing the non-enzymatic lipid peroxidation of rat liver homogenate [17]. These studies suggest that EOs can be used to prevent several degenerative diseases because they are a high source of natural antioxidants. Table **1** consists of a list of plants that produce essential oils as well as their anticancer characteristics.

Table 1. List of plants that produce essential oils as well as their anticancer characteristics.

Plant Name	Important Ingredients	Part of the Plant Used	Working Mechanism	References
Achillea ligustica	Sabinol, borneol and Santolina alcohol,	Flowering part	Antioxidant activity	[18]
Agastache rugosa	Methyl chavicol	Herbal portion	Antiproliferative effect and Antimutagenic activity	[19]
Anisomeles malabarica	α-Thujone and terpenyl acetate	Leaves	Antiproliferative effect which also includes apoptosis	[20]
Astrodaucus orientalis	α-thujene,Sabinene and α-pinene	Leaves	Cytotoxic effect	[21]
Boswellia sacra	Myrcene ,α-pinene and α-Thujene	gum-resin part	SpecificicallyTumour cell-apoptosis	[22]
Calamintha origanifolia	Tetradecanoic acid, (*Z,Z*)-9,12-octadecadienoic Acid andhexadecanoic acid	Bark and wood	Antiproliferative property	[23]
Callicarpa americana	α-Humulene and 7-epi-α-eudesmol	Fruiting body and leaves	Cytotoxic effect	[24]
Capparis spinosa	isothiocyanate, isopropyl and thymol	Herbal part	Antioxidant effect	[25]
Carum copticum	Thymol and γ -terpinene	Plant after drying	Antiproliferative action	[26]
Centipeda minima	*trans*-Chrysanthenyl acetate	Marginal portion	Apoptosis induction	[27]

(Table 1) cont.....

Plant Name	Important Ingredients	Part of the Plant Used	Working Mechanism	References
Cinnamomum zeylanicum	(*E*)-Cinnamaldehyde	barks	Cytotoxic effect	[28]
Citrus aurantifolia	Eugenol, *β*-caryophyllene	fruit	Antiproliferative effect	[29]
Commiphora gileadensis	2-Decenoic acid	Balm	Selective apoptosis Induction property	[30]
Coriandrum sativum	2-Methyl-5-hexenenitrile, 3-butenyl isothiocyanate	Leaves and seeds	Antioxidant effect	[31]
Crambe orientalis	*p*-Cymene, ascaridole	Flower and leaves	Antiproliferative effect	[32]
Croton regelianus	Epicurzerenone And curdione	Leaves	Cytotoxic effect	[33]
Curcuma zedoaria	*α*-Cadinol, caryophyllene oxide, *α*-muurolol	Dried plant	Anti-tumour effect	[34]
Cyperus kyllingia	*syn*-7-Hydroxy-7-anisylnorbornene, pregeijerene	Aerial portions	Cytotoxic effect	[35]
Dictamnus dasycarpus	*cis*-*α*-Terpineol, 6,11-oxidoacor-4-ene, citronellol	Roots And bark	Cytotoxic effect	[36]
Eucalyptus benthamii	Limonene	leaves	Cytotoxic effect and Antiproliferative effect	[37]
Foeniculum vulgare	1,8-Cineole	Seeds	Antioxidant effect	[38]
Genista sessilifolia and *Genista tinctoria*	(*E*)-*β*-Ionone, hexahydrofarnesylacetone	Aerial parts	Antiproliferative effect, Cytotoxic effect	[39]
Helichrysum gymnocephalum	*β*-Caryophyllene, sabinene	Leaves	Cytotoxic effect, antioxidant activity	[40]
Lantana camara	1,8-Cineole, 1-*p*-menthen-8-ethyl acetate	Roots and leaves	Antineoplastic effect	[41]
Lavandula officinalis	(*Z*)-Citral, (*E*)-citral	Flowering part	Cytotoxic effect	[42]
Lindera strychnifolia	Eucalyptol	Leaves	Cytotoxic effect	[43]
Malus domestica	*α*-Gurjunene, *β*-selinene	Leaves	Synergistic effect	[44]
Mangifera indica	1,8-Cineole	Leaves	Cytotoxic effect	[45]
Matricaria recutita	*α*-BisabololoxideA, (*E*)-*β*-farnesene	Flowering part	Antioxidant activity and Antiproliferative effect	[46]
Melaleuca armillaris	Menthol	Leaves	Cytotoxic effect	[47]

(Table 1) cont.....

Plant Name	Important Ingredients	Part of the Plant Used	Working Mechanism	References
Mentha piperita and *Mentha spicata*	*α*-Phellandrene, *p*-cymene	Leaves	Cytotoxic effect	[48]
Moringa oleifera	Myrcene, limonene	Roots and Wood	Antitumour effect	[49]
Myrica gale	*β*-Elemene	Leaves	Cytotoxic effect	[50]
Nigella sativa and *Nigella damascene*	Methyl cinnamate	Seeds	Antioxidant activity	[51]
Ocimum basilicum	*E*)-Nerolidol	Leaves	Anticancer activity	[52]

3.1. Antimutagenic

The antimutagenic property of EOs is caused by a variety of factors. For example, EOs stop mutagens from getting into cells, neutralize mutagens through direct scavenging, stop radicals from being made by mutagens by capturing them with antioxidants, turn on antioxidant enzymes in cells, stop P450 from turning pro mutagens into mutagens, and turn on enzymes that get rid of mutagens. Antimutagenic substances work by either promoting or suppressing DNA repair that is error-free [53]. There hasn't been any investigation into the type of antimutagenicity involving DNA repair by terpenic and phenolic compounds from EOs since Kada and Shimoi's (1987) research on Escherichia coli (Sharma *et al.*, 2001). Chemicals taken from aromatic plants, like -terpineol, D-limonene, citronellal, camphor, terpinene, 1,8-cineole, and citral, changed the activity of hepatic monooxygenase by interacting with the biotransformation of pro mutagens or procarcinogens [54]. In the yeast Saccharomyces cerevisiae, EOs have been found to inhibit mitochondrial damage and apoptosis [55]. According to recent research, several EOs have antimutagenicity against UV light-induced mutations [56].

4. ANTI-INFLAMMATORY ACTIVITY

Immune system-improving techniques work when specific factors are considered, such as stress reduction, maintaining healthy intestinal bacteria, and promoting better blood and lymph quality. Aromatherapy is an approach that has largely been successful. The use of EOs in various media to enhance immune function is known as aromatherapy (Fig. **4**) (https://www.thearomablog.com/essential-oils-for-the-immune-system/). The improvement of immunological function is one of its key functions. It works in a variety of ways, such as by controlling the hormones the adrenal glands release, which lowers stress; by boosting the immune system by helping the lymphatic system remove toxins; by encouraging the production of immune-stimulating cells; and by promoting the eradication of pathogenic microorganisms. Citrus limonum and Lavendula angustifolia were used in one study to explore the effects of aromatherapy on the human immunological system. While inhaling lemon EOs improved mood and boosted norepinephrine release, additional immunological evidence contradicted the effectiveness of either EO [57]. Numerous diseases, such as asthma, inflammatory bowel disease, arthritis, multiple sclerosis, and atherosclerosis, frequently exhibit inflammation. It is a response to injury caused by harmful physical or chemical stimuli [58]. The synthesis of numerous soluble mediators of inflammation, reactive oxygen species, lipid mediators, proteases, and cytokines, as well as the accumulation of diverse inflammatory cells, are characteristics of this reaction, which is normally an acute phase response but can also become chronic [59].

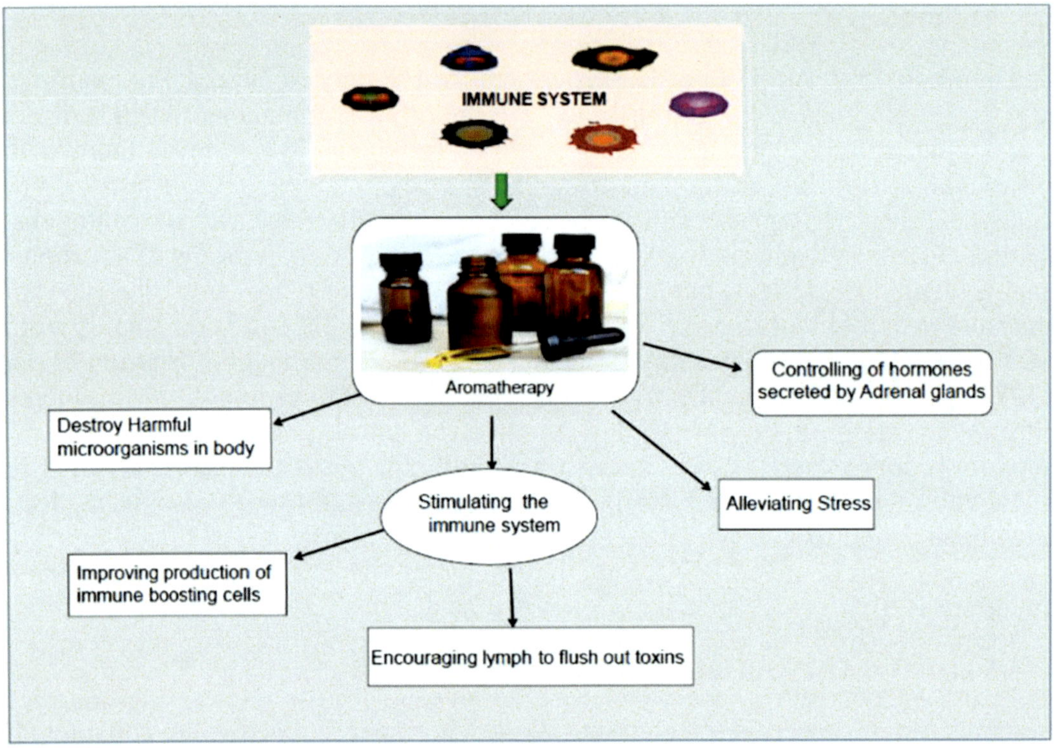

Fig. (4). How essential oils enhance immune system performance.

Additionally, macrophage cells are essential for the initiation and development of a variety of inflammatory diseases, including those brought on by septic shock and long-term inflammatory conditions. Cho *et al.*, 2009 [60] identified zedoarondiol from Curcuma heyneana, which inhibits COX-2, iNOSand pro-inflammatory cytokines by downregulating the nuclear factor NF-B pathway in LPS-stimulated murine macrophages. Eugenol, the primary constituent of many aromatic plants, was found in another study to reduce the formation of tumor necrosis factor (TNF) [61]. Japanese cryptomeria, as reported by various studies, EOs can reduce the amount of NF-B activation caused by LPS, which is crucial for the maximum production of several cytokines like TNF, IL-8, IL-1and IL-6, which are crucial for the emergence of acute inflammatory responses [62].

5. EFFECT OF ESSENTIAL OILS ON THE RESPIRATORY SYSTEM

The essential oil obtained from the plant Mentha piperita, also known as "hortel-pimenta" in Brazil, is utilized in traditional medicine for its anti-inflammatory, antispasmodic, expectorant, and anti-congestive properties. Prostaglandins and nitric oxide synthase were involved in the antispasmodic effects of peppermint oil from Mentha piperita on the rat trachea [63]. One-third of the global population is afflicted with Mycobacterium tuberculosis. Tuberculosis kills more people than any other infectious disease, and its successful management is primarily dependent on the delivery of the correct drugs. Natural products present an attractive alternative in the search for novel antimycobacterial agents [64].

The hexane extracts of *Artemisia ludoviciana*, *Chamaedora tepejilote*, *Lantana hispida*, and *Malva parviflora* were active against *M. tuberculosis* at 200 µg/mL. *J. communis* hexane extract showed activity against M. tuberculosis at 100 µg/mL. The methanol extracts of *A. ludoviciana* and *J. communis* were active against M. tuberculosis at 200 and 100 µg/mL, respectively. Activity against *M. avium* was less frequent, only J. communis hexane extract and *M. parviflora* methanol extract inhibited the bacteria at 200 and 100µg/mL, respectively [64]. The following Table **2** contains the list of important plants that are used in the treatment of respiratory diseases.

By inhalation of various gases, such as the odorless, irritating, and smelly formaldehyde,the respiratory system is affected by the gas. Being a member of the aldehyde family, formaldehyde is naturally occurs and can be found in home air, cigarette smoke, and the polluted atmosphere of cities as a result of incomplete organic combustion, photochemical smog, and chemical product release [65]. It tends to combine with protein, DNA, and RNA, which has harmful effects. It has been shown to hurt the digestive, respiratory, and central nervous systems [66]. It is increasingly being used in laboratories for anatomy, histology, and pathology. Additionally, it is employed in the creation of commercial and cosmetic goods. Its exposure through breath is thus conceivable at any time [67].

Rose oil, which is clear and light yellow and notably aromatic, predominantly comprises acyclic terpenic compounds, with citronellol accounting for 40-50 percent of the oil and geraniol accounting for 20 percent. Geraniol is responsible for the rose's distinctive scent [68]. Rose oil is utilized in aromatherapy and cosmetics as an alternative treatment. Its medical effects have also been demonstrated through numerous experiments. Various studies indicate that rose oil inhalation protects against formaldehyde-induced testicular injury [69].

Table 2. List of plants used to treat respiratory conditions.

Species and Family Names	Local Names	Part of the Plant Used	Useful in the Treatment of
Acanthus montanus (Nees).T. Anders (Acanthaceae)	Acninuwi-sechen (Bambili)	Leaf	Pneumonia
Eremomastax speciosa (L.) Juss. (Acanthaceae)	Banjam-moh (Bambui)	Leaf	Cough
Mangifera indica (Linn.) R. Br. (Anacardiaceae)	Mangro (Bambili)	Leaf	Cough and Sore throat
Xylopia aethiopica (Dunal.) A. Rich. (Annonaceae)	Kii (Bambili)	Fruiting body	Cough
Centella asiatica (Linn) Urb. (Apiaceae)	Lelapse (Balesing)	Leaf	Cough/ Hiccup
Ageratum conyzoides Linn. (Asteraceae)	Dsehshi (Bambili)	All parts of the plant	Cough/Asthma/Catarrh
Chromolaena odorata (Linn.)King.& Robinson (Asteraceae)	Christmas Bush	Leaf	Cough
Conyza sumatrensis H.B. and K. (Asteraceae)	Sidji (Lamso)	Leaf	Catarrh / Nasal congestion
Dichrocephalaintergrifolia L. (Asteraceae)	Tsishi (Kedjom-Ketingoh)	Leaf	Cough
Emilia coccinea A. Don. (Asteraceae)	Mbode (Bambili)	Leaf	Asthma/Cough
Spilanthesfilicaulis (Shum. and Thon.) C.D. Adams (Asteraceae)	Titege-nwi (Bambili)	Flower	Pneumonia
Asclepias curassavica Linn. (Asclepiadaceae)	Touhii (Kedjom-Ketingoh)	Leaf	Cough
Polyscias fulva J. R. and Forst (Araliaceae)	Ake-kwe (Bambili)	Leaf	Pneumonia
Kigeliaafricana (Lam.) Benth. (Bignoniaceae)	Etenge (Bambui, Bambili)	Stem	Pneumonia
Cordia platythyrsaBak. (Boraginaceae)	Cordia	Leaf	Cough
Ananas comosus Linn. (Bromeliaceae)	Pineapple	Fruiting body	Cough
Canarium shweinfurthii L. (Burseraceae)	Imboh (Bambili) Imbeh (Bambui)	Resin	Catarrh
Dacryodes edulis Eng. (Burcsraceae)	Atzoh (Bambui)	Resin	Catarrh

(Table 2) cont.....

Species and Family Names	Local Names	Part of the Plant Used	Useful in the Treatment of
Carica papaya Linn. (Caricaceae)	Pawpaw	Leaf	Asthma / cough
Garcinia kola Haeckel. (Clusiaceae)	Bitter kola	Seed	Cough
Bryophyllumpinnatum (Lam.) Oken (Crassulaceae)	Fezoh (Bambui) Niwuh (Bambili)	Leaf	Asthma / Nasal congestion
Brassica oleracea L. (Cruciferae)	Cabbage	Leaf	Sore throat
Cupressus semperivens Mills. (Cupressaceae)	Cypress	Resin	Catarrh
Euphorbia hirta Linn (Euphorbiaceae)	Asthma plant	All parts of the plant	Asthma
Arbrusprecatorius L. (Fabaceae)	Nzo-zurang (Babessi)	Leaf	Cough
Ocimumgratissimum L. (Lamiaceae)	Masepo (all four villages)	Leaf	Cough
Thymus vulgaris L. (Lamiaceae)	Thyme	All parts of the plant	Cough/ catarrh
Allium cepa Linn. (Liliaceae)	Nioshi (Bambili, Bambui)	Bulb	Cough / Asthma
Allium sativum Linn. (Liliaceae)	Garlic	Bulb	Cough
Aloe barbadensis Linn. (Liliaceae)	Aloe vera	Leaf	Asthma / bronchitis catarrh
Hibiscus rosa- sinensis. L. (Malvaceae)	Hibiscus flower	Flower	Throat infection
Hibiscus vitifolius L. (Malvaceae)	Wild Hibiscus	Leaf and flower	Pneumonia
Hibiscus asper Hook.F.E (Malvaceae)	Nchone (Bambili)	Leaf	Pneumonia
Pavoniaburchelli (D.C.) R.A.Duer. (Malvaceae)	Igebuo (Bambili)	All parts of Plant	Cough/ Asthma
Ficus exasperata Val. (Moraceae)	Achwini (Bambui)	Leaf	Cough/ catarrh
Ensetegilletti Linn. (Musaceae)	Tonguo (Bambili)	Root	Tuberculosis
Musa paradisiaca Walker &Sillans. (Musaceae)	Akodong (kedjom-keku)	Fruiting body and flower	Cough / asthma
Eucalyptus globulus Libille. (Myrtaceae)	Fosigar (Kedjom-keku)	Leaf and flower	Cough/catarrh/ asthma
Psidium guajava L. (Myrtaceae)	Ngabang (Bambui)	Leaf	Cough/catarrh/ bronchitis
Elaeisguineensis Jacq. (Palmae)	Njanbih (Bambili)	Cones and oils	Cough
Raphia hookeri A. Don. (Palmae)	Atoh (Bambui)	Sap	Various ailments

(Table 2) cont.....

Species and Family Names	Local Names	Part of the Plant Used	Useful in the Treatment of
Piper umbellatum Torr. (Piperaceae)	Mbode (Bambui)	Leaf	Cough
Cymbopogon citratus (D.C) Staph. (Poaceae)	Fever grass	Leaf	Catarrh/colds

6. EFFECT OF ESSENTIAL OILS ON THE NERVOUS SYSTEM

Essential oils have a long history of medicinal usage. The Bible mentions them for "mental, spiritual, and physical healing," and they're still relevant today. Odorants' pharmacological and psychological effects are now well known and frequently, the interaction of both plays a crucial role [70]. However, there are many other places where EOs are used. They are utilized as a supplement in alternative medicine, aromatherapy, massages, Chinese medicine [71], school medicine, folk medicine, the cosmetics and perfume industries, as well as in food flavorings and cleaning goods (http://en.wikipedia.org/wiki/Essential_oil). There is numerous research that discusses how EOs affect the central nervous system (CNS) [72]. The scientific literature also describes several pharmacological properties, such as antioxidative activity, antiphlogistic effects, peripheral antinociceptive effects, antiviral activity, anticancer effects, and penetration enhancement [70]. Adorjan and Buchbauer have lately explored in depth an update on these themes [73]. The goal of the current overview is to provide a similar update regarding the activities of EOs on the central nervous system (CNS), including their analgesic, anxiolytic, effects on learning, stress-relieving, memory, attention, and arousal, effects on relaxation, sedation, and sleep, effects on mood, behavior, and perception, anticonvulsive and epilepsy-treating properties and finally, effects on the treatment of Alzheimer's disease and Parkinson's [74].

6.1. Analgesic Action of Essential Oil (EOs)

Analgesic drugs attempt to reduce pain by having a variety of effects on the peripheral or central nervous systems. Analgesics can be categorized into two major groups. Opioids (*e.g.* morphine, codeine) connect to opioid receptors in the central nervous system (CNS), while non-opioids (*e.g.* aspirin and other nonsteroidal anti-inflammatory medications, NSAIDs) inhibit the cyclooxygenase enzyme (COX) in the periphery. Opioids are highly efficient analgesics, but they have many unwanted side effects, including depression, sleepiness, nausea, constipation, pruritus, miosis, respiratory, vomiting, and drug tolerance (https://en.wikipedia.org/wiki/Analgesic). There is research that employs EOs to investigate alternatives to opioids for the treatment of pain. The body's natural response to injury, damage, and inflammation is to experience pain, which initially serves as a warning system. Nevertheless, in many circumstances, long-lasting, unrelenting pain can become a problem because it becomes unmanageable without increasing analgesic dosage. The pursuit of an alternative (even everyday) therapy free of synthetic medications is thus an important one. EOs play a significant role in this regard.

6.2. Anxiolytic Action

The psychological and physiological condition of anxiety is described as having cognitive, physical, emotional, and behavioral components. Together, these elements provide an unpleasant emotion linked to anxiety, worry, and concern as well as unease. Anxiety is a major hindrance in daily living since it can strike unexpectedly and without any apparent trigger. The symptoms of anxiety are heart palpitations, tension, nausea, chest pain, shortness of breath, perspiration, shaking, pale complexion, papillary dilation, *etc*., as the body prepares to face a threat. During this time, the body is in "fight or flight" mode, which in extreme conditions can manifest as panic (http://en.wikipedia.org/wiki/Anxiety). Benzodiazepines are frequently used to treat generalized and ongoing anxiety, even though these medications have several side effects (such as sedation) and a significant risk of misuse. Alternatives, such as aromatherapy, are therefore required [75]. Anxiolytic essential oils include but are not limited to, lavender, rose, orange, bergamot, lemon, and sandalwood [76].

The most popular phytotherapeutics for treating anxiety are treatments containing lavender. Linalool, a monoterpene alcohol, is one of the key elements in lavender essential oil. Studies on SD (Sprague-Dawley) rats (male) were conducted to look into linalool's ability to reduce anxiety [77]. As a result, 44 rats were separated into four groups: control, linalool, midazolam (a positive control benzodiazepine), and linalool plus flumazenil (a benzodiazepine antagonist).To examine anxiolytic behavior, the elevated plus maze test (EPM) was used. Rodents are thus kept in a plus-shaped structure with two enclosed and two open arms. Because rats instinctively avoid open spaces, an increase in time spent on the open arm indicates an anxiety reduction [78]. The neurohormonal-physiological component was determined by determining catecholamine and corticosterone levels in the serum. The study's findings did not suggest that linalool induced anxiolysis *via* modifying the aminobutyric acid (GABAA) receptor, but it is likely that linalool influenced motor movements and locomotion [77].

Another randomized double-blind trial looked at the impact of orally delivered lavender essential oil on reactions to anxiety-inducing film clips. Lavender pills (100, 200, and placebo) were given to 97 people who watched neutral and anxiety-inducing film segments. The researchers examined mood, the Positive and Negative Affect Scale, anxiety, the State-Trait Anxiety Inventory, heart rate, galvanic skin response, and heart rate variation. The 2001 lavender dose could reduce anxiety, galvanic skin reaction, and heart rate while increasing heart rate variation in neutral films. In anxiety-inducing film clips, lavender was moderately effective in females (just on heart rate variation), whereas galvanic skin response increased in males. As a result, lavender demonstrated mild anxiolytic effects in people but did not affect high anxiety [79].

Patients who are terrified of surgical procedures or dental procedures frequently employ aromatherapy. Therefore, as demonstrated by several studies, lavender EO is a wise choice. In one of these research, it was examined whether using lavender oil instead of the usual treatment could help surgery patients feel less anxious before their procedures.150 adults were randomly assigned to one of three groups: a control group (standard care), an experimental group (standard care with the addition of essential oil), or a non-aroma group (standard care plus jojoba oil). The anxiety during admission and transfer to the operating room was measured using visual analog scales. As a result, the lavender group demonstrated much less anxiety after transfer to the operating room, indicating that lavender was a simple, inexpensive, and safe alternative that helped alleviate pre-operative anxiety and improved patient satisfaction. The authors noted that additional research on the usage of lavender in the postoperative period is welcome [80]. An optimal soothing environment (OSE), a novel non-pharmacological strategy, was studied by Hoya *et al.* to reduce anxiety in patients undergoing gastroscopy [81].

50 participants were randomized randomly into an OSE group and a control group, each of which had 24 patients (26 patients). The 6-month trial was conducted in a 150-bed acute care facility in Japan. The Face Scale score was used to gauge the level of patient anxiety. Systolic blood pressure was checked on each patient before and after a gastroscopy, and the results were compared to the reading taken when they first arrived at the hospital. The patients waiting for gastroscopy were given a safe essential oil burner with a lavender scent for the OSE as well as the digital video disc application Flow (produced by NHK software) [81].In a cluster randomized controlled study, the effects of lavender smell on dental patients' anxiety levels were studied [82]. When 340 patients waited for dental treatment, anxiety was assessed either while they were under the influence of lavender or not at all. Both overall dental anxiety and current anxiety were measured using the Modified Dental Anxiety Scale and the State-Trait Anxiety Indicator, respectively. The examination revealed equivalent moderate levels of global dental anxiety in both groups, but only the lavender group had significantly lower levels of current worry than the control group. Even if concern

about future dental visits cannot be avoided, lavender smells may help dental patients feel less anxious [82].

Researchers Woelk and Schläfke conducted a controlled clinical experiment to compare the efficacy of Silexan, a new oral lavender oil capsule formulation, to a benzodiazepine [75]. For six weeks, adults are required to take lorazepam or silexan. The Hamilton Anxiety Rating Scale (HAMA total score) was used to scientifically gauge the level of anxiety between baseline and week 6. Silexan was able to decrease generalized anxiety and was comparable to a popular benzodiazepine such as lorazepam, it was determined after the study. Two HAMA subscores, 'somatic anxiety' and 'psychic anxiety,' were reduced in both groups. Other subscores, such as the Selfrating Anxiety Scale, the Penn State Worry Questionnaire, the Clinical Global Impressions of Severity Disorder, and a sleep diary, revealed that the two drugs had equal good benefits. Overall, these findings demonstrated that Silexan was as efficacious in adults as lorazepam. It exhibited no sedative effects or drug abuse potential, suggesting that it could be a safe and well-tolerated alternative to benzodiazepines in the treatment of generalized anxiety [75].

In a subsequent investigation, the pharmaco-physio-psychological effects of Shirodhara with medicated sesame oil supplemented with lavender essential oil (EO) were studied. Shirodhara is a popular Ayurvedic oil-dripping treatment that employs medicated herbal sesame oils. Shirodhara with plain sesame oil had previously been demonstrated to have anxiolytic effects and induce an altered state of consciousness (ASC) in healthy participants. Sesame oil Shirodhara (simple Shirodhara), lavender Shirodhara (0.3vol percent), or a control group in the supine position were given to a total of 16 healthy volunteers. A robotic oil-dripping device was used to apply the oil. Anxiety levels, skin temperature on the backs of the hands and feet, heart rate, and other psychophysiological changes were all tracked during the study. When it came to anxiolytic effects, ASC, and foot skin temperature elevation, aromatherapy was the most effective. All three groups had similar results in terms of anxiolysis, ASC, psychological impacts, and raised foot skin temperature, but aroma Shirodhara's results were more significant. Three mechanisms were proposed by the authors as the basis for the psychiatric and physiological effects of lavender Shirodhara: first, the well-known sedative effects of lavender Eos, which are mediated by olfactory nerves; second, the pharmacological effects of substances when absorbed through the skin in the sesame or lavender oil; and third, the physiological effects of sesame oil dripping on the forehead, which is induced by the somatoautonomic reflex through Future treatments may be based on the complex pharmaco-physio-psychological effects of Ayurvedic oil dripping therapy [83].

Linck and his Brazilian colleagues conducted studies on the effects of breathed linalool on anxiety, social relationships, and aggressive behavior in mice [84]. Additionally, the effect on memory was evaluated. Linalool improved social relationships while decreasing hostile behavior. Anxiolytic effects were validated by the light/dark test, which involved watching whether animals stayed in the lit chamber or the dark one. The latter symbolizes anxiolysis because mice have a natural aversion to brightly lit settings. Higher linalool doses were the only ones that harmed memory. These results were taken as showing that linalool induces anxiolysis and relaxation [84].

For its anxiolytic properties, Neroli EO is a popular choice. Essential oil made from the blooms of bitter oranges is called neroli oil (*Citrus aurantium* L., Rutaceae) (https://en.wikipedia.org/wiki/Neroli). When breathed, it has anxiolytic effects on gerbils. Measurements of forced swimming tasks and locomotor activity were taken to determine anxiety levels. To compare the forced swimming test's duration time between the fragrance group and the control group, it was compared to the total distance as well as the duration time in the central and peripheral regions. The positive control was the 1,4-benzodiazepine derivative anxiolytic Xanax® (in the US; Alprazolam in Europe). In the behavioral tests, both the inhalation of neroli oil and medication with Xanax® exhibited anxiolytic effects; however, the mechanisms underlying their anxiolytic effect responses were not understood. Nonetheless, this study supports the use of neroli in the treatment of anxiety.

When anxiety, depression, and stress are linked to hormonal imbalances in women, the EO of shell flower leaves (*Alpinia zerumbet* [Pers.] B.L. Burtt and R.M. Sm, Zingiberaceae, EOAZ) is used in phytotherapy to alleviate the symptoms. Black cumin seeds (*Nigella sativa* L., Ranunculaceae) have been linked to CNS effects in pharmacological trials. The EPM and the open-field test were used by [85] to evaluate its anxiolytic effects in rats. Rats' open-field activity increased, and antianxiety benefits were also seen in the EPM after four weeks of daily administration of the oil. While the concentration of 5hydroxyindoleacetic acid, the primary metabolite of serotonin in the human body, was increased by orally administering black cumin oil, the concentration of serotonin was decreased. Increased amounts of tryptophan were found in both the brain and the plasma. Anxiolytic properties of black cumin oil were demonstrated in this study [85]. Cancer patients who receive aromatherapy massages report less anxiety. Approximately 13.9-25 percent of cancer patients also have anxiety issues. Most of these anxiety disorders are not pathological, but they can have a significant impact on one's quality of life [86]. Recently, an Italian study group published on the neuro pharmacology of *Citrus bergamia* Risso's essential oil (Rutaceae, BEO). This oil is frequently used in aromatherapy to ease the symptoms of cancer pain, moderate mood problems, and anxiety caused by stress. The study's findings demonstrated that BEO produced distinct amino acids with neurotransmitter function in the mammalian hippocampus through exocytotic and carrier-mediated mechanisms. This confirmed the hypothesis that BEO could affect both healthy and unhealthy synaptic plasticity. Additionally, there was some neuroprotection during experimental brain ischemia and pain. These findings clarify the widespread application of BEO in complementary medicine, although more investigation and application to clinical settings are required [87].

6.3. Effects of the Treatment of Stress

Hans Seyle was the first to use the word "stress" in a scientific context in 1930. Psychology and biology refer to instances when an organism can't handle emotionally or physically demanding situations, whether they are actual or imagined, as 'stress.'" (http://de.wikipedia.org/wiki/Stress.). Both people and animals are concerned by chronic stress since it can lead to physical and mental health problems. Increased alarm and adrenaline production, excessive weariness, tense muscles, excitement, and difficulty with attention are among the symptoms. There are also various physiological reactions such as headache and elevated heart rate (http://en.wikipedia.org/wiki/Stress). According to Toda and Morimoto, the lavender scent affects salivary endocrinological stress indicators [88]. Since the study's title implies, the team's focus was on lavender essential oil's potential to reduce stress, therefore they tested the stress-sensitive salivary endocrinological markers cortisol and chromogranin A. (CgA) [89]. Thirty healthy students were divided into an aroma group and a control group, and they were required to do math exercises for 10 minutes before taking a 10-minute break. The test subjects in the scent group (16 students) were exposed to an airborne lavender essential oil (EO). An enzyme-linked immunosorbent assay was used to measure the levels of cortisol and CgA in the saliva before, after, and five and ten minutes after the arithmetic tests. It was shown that CgA levels in the aroma group were considerably lower ten minutes after task completion compared to levels measured immediately following task completion, whereas no such changes were found in the control group. Cortisol levels did not differ between the two groups. As a result, the researchers concluded that lavender essential oil has anti-stress properties [88].

Limes are used to make lime essential oil (LEO). LEO is derived from the peel (*Citrus aurantifolia* [Christm.] Swingle, Rutaceae). Many tropical countries cultivate the lime plant. LEO's key ingredients are limonene and citral, and it's used to cure stress, infection, inflammation, cancer, and exhaustion, among other things [90] used 40 healthy office women between the ages of 25 and 45 to analyze the impact of aromatherapy massage with LEO on stress. To the control group or the therapy group, all probands were randomly assigned. The placebo group received non-volatile sweet almond oil as a carrier oil, whereas the 10% LEO group received the non-volatile sweet almond oil. We studied the benefits of a single 1-hour LEO massage as well as the cumulative effects of four 1-hour LEO massage sessions spread out over four weeks. Before and after the massage, stress markers such as cortisol levels, blood pressure, heart rate, and body temperature were examined. It was also utilized to examine mental health factors using the Thai General Health Questionnaire (GHQ28). Before the aroma massage, there was no significant difference between the aroma group and the placebo group in terms of cortisol levels and blood pressure. Nevertheless, a single LEO massage significantly decreased blood pressure compared to the control group, perhaps due to the stimulation of parasympathetic activity. In contrast, frequent LEO massages decreased GHQ28 levels almost as much as the control group [90]. The impact of aromatherapy before and after social skill training (SST), a crucial component of psychiatric treatment.. During the SST, some patients experience intense stress and tension. Six patients with either schizophrenia or depression took part in the study. Hand baths, aroma massages, and fragrance inhalation (10 min) were used to ease stress throughout a one-hour SST session. One of six distinct mixtures was utilized for massage and inhalation. Cortisol and immunoglobulin A (IgA) levels were determined by taking saliva samples. Cortisol levels can rise in stressful conditions, but whether or not IgA levels alter (increase or decrease) is dependent on the stressor being adjusted. An increase in saliva cortisol levels was observed during an SST, but this rise was reduced by pretreatment with EOs.Subjects who received aroma massage or inhalation had higher Ig A levels than those who did not receive aroma massage or inhalation. This study demonstrated that EOs exhibit anti-stress and calming properties, although additional research is required to corroborate these results [91].

6.4. Influence on Learning, Memory, Attention, and Arousal

In this part, the central nervous system-stimulating effects of essential oils will be described. As an example, how probands can concentrate on challenging exercises, their attention while performing activities, and their impact on performance will be a major focus of this research. Numerous studies have demonstrated the psychophysiological features of odors, but the cognitive functions remain little known. Flavors were tested to see how they affected the ability to maintain attention in a vigilance task [92]. Long-term alertness is defined as "vigilance," which is the ability to remain alert for an extended period. In the worst-case scenario, a lack of attention to safety can lead to tragic incidents in the course of normal daily activities. There were three alternative scenarios in the study: two of them had odors, either from the essential oils of *Lavandula angustifolia* Mill. (Lamiaceae) or *Eucalyptus globulus* Labill. (Myrtaceae); the third didn't have any odors at all (control). The smell was provided to the subjects *via* a constant flow olfactometer while they were doing the vigilance task; in the control scenario, there was no smell present. An observer's reaction time could be assessed by asking them to keep track of the target number '0,' while simultaneously keeping track of other distracting numbers, for 30 minutes. When compared to the control group, the reaction time of those exposed to the lavender aroma was dramatically reduced. It was concluded that lavender essential oil was able to help students keep their focus during long and hard workouts [92].In the same year, the same researchers conducted a follow-up study in which they studied the effects of lavender and eucalyptus odors on human vigilance. If you're doing an activity that requires a high level of alertness, calming fragrances like lavender are more helpful than stimulating odors. In contrast, stimulating odors are more advantageous for less demanding activities since they assist workers in remaining alert. In the study, two different pure essential oils (lavender and eucalyptus, as previously mentioned) as well as the major constituents of lavender (linalyl acetate) and peppermint (-) menthol, *Mentha piperita* L., Lamiaceae) were presented *via* a direct odor delivery system to maintain the inhalation volume as much as possible [93]. Expectation has a crucial role and may have a significant impact on the actual effectiveness of a medication, as is well-known. Robbins and Broughan conducted a study because the effects of changing a proband's expectations about an essential oil on memory have yet to be properly examined [94]. The essential oil of Spanish sage (*Salvia lavandulifolia* Vahl, Lamiaceae) was employed for the experiment. It is not often used in commercial cosmetic products, although its memory-enhancing properties are well-known. In the study, 60 participants between the ages of 19 and 45 were randomly assigned to one of three groups and were required to complete a memory test before and after receiving group-specific instructions. The first group, the "negative expectancy group," was told that Spanish sage oil would impair their memory in the second test compared to the first (which was odorless). Those in the second group dubbed the "positive expectancy group," were made to assume that Spanish sage oil would improve their recall. Because of this, the second memory test should yield a better result. There were no benefits of using Spanish sage oil for the control group to serve as a baseline. After the test, participants were told they had to complete a second memory assignment that was comparable to the one they had just completed. Second memory test scores were lower for the "negative expectancy" group than for the first memory test. The "positive expectancy group" did better in the second memory test than in the first, as was to be predicted. Surprisingly, in contrast to expectation, individuals in the control group who were not given a verbal suggestion during the second memory exercise did not recall a greater number of words. These findings demonstrate that psychological processes, particularly expectancies, which could be seen explicitly in areas of manipulating expectations, were a part of how aromatherapy worked [94].

6.5. Action on Relaxation, Sedation, and Sleep

Relaxation is an emotional state in which arousal produced by fury, fear, or worry is absent. Because of this, it is a state of reduced stress. Medical sedation is the use of sedative medicines to reduce the activity of the central nervous system (http://en.wikipedia.org/wiki/Sedation). A natural recurring state without consciousness is referred to as sleep, during which sensory and motor functions are momentarily suspended. Although there is less ability to respond to stimuli than in a coma, awakening is still easier (http://en.wikipedia.org/wiki/Sleep). Benzodiazepines are commonly used as sedatives or hypnotics to achieve a state of relaxation or drowsiness or to induce sleep. To put it another way, a single medication might have a plethora of effects. Some overlap exists between the terms "sedative" and "hypnotic," and it should be noted (http: //en.wi kip edia.o rg/wi ki/S ed ati ve).

In this section, the use of essential oils in addition to or in place of conventional medication will be discussed. Hongratanaworakit researched the soothing effects of rose oil (Rosa damascena Mill., Rosaceae) on humans. The EO was applied to the skin and the effects on the autonomic and emotional systems of 40 healthy volunteers were studied after it had been absorbed through the skin. The test subjects were required to wear breathing masks to prevent inhalation of the odor and potential olfactory stimulation. To evaluate the autonomic parameters, blood pressure, breathing rate, blood oxygen saturation, pulse rate, and skin temperature were measured. We employed rating scales to evaluate emotional responses. Compared to a placebo, rose oil significantly decreased autonomic parameters such as breathing rate, blood oxygen saturation, and blood pressure, indicating a reduction in autonomic arousal. In terms of emotional dimensions, the odor group felt more relaxed and peaceful, but less watchful than the non-odor group. These findings persuaded the author of the calming properties of rose oil and supported its use in aromatherapy, even for the treatment of depression or stress in humans [95]. The lavender essential oil has a reputation for promoting relaxation, although there is conflicting empirical evidence to support this claim. Several earlier research, according to [96], may have been influenced by anticipation. Therefore, these scientists devised a study to evaluate whether lavender (Lavandula angustifolia Mill., Lamiaceae) scent, anticipation, or both influence post-stress relaxation. In a double-blind, placebo-controlled trial, 96 healthy female college students participated. After an exhilarating cognitive exam, the probands were exposed to the lavender aroma, a placebo, or no aroma while they relaxed. When the scent was introduced, the student's expectations were modified so that they believed the aroma would influence their ability to relax. Consequently, the scent did not affect the galvanic skin responses observed during relaxing. However, the authors hypothesized that prior associations of lavender aromatherapy with relaxation were probably driven by expectations; they are susceptible to manipulation [96].

6.6. Anticonvulsive Action and Treatment of Epilepsy

Epilepsy is a chronic, recurrent condition characterized by paroxysmal manifestations of its symptoms. It is brought on by an increase in neuronal activity and a lowering of the seizure threshold in the central nervous system [97].One theory put out is that neurons can release large amounts of the excitatory neurotransmitter glutamate, which can bind to glutamatergic neurons and lead to an excessive calcium release in the postsynaptic cells. Another hypothesis is that mutations make GABA (an inhibitory neurotransmitter) less effective in its function.There are over 40 distinct forms of epilepsy, each with its own set of seizure characteristics, typical onset age, EEG finding, treatment, and prognosis. Epilepsy affects an estimated 50 million individuals globally. Epilepsy can be treated but not cured with medication; nonetheless, 30% of people still experience uncontrolled seizures even if they are taking the finest available drugs (http://en.wikipeida.org/wiki/Epilepsy). Pathan *et al.*, [98] investigated the anticonvulsant effect of safranal in mice with status epilepticus (SE). SE is a unique kind of epilepsy that is defined by continuous seizure activity for more than 30 minutes or by discontinuous seizure activity and unconsciousness for more than 30 minutes and is also related to death. Natural bioactive compounds are in high demand due to the prevalence of unwanted side effects in synthetic medicines. Safranal, a monoterpene aldehyde, is the active component of *Crocus sativus* L. stigma extract (Iridaceae) and is responsible for the saffron aroma. This volatile oil's agonistic activity on GABAA receptors is ascribed to its anticonvulsant properties. For an experiment, SE was generated in mice by administering phenytoin (50 mg/kg) intravenously and pentylene tetrazole (PTZ, 100mg/kg) subcutaneously two hours later. 36 animals were divided into one of six groups.The first group received normal saline as a control, the second group received diazepam as a positive control, the third, fourth, and fifth groups were supplied safranal at varying doses (0.1, 0.2, or 0.4 ml/kg), and the final group was treated with sesame oil as vehicle control. Only diazepam provided complete protection against PTZ-induced SE, whereas normal saline and sesame oil exhibited no action. At lower doses, safranal did not exhibit an anticonvulsive effect, but at greater levels, considerable protection was seen. Due to these data, the authors hypothesized that safranal protected rats against PTZ-induced SE and mortality in a dose-dependent manner. In light of this, safranal could be a viable future adjunct medication for the treatment of SE [98]. Terpinen-4-ol, a monoterpenoid alcohol, is a component of several EOs from various plants. According to a study, similar monoterpenoid alcohols have already demonstrated their anticonvulsant efficacy in animal models [99]. When they administered terpinene-4-ol to mice, they noticed a notable decrease in spontaneous motor activity, an increase in the time before seizures induced by PTZ and convulsions brought on by picrotoxin, as well as a decrease in the number of tonic hind paw convulsions [99]. Wahab and his team used common animal seizure models, such as the maximal electroshock model or the PTZ, strychnine, and bicuculline test, to analyze the anticonvulsant effects of the volatile oil of nutmeg (*Myristica fragrans* Houtt., Myristicaceae). Although the anticonvulsive effect of nutmeg oil did not last very long, it was significantly anticonvulsant effective in the MES model. When PTZ-induced jerks were used to generate it, it even exhibited dose-dependent anticonvulsive action. The trials demonstrated that nutmeg EO could postpone the onset of strychnine-induced seizures in the extensor muscles of the hind limb. At higher doses, weak pro-convulsant action against PTZ and bicuculline was seen despite the results pointing to an anticonvulsive potency at lower doses. However, nutmeg oil exhibited a broad therapeutic index because, in the neurotoxicity test, dosages up to 600µl/kg did not decrease locomotor activity. Additionally, the LD50 value (2150µl/kg) was significantly larger than the amounts required to have an anticonvulsant effect (50–300µl/kg). Based on these findings, the scientists hypothesized that nutmeg oil could potentially be used to treat grand mal and partial seizures, as it prevented convulsions in conventional animal models. Due to a modest enhancement of clonic seizure activity, nutmeg volatile oil cannot be recommended for the treatment of myoclonic and absence seizures [100]. The volatile oil of half a bar (*Cymbopogon proximuschst.* ex A. Rich., Poaceae) was analyzed for its chemical and pharmacological properties [101]. Folk medicine in Egypt uses this herb as an antispasmodic and diuretic. Hydro distillation was used to extract the EO, which was then analyzed using GC/MS. Piperitone was the most prominent peak in the chromatogram, which showed eight peaks based on the eight principal components (72.4 percent). It was shown that the oral absorption of the EO ranged from 80 to 90 percent in rats and mice that were given it orally and intravenously. In anesthetized rats, intraperitoneal administration of volatile oil lowered arterial blood pressure in a dose-dependent manner. There were no significant changes in the heart rate except in the highest dose, where a 16 percent drop was observed. Atropine and mepyramine could not reverse these declines, but indomethacin could. The electrocardiogram (ECG) did not show any significant shifts. In the seizure tests, EO was administered i.p. (1,2ml/kg) to mice, followed by electric shock, PTZ, picrotoxin, or strychnine to induce convulsions. Only 100% protection against electrically induced convulsions was reported. Additionally, oil provided to pigeons at doses between 0.4 and 0.8 ml/kg was able to prevent ouabain-induced vomiting. In conclusion, the essential oil demonstrated cardio-depressant, antiemetic, and anticonvulsant properties [101].

6.7. Action on Dementia and Alzheimer's Disease

Alzheimer's disease (AD), the most common neurodegenerative condition, is characterized by a deficiency in cholinergic-mediated neurotransmission that contributes to cognitive dysfunction and memory loss. Treatment with AChEIs such as tacrine, donepezil, rivastigmine, or galanthamine can help alleviate the symptoms of Alzheimer's disease. Weakening of AChE, which hydrolyzes the neurotransmitter Acetylcholine (AChE), can be prevented by binding to the enzyme's active site reversibly (ACh). As a result, the synaptic cleft's ACh content rises, alleviating symptoms of Alzheimer's disease. Rivastigmine, the only inhibitor of butyrylcholinesterase (BuChE), which hydrolyzes ACh in the peripheral nervous system, might elicit peripheral cholinergic-related adverse effects [102]. (Okello *et al*., 2008) [102] examined the *in vitro* suppression of human acetyl and butyrylcholinesterase by *Narcissus poeticus* L. flower absolute, also a part of the Amaryllidaceae family. The GC/MS analysis of the floral absolute revealed three significant constituents: benzyl alcohol (11.0 percent), phenylethyl alcohol (17.5 percent), and benzyl benzoate (19.0 percent). Geranial, neral, linalool, cymene, and 1,8-cineole were detected at significantly lower concentrations, and these individual scents inhibit cholinesterase. Several dilutions of the absolute were made before the start of the testing in 80 percent ethanol. Ellman's innovative colorimetric approach for 96-well microtitre plates was utilized to measure the inhibition of cholinesterase. This reaction was initiated by mixing the various components in the microtiter plates, including human erythrocyte AChE and human serum BuChE dilutions, and then incubating everything for a while. At a wavelength of 405 nm, the change in absorbance kinetic mode was observed, and two controls were included for comparison. Doses of 0.1 mg/ml or more of AChE and BuChE were found to inhibit both enzymes by 39.1 percent. The authors concluded that it was unclear whether or not *N. poeticus* L. could be used therapeutically. Narcissus species extracts are infrequently utilized in aromatherapy but are commonly employed in the perfume industry. *N. poeticus* L. absolute, as stated, had mostly behavioral effects, therefore it might be used in additional cognitive domains. Additional research must be conducted [102]. In persons suffering from severe dementia, agitation is the most common symptom. It is characterized by agitation and aggressive behavior, which can be hazardous to family members or nursing personnel. Although the efficacy is not satisfactory and there are several negative effects, neuroleptic medications are commonly used. As a result, the potential of EOs derived from *Melissa officinalis* L. and *Lavandula angustifolia* Mill., both

Lamiaceae, in the treatment of agitation in persons suffering from severe dementia were studied [103]. Both have been shown to have relaxing and sedative characteristics, as well as the ability to improve memory. In addition, radioligand binding was performed to determine the receptor binding characteristics. Balm oil (EO of *M. officinalis*) and lavender both decreased radioligand binding to muscarinic M1, 5HT2A, histamine H3, and GABAA receptor channel sites, according to the results. Compared to lavender oil, melaleuca oil had a larger range of receptor binding properties, and it even had the potential to influence the affinity of 5HT1A receptors and the agonist site of the GABAA receptor for agonists. Because lavender and balm oil interactwith several neurotransmitter receptors, they can be utilized to alleviate agitation symptoms, as indicated by radioligand binding. But balm oil can also help patients spend more time engaged in productive tasks, thereby reducing the amount of time they are socially isolated [103].

With a focus on ligand-gated ion channels, a dual radioligand binding and electrophysiological study was conducted by [104]. To evaluate the pharmacological makeup of the EOs derived from the plants just now covered. Both, as was previously indicated, are clinically effective in the management of agitations. The rat forebrain GABAA receptor channel was suppressed by lavender oil's ability to bind TBPS (tbutylbicyclophosphorothionate), but it did not affect NMDA, AMPA, or nicotinic acetylcholine receptors. Flunitrazepam binding could be inhibited by combining both EOs (50:50), while single oils had no impact. Lavender oil reversibly suppressed GABA-induced currents in a dose-dependent manner, according to electrophysiological experiments with rat cortical cultures, but it did not affect NMDA or AMPA-induced currents. On neurotransmission, the lavender essential oil has a depressing impact [104]. There were no effects on GABAA or NMDA-induced currents when the EO of *Melissa officinalis* L. (Lamiaceae) was used, as was the case with lavender fragrance. In this article, we discussed the pharmacological characteristics of various essential oils (EOs) [105]. Patients with dementia were also studied for the effects of *L. angustifolia* ill. on their agitated behavior [106]. The crossover randomized clinical experiment included seventy Chinese old people who had either Alzheimer's disease, vascular dementia, or another form of dementia. Groups of people were splintered into two. The scent group had to inhale lavender EO for three weeks, then switch to the control group, which received an odorless sunflower mixture to inhale for another three weeks; the other group did the opposite. Clinical response was evaluated using the Chinese version of the Cohen–Mansfield Agitation Inventory (CCMAI) and Neuropsychiatric Inventory (CNPI). As a result, the mean CCMAI and CNPI scores decreased following lavender aromatherapy. In conclusion, lavender therapy was well tolerated throughout the research and indicated a significant reduction in dementia agitation. Therefore aromatherapy with lavender could be a significant complement or substitute for psychotropic drugs [106].

7. EFFECT OF ESSENTIAL OILS ON THE SKIN

Massage with EOs increased circulation, allowing new nutrients and waste products to reach the tissues. Softer, more supple skin thanks to enhanced elasticity that helps to repair scar tissue more quickly, as well as decrease stretch marks. Faster desquamation promotes new cell growth and a healthier, more radiant complexion. Acne is a prevalent skin condition that can afflict anyone at any stage of life, from puberty to adulthood [107]. Regardless of the patient's age, both the initial lesions of acne—papules, pustules, and comedones—and the secondary lesions—post-inflammatory hyperpigmentation, erythema, and scarring—can have a significant psychosocial impact [108]. In many fields of medicine, including dermatology, complementary and alternative medicine (CAM) is well-liked by patients and consumers. This is largely because these treatments are thought to be more "natural" than allopathic prescription drugs, which makes them safer and thought to have fewer side effects [109]. Some of the most frequent complementary and alternative medicine (CAM) methods used in dermatology include topical agents (usually plant extracts), essential oils/aromatherapy, herbal therapy, and acupuncture [110]. Psoralens, capsaicin, indigo, and podophyllin are only a few examples of well-known single-compound botanicals in dermatology. Green tea extract and aloe vera leaf oil are two complex polyphenol phytochemical botanicals that have been researched for the treatment of acne [111].

7.1. Essential Oils and Aromatherapy as Alternative Therapy for Acne

7.1.1. Tea Tree Oil (TTO)

Tea tree oil is the common name for the essential oil extracted from the *Melaleuca alternifolia* plant, which has been used medicinally in several nations for decades. TTO exhibits broad-spectrum antibacterial action *via* non-specific cell membrane disruption [112]. It is found in a variety of over-the-counter acne treatments (face/body washes/cleansers, soaps, toners, treatment gels or lotions, blemish sticks, and masks). An analysis of botanicals used in dermatology revealed that TTO "may have the potential to become conventional treatment" for acne [113].

7.1.2. Copaiba

Copaiba is an oleoresin extracted from the trunks of Copaifera tree species grown in South America. As a "skin-healing agent," it has been used for generations in

Central and South America, particularly in Brazil, where it is popular. The anti-inflammatory, therapeutic, and antibacterial properties of oil resin are well-known in traditional medicine. As a biological defensive mechanism for the plant against predators and disease, the diterpine chemicals in Copaiba oil are principally responsible for its medicinal effects [114].

7.1.3. Sandalwood Oil

In several Asian countries, sandalwood oil is used to treat inflammatory and skin eruptions. Concentrations as low as 0.06 percent had antibacterial effects on *S aureus*, *S epidermis*, and *P acnes*. Inhibition of COX-1 and -2 and 12-lipoxygenase pathways, as well as lipo-polysaccharide, stimulated dermal fibroblasts and keratinocyte models, are likely to be responsible for anti-inflammatory effects [115].

7.1.4. Rosemary Extract

At least three bioactive components are present in rosemary extract: rosmarinic acid, carnosol, and carnosic acid. These have distinct effects on cytokine production modulation. *In vivo*, animal models have demonstrated that inhibition/suppression of cytokine production inhibits P acnes-induced inflammation. *In vitro*, rosemary extract may also inhibit NF-kB activation and normalize TLR-2. While rosemary extract may offer anti-inflammatory properties to cosmeceutical or dermatological products, injection of rosemary extract in a mouse model was not related to skin irritation or inflammation [116].

7.1.4. Jeju Essential Oil

Thymus plants are the source of Jeju essential oil. a 2009 study found that Jeju essential oil may have antibacterial activity against the acne bacterium *P acnes*, suggesting that it could be effective in the treatment of acne [117].

7.1.5. Korean Citrus

The antibacterial efficacy of Citrus obovoides and Citrus natsuyadai essential oils against P. acnes and S. epidermidis was assessed. Possible involvement in treating acne may be suggested by lower P acnes IL-8 and TNF production [118].

8. EFFECT OF ESSENTIAL OILS ON MUSCLES, JOINTS, AND THE CIRCULATION

Oils with a rubefacient effect are beneficial for joints and muscles because they warm and promote blood flow, which brings oxygen to stiff or inflexible muscles and joints and aids in the removal of waste products like carbon dioxide and lactic acid buildup. Conditions like rheumatoid arthritis that cause persistent pain can be treated using essential oils (RA). An autoimmune illness, this type of arthritis makes your body's immune system attack your joints. It results in swelling, discomfort, and joint tissue inflammation. Rheumatoid arthritis can permanently harm joints and cartilage if it is not treated. If the patient has rheumatoid arthritis, his doctor may have recommended medications to lessen pain and inflammation. The use of essential oils is a secure complementary or alternative pain management strategy. Essential oils must be diluted with carrier oils such as coconut oil, sweet almond oil, olive oil, avocado oil, jojoba oil, argan oil, and grapeseed oil before applying topically [119].

8.1. Eucalyptus Oil

Eucalyptus oil has analgesic and anti-inflammatory properties. This oil may also improve circulation. Researchers examined the effects of eucalyptus aromatherapy on pain control following total knee replacement. The study found that after this procedure, inhaling eucalyptus oil can significantly lower inflammation, pain, and blood pressure. Applying this diluted oil or gel to the affected area will reduce inflammation and relieve discomfort if you have rheumatoid arthritis [120].

8.2. Ginger Oil

Ginger is a common remedy utilized for its anti-inflammatory and pain-relieving qualities. A 2001 study by reliable Sources examined the analgesic benefits of ginger on osteoarthritis patients' joint and knee pain. More than half of the individuals in the study reported a reduction in knee pain while consuming ginger extract as opposed to a placebo. Additionally, they used fewer medicines to alleviate their joint discomfort over time. A few drops of ginger oil can be applied topically to the affected area to treat pain. After rubbing the region with oil, apply a warm compress for extra relief. Noting that it is possible to be allergic to ginger when used topically, you should always perform a patch test first [121].

8.3. Turmeric Oil

Turmeric is a herb that has medicinal properties. Curcumin, an effective anti-inflammatory chemical, is present in turmeric. Turmeric can be used as an essential oil to lessen inflammation, increase blood flow, and enhance digestion. You can infuse turmeric essential oil into the air or apply turmeric oil directly to the affected area to treat rheumatoid arthritis. When cooking, turmeric, a spice with a strong reputation for healing, can be used [122].

8.4. Frankincense Oil

Frankincense comes from the dried sap of Boswellia trees. It has been burned as incense for a very long time. It is also known for being antiseptic, healing, and reducing inflammation. A study confirmed that frankincense could be used to treat inflammatory symptoms, especially those caused by osteoarthritis. Apply diluted frankincense oil to the area with rheumatoid arthritis to treat it [123].

8.5. Orange Oil

Essential oil from the orange fruit has antibacterial, anti-inflammatory, and antidepressant effects. Patients experiencing discomfort from fractured limbs benefited from aromatherapy using an orange essential oil. Researchers found that those who inhaled orange oil experienced less discomfort than those who did not and concluded that it might be used in conjunction with other treatments. Pain from arthritis can be relieved by applying and massaging diluted orange oil on your skin. Add a few drops of diluted orange oil to your bath to help you relax and alleviate any aches and pains you may be experiencing. Citrus essential oils should never be exposed to sunlight after applying topically. Certain essences have a specific influence on the blood and the flow of circulation in the case of the blood circulation system: High blood pressure can be effectively treated with hypotensive oils (hypertension). Lavender, Marjoram, Ylang Ylang, and Lemon are all hypotensive oils. Using hypertensive oils can assist in raisingblood pressure, which is just as harmful as having low blood pressure. Aromatic herbs such as Rosemary, Black Pepper, Eucalyptus, and Ginger are all known to raise blood pressure.

Rubefacient oils, on the other hand, have a warming impact on the skin. They aid in the reduction of edema and inflammation by constricting capillaries. Cypress, lemon, and clary sage are just a few of the many tonics available. This type of oil is known as a rubefacient, or warming oil because it warms the tissues where it's being applied. There is a more efficient flow of blood in that location because of this. Consequently, the transport of oxygen and food, as well as the evacuation of waste, aids in the healing process. Black pepper, rosemary, ginger, lemon, and eucalyptus are all rubefacients [124].

8.6. Effect of Essential Oils on the Reproductive System

The use of therapeutic plants in traditional medicine is not new. To control fertility, herbal therapies have been used safely. Dill, also known as *Anethum graveolens* L., is a plant that belongs to the Umbelliferae family and has pharmacological effects that include antibacterial action [125], effects on hyperlipidemia and hypercholesterolemia, and antiproliferative activity [125,

126]. Dill is used as a traditional treatment to help women have easier periods and increase milk supply. Rats' estrous cycle was lengthened by the plants *Calotropis procera* (Asclepiadaceae) and *Rivea hypocrateriformis* (Convolvulaceae) [127, 128]. Carvone (58.11), limonene (37.12), trans-dihydrocarvone (2.67), -phellandrene (0.83), myrcene (0.16), -pinene (0.03), and cis-dihydrocarvone (0.01) are the extract of *Anethum graveolens* L. that may affect the luteal phase of the estrous cycle [129].

Due to the increased release of chemicals into the environment, attention must be paidto a better knowledge of their toxicity in human and ecotoxicological repercussions. Numerous studies indicate that environmental toxins interfere with male reproduction and are a significant factor in the declining amount and quality of human sperm [130].

According to numerous studies, repeated exposure to pyrethrinoid can reduce fertility, degrade the quality of semen, and lead to testicular degeneration, male reproductive failure, and abnormalities in the fetuses of rodents [131, 132]. A type-II pyrethroid synthetic pesticide known as deltamethrin [(R, S)] has been used extensively to control harmful insects in horticulture, forestry, and agriculture [133]. One of the herbs with the highest antioxidant activity is known as rose-scented geranium (Pelargonium graveolens L'Hér.). The use of essential oils as folk medicine has lately spread to encompass therapy against a variety of inflammatory disorders. Many of the novel medications that have been developed in recent years come from natural sources [134]. In the past, geranium essential oil was used to cure cancer, heavy menstrual flow, inflammation, hemorrhoids, and dysentery [135]. It is a significant naturally occurring antioxidant that, by conjugating with compounds, guards against free radical damage and facilitates detoxification. It is absorbed by enzymes related to geranium under oxidative stress to detoxify the peroxides created owing to enhanced lipid peroxidation. A large dose of geranium-containing essential oil greatly reduced these effects. According to experimental findings, geranium's antioxidant properties can effectively alleviate the oxidative stress caused by deltamethrin in the mouse testis [136].

CONCLUSION

The natural extracts of plants in the form of essential oils are very beneficial for human health. Today their role is very important and becoming popular in our day-to-day life for the treatment of numerous diseases. Their role as alternative natural remedial is widely accepted all over the globe. Their use in the treatment of human health problems is growing in such a way that people are ready to accept natural aromatherapy. Its herbs and plants are planted in large numbers to fulfill the large demand for essential oils in the market. As described in the chapter, their use covers major health problems of human health like cancer treatment, immunotherapy, treatment of skin diseases, respiratory problems, reproductive problems, neurological diseases, mental stress, muscular, joint, and blood circulation-related diseases, and various other health issues.

REFERENCES

[1] Winkelman WJ. Aromatherapy, botanicals, and essential oils in acne. Clin Dermatol 2018; 36(3): 299-305.
[http://dx.doi.org/10.1016/j.clindermatol.2018.03.004] [PMID: 29908571]

[2] Kiecolt-Glaser JK, Graham JE, Malarkey WB, Porter K, Lemeshow S, Glaser R. Olfactory influences on mood and autonomic, endocrine, and immune function. Psychoneuroendocrinology 2008; 33(3): 328-39.
[http://dx.doi.org/10.1016/j.psyneuen.2007.11.015] [PMID: 18178322]

[3] Stevensen CJ. Aromatherapy in dermatology. Clin Dermatol 1998; 16(6): 689-94.
[http://dx.doi.org/10.1016/S0738-081X(98)00058-3] [PMID: 9949913]

[4] Bhalla Y, Gupta VK, Jaitak V. Anticancer activity of essential oils: A review. J Sci Food Agric 2013; 93(15): 3643-53.
[http://dx.doi.org/10.1002/jsfa.6267] [PMID: 23765679]

[5] Moon JK, Shibamoto T. Antioxidant assays for plant and food components. J Agric Food Chem 2009; 57(5): 1655-66.
[http://dx.doi.org/10.1021/jf803537k] [PMID: 19182948]

[6] Stadler RH, Markovic J, Turesky RJ. *In vitro* anti- and pro-oxidative effects of natural polyphenols. Biol Trace Elem Res 1995; 47(1-3): 299-305.
[http://dx.doi.org/10.1007/BF02790130] [PMID: 7779561]

[7] Van Houten B, Woshner V, Santos JH. Role of mitochondrial DNA in toxic responses to oxidative stress. DNA Repair 2006; 5(2): 145-52.
[http://dx.doi.org/10.1016/j.dnarep.2005.03.002] [PMID: 15878696]

[8] Azmi AS, Bhat SH, Hanif S, Hadi SM. Plant polyphenols mobilize endogenous copper in human peripheral lymphocytes leading to oxidative DNA breakage: A putative mechanism for anticancer properties. FEBS Lett 2006; 580(2): 533-8.
[http://dx.doi.org/10.1016/j.febslet.2005.12.059] [PMID: 16412432]

[9] Wei A, Shibamoto T. Antioxidant/lipoxygenase inhibitory activities and chemical compositions of selected essential oils. J Agric Food Chem 2010; 58(12): 7218-25.
[http://dx.doi.org/10.1021/jf101077s] [PMID: 20499917]

[10] Tomaino A, Cimino F, Zimbalatti V, *et al.* Influence of heating on antioxidant activity and the chemical composition of some spice essential oils. Food Chem 2005; 89(4): 549-54.
[http://dx.doi.org/10.1016/j.foodchem.2004.03.011]

[11] El-Ghorab A, El-Massry KF, Shibamoto T. Chemical composition of the volatile extract and antioxidant activities of the volatile and nonvolatile extracts of Egyptian corn silk (Zea mays L.). J Agric Food Chem 2007; 55(22): 9124-7.
[http://dx.doi.org/10.1021/jf071646e] [PMID: 17914872]

[12] Tepe B, Donmez E, Unlu M, *et al.* Antimicrobial and antioxidative activities of the essential oils and methanol extracts of Salvia cryptantha (Montbret et Aucher ex Benth.) and Salvia multicaulis (Vahl). Food Chem 2004; 84(4): 519-25.
[http://dx.doi.org/10.1016/S0308-8146(03)00267-X]

[13] Mau J, Lai EY, Wang NP, Chen CC, Chang CH, Chyau CC. Composition and antioxidant activity of

the essential oil from Curcuma zedoaria. Food Chem 2003; 82(4): 583-91. [http://dx.doi.org/10.1016/S0308-8146(03)00014-1]

[14] Mimica-Dukic N, Bozin B, Sokovic M, Simin N. Antimicrobial and antioxidant activities of *Melissa officinalis* L. (Lamiaceae) essential oil. J Agric Food Chem 2004; 52(9): 2485-9. [http://dx.doi.org/10.1021/jf030698a] [PMID: 15113145]

[15] Botsoglou NA, Florou-Paneri P, Christaki E, Giannenas I, Spais AB. Performance of rabbits and oxidative stability of muscle tissues as affected by dietary supplementation with Oregano essential oil. Arch Anim Nutr 2004; 58(3): 209-18. [http://dx.doi.org/10.1080/00039420410001701404] [PMID: 15264670]

[16] Papageorgiou G, Botsoglou N, Govaris A, Giannenas I, Iliadis S, Botsoglou E. Effect of dietary oregano oil and α -tocopheryl acetate supplementation on iron-induced lipid oxidation of turkey breast, thigh, liver and heart tissues. J Anim Physiol Anim Nutr 2003; 87(9-10): 324-35. [http://dx.doi.org/10.1046/j.1439-0396.2003.00441.x] [PMID: 14507415]

[17] Candan F, Unlu M, Tepe B, *et al.* Antioxidant and antimicrobial activity of the essential oil and methanol extracts of Achillea millefolium subsp. millefolium Afan. (Asteraceae). J Ethnopharmacol 2003; 87(2-3): 215-20. [http://dx.doi.org/10.1016/S0378-8741(03)00149-1] [PMID: 12860311]

[18] Tuberoso CIG, Kowalczyk A, Coroneo V, Russo MT, Dessì S, Cabras P. Chemical composition and antioxidant, antimicrobial, and antifungal activities of the essential oil of Achillea ligustica all. J Agric Food Chem 2005; 53(26): 10148-53. [http://dx.doi.org/10.1021/jf0518913] [PMID: 16366708]

[19] Kim MH, Chung WT, Kim YK, *et al.* The effect of the oil of Agastache rugosa O. Kuntze and three of its components on human cancer cell lines. J Essent Oil Res 2001; 13(3): 214-8. [http://dx.doi.org/10.1080/10412905.2001.9699669]

[20] Preethy CP, Padmapriya R, Periasamy VS, *et al.* Antiproliferative property of n-hexane and chloroform extracts of Anisomeles malabarica (L). R. Br. in HPV16-positive human cervical cancer cells. J Pharmacol Pharmacother 2012; 3(1): 26-34. [http://dx.doi.org/10.4103/0976-500X.92500] [PMID: 22368413]

[21] Razavi SM, Imanzadeh G, Dolati S, *et al.* Phytochemical prospection and biological activity of Astrodaucus orientalis (L.) Drude growing wild in Iran. Pharmacologia 2011; 2(10): 299-303. [http://dx.doi.org/10.5567/pharmacologia.2011.299.303]

[22] Suhail MM, Wu W, Cao A, *et al.* Boswellia sacra essential oil induces tumor cell-specific apoptosis and suppresses tumor aggressiveness in cultured human breast cancer cells. BMC Complement Altern Med 2011; 11(1): 129. [http://dx.doi.org/10.1186/1472-6882-11-129] [PMID: 22171782]

[23] Formisano C, Rigano D, Napolitano F, *et al.* Volatile constituents of Calamintha origanifolia Boiss. growing wild in Lebanon. Nat Prod Commun 2007; 2(12): 1934578X0700201213.

[24] Jones WP, Lobo-Echeverri T, Mi Q, *et al.* Cytotoxic constituents from the fruiting branches of Callicarpa americana collected in southern Florida. J Nat Prod 2007; 70(3): 372-7. [http://dx.doi.org/10.1021/np060534z] [PMID: 17279798]

[25] Kulisic-Bilusic T, Schmöller I, Schnäbele K, Siracusa L, Ruberto G. The anticarcinogenic potential of essential oil and aqueous infusion from caper (Capparis spinosa L.). Food Chem 2012; 132(1): 261-7. [http://dx.doi.org/10.1016/j.foodchem.2011.10.074] [PMID: 26434289]

[26] Yin Q, Yan F, Zu XY, *et al.* Anti-proliferative and pro-apoptotic effect of carvacrol on human hepatocellular carcinoma cell line HepG-2. Cytotechnology 2012; 64(1): 43-51. [http://dx.doi.org/10.1007/s10616-011-9389-y] [PMID: 21938469]

[27] Su M, Wu P, Li Y, Chung HY. Antiproliferative effects of volatile oils from Centipeda minima on human nasopharyngeal cancer CNE cells. Nat Prod Commun 2010; 5(1): 1934578X1000500135.

[http://dx.doi.org/10.1177/1934578X1000500135]

[28] Unlu M, Ergene E, Unlu GV, Zeytinoglu HS, Vural N. Composition, antimicrobial activity and *in vitro* cytotoxicity of essential oil from Cinnamomum zeylanicum Blume (Lauraceae). Food Chem Toxicol 2010; 48(11): 3274-80. [http://dx.doi.org/10.1016/j.fct.2010.09.001] [PMID: 20828600]

[29] Patil JR, Jayaprakasha GK, Chidambara Murthy KN, Tichy SE, Chetti MB, Patil BS. Apoptosis-mediated proliferation inhibition of human colon cancer cells by volatile principles of Citrus aurantifolia. Food Chem 2009; 114(4): 1351-8. [http://dx.doi.org/10.1016/j.foodchem.2008.11.033]

[30] Amiel E, Ofir R, Dudai N, Soloway E, Rabinsky T, Rachmilevitch S. β-Caryophyllene, a compound isolated from the biblical balm of gilead (Commiphora gileadensis), is a selective apoptosis inducer for tumor cell lines. Evid-based Complement Alternat Med 2012; 2012.

[31] Alenzi FQ, El-Bolkiny YES, Salem ML. Protective effects of *Nigella sativa* oil and thymoquinone against toxicity induced by the anticancer drug cyclophosphamide. Br J Biomed Sci 2010; 67(1): 20-8. [http://dx.doi.org/10.1080/09674845.2010.11730285] [PMID: 20373678]

[32] Razavi SM, Nejad-Ebrahimi S. Chemical composition, allelopatic and cytotoxic effects of essential oils of flowering tops and leaves of *Crambe orientalis* L. from Iran. Nat Prod Res 2009; 23(16): 1492-8. [http://dx.doi.org/10.1080/14786410802611303] [PMID: 19662570]

[33] Bezerra DP, Filho JDBM, Alves APNN, *et al.* Antitumor activity of the essential oil from the leaves of Croton regelianus and its component ascaridole. Chem Biodivers 2009; 6(8): 1224-31. [http://dx.doi.org/10.1002/cbdv.200800253] [PMID: 19697341]

[34] Chen W, Lu Y, Gao M, Wu J, Wang A, Shi R. Anti-angiogenesis effect of essential oil from Curcuma zedoaria *in vitro* and *in vivo.* J Ethnopharmacol 2011; 133(1): 220-6. [http://dx.doi.org/10.1016/j.jep.2010.09.031] [PMID: 20920565]

[35] Pyne SG, Liawruangrath B, Liawruangrath S, Garson M, Khamsan S, Teerawutkulrag A. Antimalarial, anticancer, antimicrobial activities and chemical constituents of essential oil from the aerial parts of Cyperus kyllingia Endl. Rec Nat Prod 2011; 324-7.

[36] Lei J, Yu J, Yu H, Liao Z. Composition, cytotoxicity and antimicrobial activity of essential oil from Dictamnus dasycarpus. Food Chem 2008; 107(3): 1205-9.

[37] Döll-Boscardin PM, Sartoratto A, Sales Maia BH, *et al. in vitro* cytotoxic potential of essential oils of Eucalyptus benthamii and its related terpenes on tumor cell lines. Evid-Based Complemen Alternat Med 2012; 2012.

[38] Mohamad RH, El-Bastawesy AM, Abdel-Monem MG, *et al.* Antioxidant and anticarcinogenic effects of methanolic extract and volatile oil of fennel seeds (Foeniculum vulgare). J Med Food 2011; 14(9): 986-1001. [http://dx.doi.org/10.1089/jmf.2008.0255] [PMID: 21812646]

[39] Rigano D, Cardile V, Formisano C, *et al.* Genista sessilifolia DC. and Genista tinctoria L. inhibit UV light and nitric oxide-induced DNA damage and human melanoma cell growth. Chem Biol Interact 2009; 180(2): 211-9. [http://dx.doi.org/10.1016/j.cbi.2009.02.010] [PMID: 19497419]

[40] Afoulous S, Ferhout H, Raoelison EG, *et al.* Helichrysum gymnocephalum essential oil: chemical composition and cytotoxic, antimalarial and antioxidant activities, attribution of the activity origin by correlations. Molecules 2011; 16(10): 8273-91. [http://dx.doi.org/10.3390/molecules16108273] [PMID: 21959299]

[41] Pour BM, Sasidharan S, Jegathambigai RN, Surash R. Anti-leukemia activity of methanolic extracts of Lantana camara. Pharmacognosy Res 2009; 1: 5.

[42] Zamanian-Azodi M, Rezaie-Tavirani M, Heydari-Kashal S, Kalantari S, Dailian S, Zali H. Proteomics

analysis of MKN45 cell line before and after treatment with Lavender aqueous extract. Gastroenterol Hepatol Bed Bench 2012; 5(1): 35-42.
[PMID: 24834196]

[43] Yan R, Yang Y, Zeng Y, Zou G. Cytotoxicity and antibacterial activity of Lindera strychnifolia essential oils and extracts. J Ethnopharmacol 2009; 121(3): 451-5.
[http://dx.doi.org/10.1016/j.jep.2008.06.010] [PMID: 18602979]

[44] Walia M, Mann TS, Kumar D, Agnihotri VK, Singh B. Chemical composition and *in vitro* cytotoxic activity of essential oil of leaves of Malus domestica growing in Western Himalaya (India). Evid Based Complement Alternat Med 2012; 2012: 1-6.
[http://dx.doi.org/10.1155/2012/649727] [PMID: 22619691]

[45] Simionatto E, Peres MTLP, Hess SC, *et al.* Chemical composition and cytotoxic activity of leaves essential oil from Mangifera indica var. coquinho (Anacardiaceae). J Essent Oil Res 2010; 22(6): 596-9.
[http://dx.doi.org/10.1080/10412905.2010.9700408]

[46] McKay DL, Blumberg JB. A Review of the bioactivity and potential health benefits of chamomile tea (*Matricaria recutita* L.). Phytother Res 2006; 20(7): 519-30.
[http://dx.doi.org/10.1002/ptr.1900] [PMID: 16628544]

[47] Chabir N, Romdhane M, Valentin A, *et al.* Chemical study and antimalarial, antioxidant, and anticancer activities of Melaleuca armillaris (Sol Ex Gateau) Sm essential oil. J Med Food 2011; 14(11): 1383-8.
[http://dx.doi.org/10.1089/jmf.2010.0168] [PMID: 21476932]

[48] Hussain AI, Anwar F, Nigam PS, Ashraf M, Gilani AH. Seasonal variation in content, chemical composition and antimicrobial and cytotoxic activities of essential oils from four *Mentha* species. J Sci Food Agric 2010; 90(11): 1827-36.
[http://dx.doi.org/10.1002/jsfa.4021] [PMID: 20602517]

[49] Bose CK. Possible role of Moringa oleifera Lam. root in epithelial ovarian cancer. MedGenMed 2007; 9(1): 26.
[PMID: 17435633]

[50] Sylvestre M, Legault J, Dufour D, Pichette A. Chemical composition and anticancer activity of leaf essential oil of Myrica gale L. Phytomedicine 2005; 12(4): 299-304.
[http://dx.doi.org/10.1016/j.phymed.2003.12.004] [PMID: 15898708]

[51] Edris A. Anti-cancer properties of Nigella spp. essential oils and their major constituents, thymoquinone and β-elemene. Curr Clin Pharmacol 2009; 4(1): 43-6.
[http://dx.doi.org/10.2174/157488409787236137] [PMID: 19149500]

[52] Kathirvel P, Ravi S. Chemical composition of the essential oil from basil (*Ocimum basilicum* Linn.) and its *in vitro* cytotoxicity against HeLa and HEp-2 human cancer cell lines and NIH 3T3 mouse embryonic fibroblasts. Nat Prod Res 2012; 26(12): 1112-8.
[http://dx.doi.org/10.1080/14786419.2010.545357] [PMID: 21939371]

[53] Sharma N, Trikha P, Athar M, Raisuddin S. Inhibition of benzo[a]pyrene- and cyclophoshamide-induced mutagenicity by Cinnamomum cassia. Mutat Res 2001; 480-481: 179-88.
[http://dx.doi.org/10.1016/S0027-5107(01)00198-1] [PMID: 11506812]

[54] De-Oliveira AC, Ribeiro-Pinto LF, Paumgartten JR. *in vitro* inhibition of CYP2B1 monooxygenase by β-myrcene and other monoterpenoid compounds. Toxicol Lett 1997; 92(1): 39-46.
[http://dx.doi.org/10.1016/S0378-4274(97)00034-9] [PMID: 9242356]

[55] Edris AE. Pharmaceutical and therapeutic Potentials of essential oils and their individual volatile constituents: a review. Phytother Res 2007; 21(4): 308-23.
[http://dx.doi.org/10.1002/ptr.2072] [PMID: 17199238]

[56] Bakkali F, Averbeck S, Averbeck D, Zhiri A, Baudoux D, Idaomar M. Antigenotoxic effects of three

essential oils in diploid yeast (Saccharomyces cerevisiae) after treatments with UVC radiation, 8-MOP plus UVA and MMS. Mutat Res Genet Toxicol Environ Mutagen 2006; 606(1-2): 27-38. [http://dx.doi.org/10.1016/j.mrgentox.2006.02.005] [PMID: 16678471]

[57] Seo JY. [The effects of aromatherapy on stress and stress responses in adolescents]. J Korean Acad Nurs 2009; 39(3): 357-65. [http://dx.doi.org/10.4040/jkan.2009.39.3.357] [PMID: 19571632]

[58] Rankin JA. Biological mediators of acute inflammation. AACN Clin Issues 2004; 15(1): 3-17. [http://dx.doi.org/10.1097/00044067-200401000-00002] [PMID: 14767362]

[59] Burg ND, Pillinger MH. The neutrophil: function and regulation in innate and humoral immunity. Clin Immunol 2001; 99(1): 7-17. [http://dx.doi.org/10.1006/clim.2001.5007] [PMID: 11286537]

[60] Cho W, Nam JW, Kang HJ, Windono T, Seo EK, Lee KT. Zedoarondiol isolated from the rhizoma of Curcuma heyneana is involved in the inhibition of iNOS, COX-2 and pro-inflammatory cytokines via the downregulation of NF-κB pathway in LPS-stimulated murine macrophages. Int Immunopharmacol 2009; 9(9): 1049-57. [http://dx.doi.org/10.1016/j.intimp.2009.04.012] [PMID: 19398040]

[61] Qiu J, Feng H, Lu J, *et al.* Eugenol reduces the expression of virulence-related exoproteins in Staphylococcus aureus. Appl Environ Microbiol 2010; 76(17): 5846-51. [http://dx.doi.org/10.1128/AEM.00704-10] [PMID: 20639367]

[62] Yoon WJ, Kim SS, Oh TH, Lee NH, Hyun CG. Cryptomeria japonica essential oil inhibits the growth of drug-resistant skin pathogens and LPS-induced nitric oxide and pro-inflammatory cytokine production. Pol J Microbiol 2009; 58(1): 61-8. [PMID: 19469288]

[63] Argueta A, Cano Asseleih LM, Rodarte García ME. Atlas de las plantas de la medicina tradicional mexicana 1994.

[64] Jimenez-Arellanes A, Meckes M, Ramirez R, Torres J, Luna-Herrera J. Activity against multidrug-resistant *Mycobacterium tuberculosis* in Mexican plants used to treat respiratory diseases. Phytother Res 2003; 17(8): 903-8. [http://dx.doi.org/10.1002/ptr.1377] [PMID: 13680821]

[65] Usanmaz SE, Akarsu ES, Vural N. Neurotoxic effects of acute and subacute formaldehyde exposures in mice. Environ Toxicol Pharmacol 2002; 11(2): 93-100. [http://dx.doi.org/10.1016/S1382-6689(01)00109-0] [PMID: 21782590]

[66] Sarsilmaz M, Kaplan S, Songur A, *et al.* Effects of postnatal formaldehyde exposure on pyramidal cell number, volume of cell layer in hippocampus and hemisphere in the rat: A stereological study. Brain Res 2007; 1145: 157-67. [http://dx.doi.org/10.1016/j.brainres.2007.01.139] [PMID: 17346681]

[67] Sarsilmaz M, Ozen OA. Histopathologic changes on Leydig cells of the rats ınhaled formaldehyde along subchronic period. Fırat Med J 2000; 2: 1-5.

[68] Kurkcuoglu M, Baser KHC. Studies on Turkish rose concrete, absolute, and hydrosol. Chem Nat Compd 2003; 39(5): 457-64. [http://dx.doi.org/10.1023/B:CONC.0000011120.71479.7f]

[69] Köse E, Sarsılmaz M, Taş U, *et al.* Rose oil inhalation protects against formaldehyde-induced testicular damage in rats. Andrologia 2012; 44(Suppl. 1): 342-8. [http://dx.doi.org/10.1111/j.1439-0272.2011.01187.x] [PMID: 21749434]

[70] Baser KH, Buchbauer G. Handbook of essential oils: science, technology, and applications. CRC Press 2009. [http://dx.doi.org/10.1201/9781420063165]

[71] Huang L, Yagura T, Chen S. Sedative activity of hexane extract of Keampferia galanga L. and its

active compounds. J Ethnopharmacol 2008; 120(1): 123-5.
[http://dx.doi.org/10.1016/j.jep.2008.07.045] [PMID: 18761077]

[72] Heuberger E. Effects of Essential Oils in the Central Nervous System. ESSENTIAL 2009; 28: 281.

[73] Adorjan B, Buchbauer G. Biological properties of essential oils: an updated review. Flavour Fragrance J 2010; 25(6): 407-26.
[http://dx.doi.org/10.1002/ffj.2024]

[74] Dobetsberger C, Buchbauer G. Actions of essential oils on the central nervous system: An updated review. Flavour Fragrance J 2011; 26(5): 300-16.
[http://dx.doi.org/10.1002/ffj.2045]

[75] Woelk H, Schläfke S. A multi-center, double-blind, randomised study of the Lavender oil preparation Silexan in comparison to Lorazepam for generalized anxiety disorder. Phytomedicine 2010; 17(2): 94-9.
[http://dx.doi.org/10.1016/j.phymed.2009.10.006] [PMID: 19962288]

[76] Setzer WN. Essential oils and anxiolytic aromatherapy. Nat Prod Commun 2009; 4(9): 1934578X0900400928.
[http://dx.doi.org/10.1177/1934578X0900400928]

[77] Cline M, Taylor JE, Flores J, Bracken S, McCall S, Ceremuga TE. Investigation of the anxiolytic effects of linalool, a lavender extract, in the male Sprague-Dawley rat. AANA J 2008; 76(1): 47-52.
[PMID: 18323320]

[78] Rodgers RJ. Animal models of?? anxiety??: where next? Behav Pharmacol 1997; 8(6): 477-96.
[http://dx.doi.org/10.1097/00008877-199711000-00003] [PMID: 9832964]

[79] Bradley BF, Brown SL, Chu S, Lea RW. Effects of orally administered lavender essential oil on responses to anxiety-provoking film clips. Hum Psychopharmacol 2009; 24(4): 319-30.
[http://dx.doi.org/10.1002/hup.1016] [PMID: 19382124]

[80] Braden R, Reichow S, Halm MA. The use of the essential oil lavandin to reduce preoperative anxiety in surgical patients. J Perianesth Nurs 2009; 24(6): 348-55.
[http://dx.doi.org/10.1016/j.jopan.2009.10.002] [PMID: 19962101]

[81] Hoya Y, Matsumura I, Fujita T, Yanaga K. The use of nonpharmacological interventions to reduce anxiety in patients undergoing gastroscopy in a setting with an optimal soothing environment. Gastroenterol Nurs 2008; 31(6): 395-9.
[http://dx.doi.org/10.1097/SGA.0b013e31818eb5c9] [PMID: 19077833]

[82] Kritsidima M, Newton T, Asimakopoulou K. The effects of lavender scent on dental patient anxiety levels: a cluster randomised-controlled trial. Community Dent Oral Epidemiol 2010; 38(1): 83-7.
[http://dx.doi.org/10.1111/j.1600-0528.2009.00511.x] [PMID: 19968674]

[83] Xu F, Uebaba K, Ogawa H, *et al.* Pharmaco-physio-psychologic effect of Ayurvedic oil-dripping treatment using an essential oil from Lavendula angustifolia. J Altern Complement Med 2008; 14(8): 947-56.
[http://dx.doi.org/10.1089/acm.2008.0240] [PMID: 18990044]

[84] Linck VM, da Silva AL, Figueiró M, *et al.* Inhaled linalool-induced sedation in mice. Phytomedicine 2009; 16(4): 303-7.
[http://dx.doi.org/10.1016/j.phymed.2008.08.001] [PMID: 18824339]

[85] Perveen T, Haider S, Kanwal S, Haleem DJ. Repeated administration of Nigella sativa decreases 5-HT turnover and produces anxiolytic effects in rats. Pak J Pharm Sci 2009; 22(2): 139-44.
[PMID: 19339222]

[86] Mantovan F, Rauter E, Müller I. [Massage and music therapy for relief of anxiety of cancer patients in palliative care]. Pflege Z 2009; 62(3): 164-9.
[PMID: 19348407]

[87] Bagetta G, Morrone LA, Rombolà L, *et al.* Neuropharmacology of the essential oil of bergamot. Fitoterapia 2010; 81(6): 453-61. [http://dx.doi.org/10.1016/j.fitote.2010.01.013] [PMID: 20093169]

[88] Toda M, Morimoto K. Effect of lavender aroma on salivary endocrinological stress markers. Arch Oral Biol 2008; 53(10): 964-8. [http://dx.doi.org/10.1016/j.archoralbio.2008.04.002] [PMID: 18635155]

[89] Toda M, Makino H, Kobayashi H, Nagasawa S, Kitamura K, Morimoto K. Medical assessment of the health effects of short leisure trips. Arch Environ Health 2004; 59(12): 717-24. [http://dx.doi.org/10.1080/00039890409602958] [PMID: 16789482]

[90] Saiyudthong S, Ausavarungnirun R, Jiwajinda S, Turakitwanakan W. Effects of aromatherapy massage with lime essential oil on stress. International Journal of Essential Oil Therapeutics 2009; 3(2/3): 76-80.

[91] Rhind JP. Fragrance and wellbeing: Plant aromatics and their influence on the psyche. Singing Dragon; 2013, 21.

[92] Malloggi E, Menicucci D, Cesari V, Frumento S, Gemignani A, Bertoli A. Lavender aromatherapy: A systematic review from essential oil quality and administration methods to cognitive enhancing effects. Applied Psychology: Health and Well-Being. 2022 May;14(2):663-90.

[93] Shimizu K, Gyokusen M, Kitamura S, *et al.* Essential oil of lavender inhibited the decreased attention during a long-term task in humans. Biosci Biotechnol Biochem 2008; 72(7): 1944-7. [http://dx.doi.org/10.1271/bbb.70835] [PMID: 18603803]

[94] Robbins G, Broughan C. The effects of manipulating participant expectations of an essential oil on memory through verbal suggestion. Int J Essent Oil Ther 2007; 1: 56-60.

[95] Hongratanaworakit T. Relaxing effect of rose oil on humans. Nat Prod Commun 2009; 4(2): 1934578X0900400226. [http://dx.doi.org/10.1177/1934578X0900400226]

[96] Howard S, Hughes BM. Expectancies, not aroma, explain impact of lavender aromatherapy on psychophysiological indices of relaxation in young healthy women. Br J Health Psychol 2008; 13(4): 603-17. [http://dx.doi.org/10.1348/135910707X238734] [PMID: 17845737]

[97] Thews G, Mutschler E, Vaupel P. Anatomie, Physiologie, Pathophysiologie des Menschen. Stuttgart: Wiss. Verl. Ges 1999; pp. 345-8.

[98] Pathan SA, Zaidi SM, Jain GK, Vohora D, Ahmad FJ, Khar RK. Anticonvulsant evaluation of safranal in pentylenetetrazole-induced status epilepticus in mice. Int J Essent Oil Therapeut 2009; 3(2/3): 106-8.

[99] da Fonsêca DV, da Silva Maia Bezerra Filho C, Lima TC, de Almeida RN, de Sousa DP. Anticonvulsant essential oils and their relationship with oxidative stress in epilepsy. Biomolecules 2019; 9(12): 835. [http://dx.doi.org/10.3390/biom9120835] [PMID: 31817682]

[100] Wahab A, Haq RU, Ahmed A, Khan RA, Raza M. Anticonvulsant activities of nutmeg oil of *Myristica fragrans*. Phytother Res 2009; 23(2): 153-8. [http://dx.doi.org/10.1002/ptr.2548] [PMID: 19067329]

[101] El Tahir KE, Abdel-Kader MS. Chemical and pharmacological study of Cymbopogon proximus volatile oil. Res J Med Plant 2008; 2(2): 53-60. [http://dx.doi.org/10.3923/rjmp.2008.53.60]

[102] Okello EJ, Dimaki C, Howes MJ, Houghton PJ, Perry EK. *in vitro* inhibition of human acetyl-and butyryl-cholinesterase by *Narcissus poeticus* L.(Amaryllidaceae) flower absolute. Int J Essent Oil Therapeut 2008.

[103] Elliott MS, Abuhamdah S, Howes MJ, Lees G, Ballard CG, Holmes C. The essential oils from *Melissa officinalis* L. and Lavandula angustifolia Mill. as potential treatment for agitation in people with severe dementia. Int J Essent Oil Ther 2007; 1(4): 143-52.

[104] Huang L, Abuhamdah S, Howes MJR, *et al.* Pharmacological profile of essential oils derived from <I>Lavandula angustifolia</I> and <I>Melissa officinalis</I> with anti-agitation properties: focus on ligand-gated channels. J Pharm Pharmacol 2008; 60(11): 1515-22. [http://dx.doi.org/10.1211/jpp/60.11.0013] [PMID: 18957173]

[105] Abuhamdah S, Huang L, Elliott MSJ, *et al.* Pharmacological profile of an essential oil derived from *Melissa officinalis* with anti-agitation properties: focus on ligand-gated channels. J Pharm Pharmacol 2010; 60(3): 377-84. [http://dx.doi.org/10.1211/jpp.60.3.0014] [PMID: 18284819]

[106] Lin PW, Chan WC, Ng BF, Lam LC. Efficacy of aromatherapy (Lavandula angustifolia) as an intervention for agitated behaviours in Chinese older persons with dementia: a cross-over randomized trial. Int J Geriat Psych 2007; 22(5): 405-10.

[107] Gollnick HPM, Finlay AY, Shear N. Can we define acne as a chronic disease? If so, how and when? Am J Clin Dermatol 2008; 9(5): 279-84. [http://dx.doi.org/10.2165/00128071-200809050-00001] [PMID: 18717602]

[108] Koo JYM, Smith LL. Psychologic aspects of acne. Pediatr Dermatol 1991; 8(3): 185-8. [http://dx.doi.org/10.1111/j.1525-1470.1991.tb00856.x] [PMID: 1836060]

[109] Kemper KJ, Vohra S, Walls R. American Academy of Pediatrics. The use of complementary and alternative medicine in pediatrics. Pediatrics 2008; 122(6): 1374-86. [http://dx.doi.org/10.1542/peds.2008-2173] [PMID: 19047261]

[110] Davis MP, Darden PM. Use of complementary and alternative medicine by children in the United States. Arch Pediatr Adolesc Med 2003; 157(4): 393-6. [http://dx.doi.org/10.1001/archpedi.157.4.393] [PMID: 12695237]

[111] Agnew T, Leach M, Segal L. The clinical impact and cost-effectiveness of essential oils and aromatherapy for the treatment of acne vulgaris: a protocol for a randomized controlled trial. J Altern Complement Med 2014; 20(5): 399-405. [http://dx.doi.org/10.1089/acm.2013.0137] [PMID: 23829810]

[112] Koh KJ, Pearce AL, Marshman G, Finlay-Jones JJ, Hart PH. Tea tree oil reduces histamine-induced skin inflammation. Br J Dermatol 2002; 147(6): 1212-7. [http://dx.doi.org/10.1046/j.1365-2133.2002.05034.x] [PMID: 12452873]

[113] Reuter J, Merfort I, Schempp CM. Botanicals in dermatology: An evidence-based review. Am J Clin Dermatol 2010; 11(4): 247-67. [PMID: 20509719]

[114] da Silva AG, Puziol PdeF, Leitao RN, *et al.* Application of the essential oil from copaiba (Copaifera langsdori Desf.) for acne vulgaris: A double-blind, placebo-controlled clinical trial. Altern Med Rev 2012; 17(1): 69-75. [PMID: 22502624]

[115] Busse D, Kudella P, Grüning NM, *et al.* A synthetic sandalwood odorant induces wound-healing processes in human keratinocytes *via* the olfactory receptor OR2AT4. J Invest Dermatol 2014; 134(11): 2823-32. [http://dx.doi.org/10.1038/jid.2014.273] [PMID: 24999593]

[116] Tsai TH, Chuang LT, Lien TJ, Liing YR, Chen WY, Tsai PJ. Rosmarinus officinalis extract suppresses Propionibacterium acnes-induced inflammatory responses. J Med Food 2013; 16(4): 324-33. [http://dx.doi.org/10.1089/jmf.2012.2577] [PMID: 23514231]

[117] Oh TH, Kim SS, Yoon WJ, *et al.* Chemical composition and biological activities of Jeju Thymus

quinquecostatus essential oils against Propionibacterium species inducing acne. J Gen Appl Microbiol 2009; 55(1): 63-8.
[http://dx.doi.org/10.2323/jgam.55.63] [PMID: 19282635]

[118] Kim SS, Baik JS, Oh TH, Yoon WJ, Lee NH, Hyun CG. Biological activities of Korean Citrus obovoides and Citrus natsudaidai essential oils against acne-inducing bacteria. Biosci Biotechnol Biochem 2008; 72(10): 2507-13.
[http://dx.doi.org/10.1271/bbb.70388] [PMID: 18838824]

[119] Mullins P. Massage and Reflexology. Complementary Therapies and the Management of Diabetes and Vascular Disease. John Wiley & Sons 2006.
[http://dx.doi.org/10.1002/9780470057438.ch13]

[120] Sadlon AE, Lamson DW. Immune-modifying and antimicrobial effects of Eucalyptus oil and simple inhalation devices. Altern Med Rev 2010; 15(1): 33-47.
[PMID: 20359267]

[121] Jeena K, Liju VB, Kuttan R. Antioxidant, anti-inflammatory and antinociceptive activities of essential oil from ginger. Indian J Physiol Pharmacol 2013; 57(1): 51-62.
[PMID: 24020099]

[122] Das K. Turmeric (Curcuma longa) oils. Essential oils in food preservation, flavor and safety. Academic Press 2016.

[123] Mikhaeil BR, Maatooq GT, Badria FA, Amer MMA. Chemistry and immunomodulatory activity of frankincense oil. Z Naturforsch C J Biosci 2003; 58(3-4): 230-8.
[http://dx.doi.org/10.1515/znc-2003-3-416] [PMID: 12710734]

[124] Fisher K, Phillips C. Potential antimicrobial uses of essential oils in food: Is citrus the answer? Trends Food Sci Technol 2008; 19(3): 156-64.
[http://dx.doi.org/10.1016/j.tifs.2007.11.006]

[125] Delaquis P, Stanich K, Girard B, Mazza G. Antimicrobial activity of individual and mixed fractions of dill, cilantro, coriander and eucalyptus essential oils. Int J Food Microbiol 2002; 74(1-2): 101-9.
[http://dx.doi.org/10.1016/S0168-1605(01)00734-6] [PMID: 11929164]

[126] Nakano Y, Matsunaga H, Saita T, Mori M, Katano M, Okabe H. Antiproliferative constituents in Umbelliferae plants II. Screening for polyacetylenes in some Umbelliferae plants, and isolation of panaxynol and falcarindiol from the root of Heracleum moellendorffii. Biol Pharm Bull 1998; 21(3): 257-61.
[http://dx.doi.org/10.1248/bpb.21.257] [PMID: 9556156]

[127] Circosta C, Sanogo R, Occhiuto F. Effects of Calotropis procera on oestrous cycle and on oestrogenic functionality in rats. Farmaco 2001; 56(5-7): 373-8.
[http://dx.doi.org/10.1016/S0014-827X(01)01089-8] [PMID: 11482761]

[128] Shivalingappa H, Satyanarayan ND, Purohit MG, Sharanabasappa A, Patil SB. Effect of ethanol extract of Rivea hypocrateriformis on the estrous cycle of the rat. J Ethnopharmacol 2002; 82(1): 11-7.
[http://dx.doi.org/10.1016/S0378-8741(02)00073-9] [PMID: 12169399]

[129] Monsefi M, Ghasemi M, Bahaoddini A. The effects of *Anethum graveolens* L. on female reproductive system. Phytother Res 2006; 20(10): 865-8.
[http://dx.doi.org/10.1002/ptr.1959] [PMID: 16835877]

[130] Figà-Talamanca I, Traina ME, Urbani E. Occupational exposures to metals, solvents and pesticides: Recent evidence on male reproductive effects and biological markers. Occup Med 2001; 51(3): 174-88.
[http://dx.doi.org/10.1093/occmed/51.3.174] [PMID: 11385122]

[131] Wang H, Wang SF, Ning H, *et al.* Maternal cypermethrin exposure during lactation impairs testicular development and spermatogenesis in male mouse offspring. Environ Toxicol 2011; 26(4): 382-94.
[http://dx.doi.org/10.1002/tox.20566] [PMID: 20131380]

[132] Weselak M, Arbuckle TE, Wigle DT, Walker MC, Krewski D. Pre- and post-conception pesticide exposure and the risk of birth defects in an Ontario farm population. Reprod Toxicol 2008; 25(4): 472-80.
[http://dx.doi.org/10.1016/j.reprotox.2008.05.060] [PMID: 18586452]

[133] Husain R, Husain R, Adhami VM, Seth PK. Behavioral, neurochemical, and neuromorphological effects of deltamethrin in adult rats. J Toxicol Environ Health 1996; 48(5): 515-6.
[http://dx.doi.org/10.1080/009841096161212] [PMID: 8751838]

[134] Newman DJ, Cragg GM. Natural products as sources of new drugs over the last 25 years. J Nat Prod 2007; 70(3): 461-77.
[http://dx.doi.org/10.1021/np068054v] [PMID: 17309302]

[135] Kang HY, Na SS, Kim YK. [Effects of oral care with essential oil on improvement in oral health status of hospice patients]. J Korean Acad Nurs 2010; 40(4): 473-81.
[http://dx.doi.org/10.4040/jkan.2010.40.4.473] [PMID: 20820114]

[136] Ben Slima A, Ali MB, Barkallah M, *et al.* Antioxidant properties of Pelargonium graveolens L'Her essential oil on the reproductive damage induced by deltamethrin in mice as compared to alpha-tocopherol. Lipids Health Dis 2013; 12(1): 30.
[http://dx.doi.org/10.1186/1476-511X-12-30] [PMID: 23496944]

CHAPTER 7

Therapeutic Applications and Pharmacological Practices of Essential Oils

Pragati Misra[1,*], Suchit Ashish John[2], Shailesh Marker[3], Shikha Agnihotry[4], Ajeet Kumar Srivastav[5,7], Alka Sagar[6] and **Pradeep Kumar Shukla[2]**

[1] *Centre for Tissue Culture, Technology, Jacob Institute of Biotechnology and Bioengineering, Sam Higginbottom University of Agriculture, Technology and Sciences, Prayagraj, Uttar Pradesh, India*

[2] *Department of Biological Sciences, Faculty of Science, Sam Higginbottom University of Agriculture, Technology and Sciences, Prayagraj, Uttar Pradesh, India*

[3] *Department of Genetics and Plant Breeding, Naini Agricultural Institute, Sam Higginbottom University of Agriculture, Technology and Sciences, Prayagraj, Uttar Pradesh, India*

[4] *Department of Computational Biology and Bioinformatics, Jacob Institute of Biotechnology and Bio-Engineering, Sam Higginbottom University of Agriculture, Technology and Sciences, Prayagraj (Allahabad), Uttar Pradesh, India*

[5] *Redcliffe Hygiene Private Limited, Gurugram-122016, Haryana, India*

[6] *Department of Microbiology and Biotechnology, Meerut Institute of Engineering and Technology, Meerut, UP, India*

[7] *Department of Biochemistry, Babu Banrasi Das University, Lucknow, India*

Abstract: When referring to a drug's active component as "Quinta essential," Paracelsus von Hohenheim, a Swiss physician used the word "essential oil" for the very first time in the sixteenth century. Plant oils and extracts have been utilised for a variety of purposes for thousands of years. Essential oils have long been used in traditional medicine and by practitioners of alternative rejuvenation approaches. Because of their considerable immunomodulatory and antibacterial action, they have been used for many years to treat various ailments. Many volatile chemicals generated by plant secondary metabolism combine to make essential oils. Components of essential oil may be classified into two related types on a biosynthetic level. The two primary groups are terpene or terpenoid inchoation compounds, as well as aromatic and aliphatic components. Since the Middle Ages, essential oils have been utilized for antibacterial, biocidal, anti-fungal, antiprotozoal, and antifeedant purposes, as well as painkiller, calming, anti-inflammatory, anti-spasmodic, and locally anesthetic therapy.

* **Corresponding author Pragati Misra:** Centre for Tissue Culture, Technology, Jacob Institute of Biotechnology and Bioengineering, Sam Higginbottom University of Agriculture, Technology and Sciences, Prayagraj, Uttar Pradesh, India; E-mail: pragati.misra@shiats.edu.in

Pradeep Kumar Shukla, Ajeet Kumar Srivastav, Deepti Chopra, Shikha Agnihotry, Pragati Misra and Jyoti Singh (Eds.)

However, little is understood about how essential oils function. Plant oils and extracts' antimicrobial characteristics have served as the foundation for a variety of enterprises, including pharmaceuticals, alternative medicine, and herbal treatments.

Keywords: Essential oils, Pharmacological and industrial applications, medicinal uses.

1. INTRODUCTION

Essential oil (EO) study was in its infancy until the late 1800s, the chemical nature of EOs was stated in broad groups such as terpenes, aromatic polyketides, and phenylpropanoids, or else using specialized chemical nomenclature. Following Belaiche's concept to identify chemical categories that might be trained to anticipate the biological activity of EOs, vocabulary to describe EO characteristics was later established and updated. Aromatherapie exactement, is a book written by French authors Pierre Franchomme and Daniel Penoel, that pioneered a paradigm for EO ranking, based on their structural function that is still in use today [1].

EOs have historically been used for antibacterial, biocidal, anti-parasitic, and antifeedant effects, as well as painkiller, relaxing, anti-inflammatory, anti-spasmodic, and locally anesthetic therapies (Table **1**) [2, 3]. Now there are recognized possible techniques for employing EOs or their components in medications for human or animal use [4]. Most EOs work best when applied superficially, such as in mouth rinses and deep throats, or inhalation; they are rarely ingested, despite being generally recognized as safe (GRAS) [5]. Aside from preventing and healing certain ailments, EOs have extraordinary potential for promoting and maintaining overall health. However, their poor water solubility and durability, as well as its significant volatility and deleterious effects, have restricted its application in medicines [6].

Aromatic plants and their EOs have been used for flavor and fragrance, as seasonings or spices, in treatments, as bactericidal agents, and as a protectant for perishable goods since ancient times. EOs from medicinal and aromatic plants have shown biological activity among natural compounds, and their ability to scavenge free radicals has piqued the curiosity of researchers [7, 8].

Herbal compounds fight free radicals, which have been linked to several illnesses such as cancer and neurological disorders. Furthermore, they degrade food's sanitary and sensory properties [9]. EOs have potent antimicrobial properties [10 - 12]. Because of these characteristics, they may be a beneficial source for lowering resistant bacteria. Furthermore, EOs are classified as safe substances, and some of them include chemicals that may be used as antibacterial supplements [13].

Several studies have shown that they help prevent diseases and toxins in food [14, 15]. This means that they will be used in the multigrain processing industry [10], which will address the issue of food poisoning despite increased hygiene standards [11]. As a consequence of limits on the use of synthetic antioxidants and increased interest in natural, non-toxic antioxidants, several studies on the antioxidant effects of EOs have been done. Many components of EOs in plants, such as terpenoids, monoterpenes, ethyl alcohol, ketones, acetaldehyde, and esters, work together to protect the plant against herbivores, and bacteria [16]. Due to the toxicological effect of produced goods, EOs are prioritised in the food processing, dietary supplement manufacturing, and pharmaceutical sectors. Increased efforts have been made to favor the employment of EOs as natural antioxidants and preservatives [17]. Herbal products for usage as pharmaceuticals, scents, aesthetics, and food additives are getting popular among the public at large patients and medical professionals [18]. Because of the biological advantages they provide, essential/volatile oils (VOs) have received a lot of attention among all of these natural medications [19, 20]. These applications range from employing rosewood and cedarwood for the smell to flavoring drinks with lime, fennel, or juniper berry oil [21], also to prevent the spoilage of stored food crops [22].

Table 1. Essential oils for common problems. Adapted from Ali *et al.* [6].

Condition	Essential Oils
Anxiety, agitation, stress, challenging behaviors	*Angelica archangelicarad.* (angelica), *Cistus ladaniferus* (labdanum) *Citrus aurantium* var. amarafol. (petitgrainbigarade), *Citrus aurantium* var. amaraper. (orange bigarade), *Citrus bergamia* (bergamot) *Citrus sinensis* (sweet orange) *Cymbopogon martini* (palmarosa) *Eucalyptus staigeriana* (lemon-scented ironbark), *Lavandula angustifolia* (lavender) *Litsea cubeba* (may chang) *Ocimum basilicum* (basil) *Origanum majorana* (sweet marjoram) *Pelargonium graveolens*(geranium) *Pogostemon patchouli* (patchouli) *Valeriana officinalis* (valerian)
End-of-life agitation	*Lavandula angustifolia* (lavender) *Santalum album* (sandalwood) *Boswellia carteri* (frankincense)
Fatigue	*Angelica archangelicarad.* (angelica) (nervous) *Cistus ladaniferus* (labdanum) (chronic) *Citrus aurantium* var. amara (neroli bigarade) *Citrus paradisi* (grapefruit)

(Table 1) cont.....

Condition	Essential Oils
-	(exhaustion) *Coriandrum sativum* (coriander) (including mental) *Cymbopogon nardus* (citronella) *Eucalyptus radiata* (black peppermint) (chronic) *Eucalyptus smithii* (gully gum) *Juniperus communisram.* (juniper twig) *Mentha spicata* (spearmint) (mental) *Pelargonium graveolens*(geranium) (nervous) *Pinus sylvestris* (Scots pine) *Rosmarinus officinalis* ct. cineole, ct. camphor, ct. verbenone(rosemary) *Salvia sclarea* (clary) (nervous) *Zingiber officinale* (ginger)
Insomnia	*Angelica archangelica* rad. (angelica) *Canangao dorata* (ylang ylang) *Chamaeme lumnobile* (Roman chamomile) *Citrus aurantium* var. amara (neroli bigarade) *Cistus ladaniferus* (labdanum) *Citrus bergamia* (bergamot) *C. limon* (lemon) *Citrus reticulate* (mandarin) *Citrus sinensis* (sweet orange) *Cuminum cyminum* (cumin) *Juniperus communis* fruct. (juniper berry) *Lavandula angustifolia* (lavender) *Litsea cubeba* (may chang) *Melissa officinalis* (lemon balm) *Myrtus communis* (myrtle) *Ocimum basilicum* (basil) (nervous) *Origanum majorana* (sweet marjoram) *Ravensara aromatica* (ravensara) *Thymus vulgaris* ct. geraniol, ct. linalool (sweet thyme) *Valeriana officinalis* (valerian)
Mental exhaustion, burnout	*M. piperita* (peppermint) *Ocimum basilicum* (basil) *Helichrysum angustifolium*(everlasting)
Memory loss	*Litsea cubeba* (may chang) *M. piperita* (peppermint) *Rosmarinus officinalis* ct. cineole (rosemary)

(Table 1) cont.....

Condition	Essential Oils
Pain management	*Eucalyptus smithii* (gully gum) *Lavandula angustifolia* (lavender) *Matricaria recutita* (German chamomile) *Leptospermum scoparium* (manuka) *Origanum majorana* (sweet marjoram) *Pinus mugo* var. pumilio (dwarf pine) *Rosmarinus officinalis* ct. camphor (rosemary) *Zingiber officinale* (ginger)

EOs are fascinating natural chemicals with a wide range of biological effects. An EO may include a variety of chemical components, most notably mono- and sesquiterpenoids and phenylpropanoids. They are administered therapeutically by inhalation, oral administration or by transdermal application such as eucalyptus oil, peppermint oil, and rosemary oil. Thyme and clove oils have antibacterial properties due to their high phenol content. Because of their vast and diverse effects, such as antibacterial, antibiotic, anti-inflammatory, broncho-dilator, mucolytic, and so on, they can be essential materials in the treatment of many respiratory tract illnesses. Some EOs are only utilized in applications with long-term usage, while others may be used in applications with well-established usage [23].

2. THERAPEUTIC APPLICATION OF ESSENTIAL OILS

Although EOs and their constituents have been investigated for their antibacterial, antifungal, and antiviral properties, little is known about how do they work. It is vital to identify the active elements in EOs (Table **2**) and understand their modes of action in conjunction with the various EOs. To get the best and most active composition of EOs, and suitable growth circumstances for harvesting and extraction will be required. After the active element is identified during inclusion, synthetic alternatives can be created and prepared. In terms of manufacturing reproducibility and cost feasibility, these synthetic components would be easier to regulate. It has been reported that when EOs are breathed or applied directly to the skin, they alter the function of calcium and potassium ion gates by acting on the lipid components of the cellular membrane *via* their lipid soluble components [24, 25]. When certain doses of EOs are supplied, the membranes become saturated and interact with cell membranes in ways that depend on the structure and physicochemical qualities of the components [26]. These components include transport systems, enzymes, ion channels, receptors, *etc* [27].

Aromatherapy is a complementary therapy that uses essential oils as the primary therapeutic agent to treat a range of ailments. Several processes are used to extract

EOs/VOs from the plant's flowers, resins, twigs, leaflets, roots, fruits, and other parts [28]. They were developed when scientists found that EOs had antibacterial and skin permeability capabilities. These oils are usually delivered to the human skin surface by inhalation, topical application, and soaking in aromatherapy. Once in the system, the oils re-modulate and act efficiently at the problem site or in the affected area. This sort of treatment employs a variety of permutations and coalescences to provide relief from a wide range of ailments, including anxiety, gastritis, migraine, insomnia, stomach discomfort, respiratory troubles, skin disorders, inflamed knees, renal problems, and so on. When other components of life and diet are taken into account, EOs are shown to be more neutral. Medical, pharmacologic, cosmetic, neurological, sensory, and physiotherapy applications of several aromatherapy herbs have already been examined and documented [6].

Table 2. Primary chemical components (*i.e.*, >2.0%) of the studied ten essential oils. Adapted from Han [39].

Essential Oil	Chemical Components (%)
Bergamot	Limonene (35.8), Linalyl Acetate (33.0), gamma-Terpinene (9.0), Linalool (7.5), beta-Pinene (7.0)
Cilantro	trans-2-Decenal (30.0), trans-2-Decen-1-ol (15.8),Linalool (15.5), trans-2-Dodecenal (7.0), Decanal (4.7), Decanol (4.6), Tetradecanol (3.0), gamma-Terpinene (2.2)
Geranium	Citronellol (38.3), Citronellyl formate (11.6), 6,9- Guanidiene (7.4), Geraniol (6.4), Menthone (3.3), Isomenthone (3.3), Linalool (3.3), cis-Rose Oxide (2.0)
Helichrysum	Neryl acetate (35.5), gamma-Curcumene (13.9), alpha-Pinene (8.9), alpha-Curcumene (4.3), Italicene (4.0), Limonene (3.6), Neryl Propionate (3.1), Eucalyptol (2.3), Copaene (2.2)
Patchouli	Patchoulol (39.6), alpha-Bulnesene (19.1), Aromadendrene (17.8), alpha-Guaiene (13.4), alpha- Patchoulene (4.8), Aciphyllene (2.7), beta-Patchoulene (2.7), beta-Caryophyllene (2.3)
Petitgrain	Linalyl acetate (50.3), Linalool (23.9), alpha-Terpineol (6.7), Geranyl Acetate (4.1), trans-beta-Ocimene (2.3), Neryl Acetate (2.5), Myrcene (2.0)
Sandalwood	cis-alpha-Santalol (48.4), cis-beta-Santalol (22.0), cisalpha-trans-Bergamotol (6.8), cis-epi-beta-Santalol (3.9), cis-Lanceol (3.2), cis-Nuciferal (2.0), beta- Santalene (2.0)
Spikenard	beta-Gurjunene (11.3), Jatamansone (9.5), Spirojatamol (8.7), 6,9-Guanidiene (7.5), Valencene (5.6), Valerena- 4,7(11)-diene (5.6), Seychellene (3.8), 7-epi-alpha- Selinene (2.9), gamma-Vetivenene (2.6), beta-Pinene (2.5), alpha-Aristolenol (2.4), ( )-alph- -Gurjunene (2.2), beta-Patchoulene (2.0)
Ylang Ylang	Germacrene D (23.2), beta-Caryophyllene (14.7), Geranyl Acetate (6.4), Benzyl Benzoate (6.1), Linalool (5.1), delta-Cadinene (4.3), alpha-Humulene (3.9), paramethyl-Anisole (2.9)

(Table 2) cont.....

Essential Oil	Chemical Components (%)
Immortelle blend	alpha-Pinene (23.1), cis-alpha-Santalol (10.2), Limonene (6.8), Linalyl Acetate (6.3), Linalool (4.7), cis-beta-Santalol (4.4), alpha-Thujene (4.1), beta-Caryophyllene (3.8), Curzerene (3.6), Octyl Acetate (3.3), beta-Pinene (3.1), Furanoeudesma-1,3-diene (2.5), Sabinene (2.0)

For thousands of years, phytoconstituents and oils have been used for a variety of purposes. Sandalwood and cedar oil are used for aroma, while lemon, fennel, or juniper berry oil is used to flavor beverages, and lemongrass oil is used to keep stored food crops from decaying [21, 22]. Plant extracts' antibacterial properties have been used in a range of applications, including medicine, naturopathy, and alternative remedies, as well as raw and processed food [29 - 31]. The use of EOs for therapeutic, aesthetic, fragrant, and religious purposes is becoming more widespread [32, 33]. Saturated and unsaturated hydrocarbons, ethanol, aldehydes, ketones, acetone, oxides, quinones, and terpenes make up EOs [34, 35]. They are odorless, achromic liquids with a high refractive index. These oils operate on pressure points and rejuvenate since they are so intense and concentrated. Aromatherapy is a natural and harmless gift given to mankind by nature. Aromatherapy not only treats sickness symptoms, but it also regenerates the entire body. In the early stages of life, aromatherapy governs physiological, spiritual, and psychological upliftment. This treatment is useful for both acute and chronic illnesses. Pharmaceutical businesses are seeking environmentally safe, complementary, and natural treatments for infections and metabolic diseases. By using these EOs, it may be possible to increase the bioavailability and response time of medications [6]. Because of their pleasantness and cost effectiveness, EO treatments have been given special consideration among alternative medicine methods. Because aromatherapy is usually mixed with other therapies, such as physiotherapy, it is difficult to isolate the effects of aromatherapy when applied topically. However, some clinical scientific evidence supports the use of EOs in various pre- and postoperative phases. It should be emphasized that this method also works effectively in developing countries when the public healthcare system can sustain the medication's medium- to low-cost [36, 37]. Current researchs, which supports the elimination of particular EO concentrations, can explain their previously documented biological function. As a result, rosemary EO has been utilized in aromatherapy for some years, however, little study on its effects on the human body, namely, the nervous system, has been conducted. In one study with 20 healthy volunteers who inhaled rosemary EO, the participant's feelings, as well as objective measures of body temperature, heart rate, rate of breathing, and blood pressure, were recorded. Participants in the research also had their electroencephalograms obtained before and after inhaling the EO, and quantifications were performed. Aromatherapy dramatically increased blood pressure, heart rate, and breathing rate, based on the findings. The volunteers stated that they felt more rested. In comparison to the control group, participants in the study recalled more photos after consuming rosemary and lavender EOs. Moreover, a significant statistical difference in quick numerical memory was identified between the "Rosemary" and "Lavender" groups. Our findings add to the body of information on the effects of EOs on the expression of a person's cognitive abilities [38].

2.1. Modes of EO Application

Buchbauer *et al.* [40] comprehensively examined the consequences of biological processes in the context of EOs application [41]. A paradigm change is occurring in the biological investigation of EOs as a result of the large quantity of data now accessible on biological activity. Due to growing concerns about the translation of *in vitro* results to *in vivo* use, various studies have been conducted to adapt the way essential oils are supplied in the human or animal model to mirror *in vitro* outcomes. Concerns for vaporization, solubility, and assimilation are particularly persistent in the case of EOs [42].

2.1.1. Ingestion

As part of efforts to enhance EOs encapsulation, EOs may be encapsulated into various substrates, such as chitosan-coated microspheres, to reduce evaporation and boost antimicrobial activity [43]. Another method is to encase EOs in dissolved cyclodextrins, which may be used as a food component to mask flavor while also preventing EO evaporation and therefore extending the shelf life of topical creams and lotions [44]. Furthermore, effective perforation studies were carried out using EOs as a transporter for antimicrobial medicine, which may be related to how the oils interact with skin lipid crystallines [41].

2.2. Inhalation

Aromatherapy by inhalation of EOs was effective in reducing feelings of tension and hopelessness and improving the quality of sleep. The outcomes of this study using EO inhalation revealed that while the participants were effective at reducing subjective stress and depression and increasing sleep quality, they were ineffective at reducing the objective stress index and improving immune function. Its immunity-boosting properties, however, were not confirmed and need to be thoroughly investigated [45]. One of the most popular nonpharmaceutical treatments is aromatherapy. It is considered a holistic nursing intervention and can help nurses achieve their goals [46, 47]. Additionally, it benefits these patients since it reduces problems and expenditures [47, 48]. This can then cause physiological reactions in the nervous, endocrine, or immune systems [49, 50]. Herbal EOs may be absorbed by the body in a variety of methods, including massage, inhalation, compresses, aromatherapy, spas, and shower baths [47]. A professional therapist blends numerous EOs and employs them in aromatherapy massage to alleviate pain, stiffness, and spasms while also encouraging relaxation [49, 50]. Aromatherapy is a potentially relaxing and therapeutic treatment that has been demonstrated to be especially effective in relieving tension and anxiety. It has been shown to lower blood pressure, calm breathing, and restore hormonal balance [49].

2.3. Novel Methods of EO Application

EOs are most often extracted from a plant's flowers, nuts, leaves, fruits, and stems using distillation or solvent extraction. EOs are volatile byproducts of plant secondary metabolism. There are roughly 3,000 EOs, with approximately 200-300 being the most vital for industry [11]. Some of those identified to have antibacterial qualities include mint oil, basil, jasmine, eucalyptus, cardamom, green tea, oregano, camphor, and citronella; however, only lemongrass, oregano, and bay EOs displayed antimicrobial activity at concentrations less than 2% [31, 51]. Antifungal and antibacterial effects of sodium alginate-based film with 9 distinct EOs mixed in three concentrations were evaluated. The loaded films revealed the potential to suppress bacteria and fungus development depending on the kind and concentration of the EO, making them appropriate for use as cutting-edge antibacterial surgical sutures. Oregano oil was effectively mixed with chitosan to produce antimicrobial and transparent wound regeneration films [52].

Thyme oil's antimicrobial effects were favorable against both Gram-negative and Gram-positive microbes, and its effectiveness as a safe source of naturally antibacterial and antioxidant agents was further demonstrated by its incorporation into gelatin films and N-carboxy butyl chitosan/agarose foam using hypercritical carbon dioxide [53], to create antibacterial wound dressings, geraniol and citronellal were doped with nanofluid-based ferrous-ferric oxide/magnetite [54, 55]. *Garcinia mangostana* (mangosteen) extracts were added to chitosan electrospun nanofibers, which revealed the capacity to suppress the growth of *Escherichia coli* and *Staphylococcus aureus* [56]. However, due to their hydrophobicity, EOs have a poor distribution, and separation may occur either in solution or in the final dried films. Emulsifiers must be administered often to avoid these events and increase EO dispersion and stability. To produce a uniform distribution of tea tree oil in an alginate hydrogel, Catanzano *et al.* [57] employed a novel strategy and proposed utilizing a microemulsion as a carrier.

3. PHARMACOLOGICAL PRACTICES AND PROPERTIES OF ESSENTIAL OILS

3.1. Expectorants and Diuretics

Antitussives can be classified as therapeutic drugs that suppress coughing. They operate by central or peripheral processes, while some operating *via* both [58]. Previously, the authors showed the cough suppressant activity of an ethanol extract *Picralima nitida* (PNE), extracted from seeds [59]. However, the mechanism of action of cough medicine might be caused by at least five factors, pharmacological, physiological, true mimic, psychosocial, and non-categorical activity. Plant products having cough suppressant effects may exert these therapeutic effects in a variety of ways [60, 61]. *P. nitida* ethanolic seed extract has demonstrated highly substantial antioxidant, antimicrobial, mucus-suppressant, anxiolytic, and antitussive properties [62].

3.2. Antibacterial and Antifungal Actions

The quorum sensing (QS) technique of microbial interaction allows individual bacterial cells to join and operate as a singular entity, protecting them from several dangerous circumstances [63, 64]. The QS controls regulon a diverse collection of genes, many of which are involved in bacterial pathogenicities, such as exoenzyme production and biofilm formation [65, 66]. Because quorum sensing inhibition (QSI) would diminish the virulence of aggressive pathogens, thereby making them more vulnerable to the applied therapeutic intervention, it has been advocated that QSI be the first target for the development of long-term anti-infective medicines [67]. The antibiofilm action of lavender, tea tree, and chamomile EOs has been demonstrated using *S. aureus* and *E. coli* as test strains [68]. Furthermore, Schillaci *et al.* [69] discovered that two EOs of *Boswellia* sp. (Frankincense oil) may diminish biofilms constituted of two *Staphylococcus* species and *Candida albicans*. Furthermore, peppermint EOs have been observed to reduce *C. albicans* colony development [70]. Lemongrass and grapefruit EOs were discovered to be antibiofilm effective against five strains of *Staphylococcus aureus* [71]. The antibiofilm activity of known essential oil sophorolipids (EOSLs), but not EOs has been investigated since they are thought to have changed capacities to limit the initial adhesion of microorganisms to the solid surface due to their flocculating, antimicrobial, and QSI properties. These EOSLs were capable of preventing microbial adhesion to the glass surface as well as detecting the commencement of biofilm formation. Because the genes required for the production of exopolysaccharide (EPS) are under QS regulation, the QSI ability of these EOSLs has already been shown, and this may be the reason for the considerably decreased biofilm matrix. EPS is a critical component in the formation of a bacterial communities. Basil oil and ylang-ylang oil both have strong anti-biofilm properties when studied under a microscope. Furthermore, the tested strain *V. cholerae* is crucial from the standpoint of the Indian subcontinent since cholera is a prevalent problem there, and the biofilm it produces is a key component of the disease's pathophysiology [72].

The rising growth and proliferation of multidrug-resistant (MDR) bacteria, notably methicillin-resistant *S. aureus* (MRSA), as well as associated biofilms, has hampered the treatment of bacterial infections. Biofilms are difficult to eradicate with traditional antimicrobial treatments due to their greater level of resistance to antibiotics than free-living cells. Isolated *S. aureus* biofilm growth was measured using microtube and microdilution plate testing. Among the molecules contained in EOs, geraniol, citronellol, carvacrol, and eugenol all displayed variable degrees of antibacterial activity, and subMIC doses of these compounds efficiently inhibit *Staphylococcus aureus* strains from developing biofilms. *Thymus vulgaris*>*Syzygium aromaticum*>eugenol> cinnamaldehyde> citral> *Cymbopogon citratus*>*Cymbopogon martini*> geraniol>*Cymbopogon nardus* was shown to be in the order of antimicrobial properties. *T. vulgaris* and geraniol showed antibiofilm activity at 2x (MIC) minimal inhibitory action values or concentration, suggesting that they might be used therapeutically alone or in combination with antibiotics to treat clinical issues caused by *Staphylococcus aureus* that are associated with biofilms [86].

In-vitro bactericidal activities of 18 EOs chemical components from aromatic plant extracts against *S. pyogenes* were investigated. The disc diffusion technique was used to study the bactericidal activity of EOs. The MIC of EOs with related antibacterial activity was determined using the broth dilution technique. 14 of the 18 EOs were positive for antimicrobial activity against *S. pyogenes. C. verum, C. citratus, T. vulgaris, O. compactum, and S. Montana* EOs exhibited the strongest antibacterial action. According to the *in vitro* results, these EOs, which are considered potent antibacterial agents, should be recommended for individuals suffering from bacterial throat infections [87].

The strength of their composition and activities, such as antioxidant (preventing lipid oxidation) and antimicrobial properties, are essential considerations in the utilization of plant extracts in the pharmaceutical and food industries. Sesquiterpene and oxidized sesquiterpene prevail in the high extraction yield EO extract from *E. globulus* fruit. The EO extracts from the *E. globulus* fruit confirmed cases of unique antibacterial activity against infectious and rotten microbes, which might be attributed to their low antioxidant compounds. The results showed that all organisms, including antibiotic-resistant *S. aureus* and *P. aeruginous*, were responsive to EO extracts from *E. globulus* fruit. As a result of their high production and antibacterial activity, the studied EO extracts from *E. globulus* fruit were promising alternatives for usage in the food and pharmaceutical sectors [88]. EOs are complex mixtures of secondary metabolites (SMs) with antibacterial capabilities, which give themselves to applications for digestion improvement by selecting for or against certain communities of bacteria, which bovine dietitians are interested in. It is uncertain that what factors affect the antibacterial action of SMs.; nevertheless, the presence of oxygen and sulfur in the chemical structure appears to be important. Antibacterial characteristics may be exhibited by various hydrocarbons, such as p-cymene, terpinene, and limonene [89 - 92]. SMs containing oxygen, such as phenols and sulfides, are more likely to have strong antibacterial properties [93, 94]. The hydroxyl group is expected to be important in blocking the ordinary transport of ions across the cell membrane and deactivating biocatalysts [11, 95].

It has been claimed that phenylpropene eugenol, the main component of clove EO, functions as an effective antibacterial by suppressing glycogen synthesis, enzymatic activity, preventing the bacterium from utilizing intracellular carbohydrates [110]. Bacteria exposed to eugenol have higher amounts of fat in their cellular membrane and release potassium ions [111]. Because they were unable to detect changes in the amounts of external adenosine triphosphate in bacteria exposed to eugenol. Gill and Holley [110] ruled out these effects as the origin of the substance's biocidal effects. Because of the disruption of the cell membranes, phenylpropene cinnamaldehyde, the main component of cinnamon oil, is considered to have antimicrobial characteristics [112]. These result in intracellular ATP depletion, decreased glucose intake, and bacteriocin [11, 110]. Gram negative bacteria exposed to cinnamaldehyde showed no evidence of cell wall degradation [113]. The S-allyl molecule of allicin has been demonstrated to interact with thiol (-SH) groups in amino acids and proteins, potentially affecting biological activities [114]. While diallyl sulphides frequently act in the same way, various other mechanisms have been proposed [115].

The presence of alkaloids, phenols, terpene derivatives, and other antibacterial components in EOs provides them a more precise mechanism of action against a wide spectrum of pathogenic germs. EOs may be utilized as improved supplements or alternatives to fight harmful microorganisms. Most medicinal herbs contain antibacterial effects due to the presence of EOs. The type, structural composition, and functional groups of EOs are important variables in determining their antibacterial activity. Terpenoids and terpenes, phenol-derived aliphatic and aromatic compounds with biocides, antifungal, and antibacterial properties, are among the volatile molecules found in EOs and have a direct impact on the pathogenic bacterium's cellular membrane by increasing permeability and causing the leaking of essential subcellular components. They also undeniably suppress microbial enzyme synthesis and cell respiration. They also displayed cytotoxic effects on living cells under various concentration and composition. Consequently, it has been suggested that EOs extracts from medicinal herbs might be employed as alternative potent antimicrobial components, as well as play an important role in the creation of novel antibiotics (Tables **3** & **4**) [73]. EOs' antimicrobial properties are often connected to their lipophilicity and functional groups [91]. Volatile chemicals interact with lipid bilayer processes such as electron transport, ion flux, protein transportation, phosphorylation, and other enzyme-dependent mechanisms, enhancing bacterial permeability of the membrane [11, 75, 91, 116].

Table 3. Effects of essential oils extracted from medicinal plants on pathogenic microorganisms. Adapted from Akhtar *et al.*, [73].

Plant	Part Used	Chemical Compound	Inhibited Microorganism	References
Cymbopogon citrates	Fruit	Ethanolic compounds	*Enteriobacteriacae, S. aureus*	Grohs and Kunz [74]
Allium sativum	Bulb	Isothiocynate	*Enteriobacteriacae, Candida* spp.	
Thymus vulgaris	Arial part	Thymol, Linalol, Carvacrol	*L. monocytogens, E. coli, S. typhimirium, S. aureus*	Lambert *et al.* [75]
Pimpinella anisum	Seed	Trans-anethole	*S. typhimirium, E. coli*	Elgayyar *et al.* [76]
Origanum vulgare	Arial part	Carvacrol, Thymol, γ-Terpinene	*L. monocytogens, E. coli,* Adeno virus, Polio virus	Ultee and Smid [77]
Feoniculum vulgare	Seed	Trans-anethole	*Alternaria alternata, Fusarium oxysporium, Aspergillus flavus*	Hammer *et al.* [78]
Cinnamomum zelancium	Bark	Cinnamaldehyde	*Enterobacteriacae*	Hood *et al.* [79]
Amomum kerervanh	Seed	Ethanolic compounds	*Enteriobacteriacae*	Burt [11]
Syzygium aromaticum	Flower bud	Eugenol, Eugenylacetate	*Eneriobactericae, A. fumigatus, Candida* spp.,	Lanciotti *et al.* [80]
Zingiber officinale	Rhizomes	Ethanolic compounds	Adeno virus, Polio virus *Enteriobacteriacae*	
Artemisa arborescens	Leaves	β-Triketone	*Herpes simplex* virus	Sinico *et al.* [81]
Rosmarinus officinalis	Flower	Benzaylacetate, Linalool, α-pipene	*E.coli, S. typhimurm, B. cerus, S. aureus*	Oussalah *et al.* [82]
Thymus vulgaris, Mentha piperita	Arial part	1,8- Cineole, Eugenel	*S. aureus, S. typhimirium Vibrio parahaemolyticus*	Sokovic *et al.* [83]

(Table 3) cont.....

Plant	Part Used	Chemical Compound	Inhibited Microorganism	References
Salvia officinalis	Arial part	1,8-Cineole-caphure, α-pipene	*S. aureus, E. coli*	Mulyaningsih *et al.* [84]
Verbana officinalis	Arial part	Borneol, Geranoil	*S. aureus, E. coli, S. typhimirium, L. monocytogens*	Shan *et al.* [85]

Table 4. Combinations of Essential oil and its components and their antimicrobial interactions with several microorganisms. Adapted from Bassolé *et al.* [96].

Pair	Organism	Methods	Interaction	References
Thymol/carvacrol	*Staphylococcus Aureus, Pseudomonas. Aeruginosa*	Half dilution	Additive	Lambert *et al.* [75]
	Escherichia Coli	Checkerboard	Synergism	Pei *et al.* [97]
	S. aureus, Bacillus. cereus, E coli	Checkerboard	Antagonism	Gallucci *et al.* [98]
	S. aureus, P. aeruginosa	Mixture	Additive	Lambert *et al.* [75]
	E. coli	Checkerboard	Additive	Rivas *et al.* [99]
	Salmonella typhinurium	Mixture	Synergism	Zhou *et al.* [100]
Thymol/eugenol	*E. coli*	Checkerboard	Synergism	Pei *et al.* [97]
Carvacrol/eugenol	*E. coli*	Checkerboard	Synergism	Pei *et al.* [97]
	S. aureus, B. cereus, E coli	Checkerboard	Antagonism]	Gallucci *et al.* [98]
Carvacrol/myrcene	*S. aureus, B. cereus, E coli*	Checkerboard	Antagonism	Gallucci *et al.* [98]
Carvacrol/Cymene	*B. cereus*	Mixture	Synergism	Ultee *et al.* [101]
Carvacrol/linalool	*Listeria monocytogenes,*	Checkerboard	Synergism	Bassole *et al.* [101]
Eugenol/linalool	*Enterobacter aerogenes,*	-	-	-
Eugenol/menthol	*E. coli, P. aeruginosa*	-	-	-
Menthol/Geraniol Menthol/Thymol	*S. aureus, B. cereus*	-	Synergism	Gallucci *et al.* [98]
Cinnamaldehyde/	*E. coli*	Checkerboard	Additive	Pei *et al.* [97]
Carvacrol	*S. typhinurium*	Mixture	Synergism	Zhou *et al.* [100]
Cinnamaldehyde/	*E. coli*	Checkerboard	Synergism	Pei *et al.* [97]
Thymol	*S. typhinurium*	Mixture	Synergism	Zhou *et al.* [100]
Cinnamaldehyde/	*E. coli*	Checkerboard	Synergism	Pei *et al.* [97]
Thymol	*S. typhinurium*	Mixture	Synergism	Zhou *et al.* [100]
Cinnamaldehyde/	*Staphylococcus sp.,*	Mixture	Additive	Moleyar and Narasimham [102]

(Table 4) cont.....

Pair	Organism	Methods	Interaction	References
Eugenol	*Micrococcus sp., Bacillus sp., and Enterobacter sp.*	-	-	-
1,8-Cineole/	*methicillin-resistant*	Checkerboard	Additive	Mulyaningsih *et al.* [84]
Aromadendrene	*S. aureus (MRSA) and vancomycin-resistant enterococci (VRE) Enterococcus faecalis*	-	-	-
Limonene/ 1,8-cineole	*S. aureus, P. aeruginosa*	Mixture	Synergism	van Vuuren and Viljoen [103]
α-pinene/ Limonene	*Saccharomyces cerevisiae*	Checkerboard	synergism, additive	Tserennadmid *et al.* [104]
α-pinene/Linalool Linalool/ Terpinen-4-ol	-	-	-	-
O. vulgare/ Rosmarinus officinalis	*L.monocytogenes, Yersinia enterocolitica, Aeromonas hydrophilla, P. fluorescens*	Mixture	synergism	de Azeredo *et al.* [105]
O. vulgare/T. vulgaris	*P. fluorescens*	Mixture	Additive	-
Lippia multiflora/ Mentha piperita	*E. coli, E. aerogenes, Enterococcus faecalis, L. monocytogenes*	Checkerboard	Synergism, additive	Bassole *et al.* [101]
L. multiflora/ O. basilicum	*P. aeruginosa, Salmonella enterica, S. typhimurium, Shigella. dysenteriae, S. Aureus*	-	-	-
M. piperita/ O. basilicum	*E. coli, E. aerogenes, E. faecalis, L. monocytogenes, P. aeruginosa, S. enterica, S. typhimurium, S. dysenteriae, S. aureus*	-	-	-
S. aromaticum/ R. officinalis	*Staphylococcus. epidermidis, S aureus, B. subtilis, E. coli, Proteus vulgaris, P. aeruginosa*	Mixture	Additive	Fu *et al.* [106]
-	*Candida albicans*	-	Synergism	-
-	*Aspergillus niger*	-	Antagonism	-

(Table 4) cont.....

Pair	Organism	Methods	Interaction	References
C. zeylanicum/ S. aromaticum	*E. coli Y. enterocolitica, L. monocytogenes, B. Cereus*	Mixture Mixture	Antagonism Synergism	Goni *et al.* [107]
O. vulgare/O. basilicum	*B. Cereus, E. Coli, P. Aeruginosa*	Checkerboard	Additive	Gutierrez *et al.* [108]
O. vulgare/ Melissa officinalis	*B. cereus*	-	-	-
O. vulgare/O. majorana	*B. cereus, E. coli*	-	-	-
O. vulgare/R. officinalis	*B. cereus*	-	-	-
O. vulgare/T. vulgaris	*Enterobacter cloacae, P. fluorescens, Listeria Innocua*	Checkerboard	Additive	Gutierrez *et al.* [108]
O. vulgare/ Salvia triloba	*B. cereus*	-	-	-
O. vulgare/T. vulgaris	*B. cereus, P. aeruginosa*	-	-	-
O. vulgare/T. vulgaris	*Enterobacter cloacae, P. fluorescens, Listeria Innocua*	Checkerboard	Additive	Gutierrez *et al.* [108]
T. vulgaris/O. majorana	*E. cloacae*	-	-	-
T. vulgaris/ M. officinalis	*L. innocua*	-	-	-
Cymbopogon citratus/ C. giganteus	*E. coli, E. aerogenes, L. monocytogenes, S. typhimurium, S. dysenteriae, S. aureus*	Checkerboard	Synergism, additive	Bassole *et al.* [109]

Numerous Gram-negative bacterial strains use the QS mechanism to monitor population density *via* signaling molecules such as N-acyl homoserine lactones (AHLs) [117]. It happens when AHLs bind to cellular receptors and activate many target genes, including those involved in virulence, antibiotic resistance, biofilm formation, bioluminescence, movement, and flocking [118]. The QS is a new method for creating early strategies to combat MDR illnesses [118]. Because of their ability to inhibit lipid oxidation and neutralize free radicals, the EOs from *E. globulus and E. radiata* may be suitable alternatives for synthetic drugs. When the two oils were mixed, they demonstrated outstanding antibacterial activity against a variety of Gram-negative bacteria as well as a combinatorial interaction with a variety of popular antibiotics against *A. baumannii* bacteria. These findings, together with the established anti-QS properties, showed that these oils might be a viable alternative to traditional antibiotics and disinfectants [119].

The EO from *E. globulus* leaves displayed antibacterial action against periodontist pathogenic bacteria. This EO has been found to have increased antioxidant activity and to be more efficient against Gram-negative microbes. The chemical characterization of the numerous chemicals that comprise the *E. globules* EO revealed the presence of oxidized terpenoids, which have the potential to function as antibacterial agents induced by microbial rupture of membranes. Because of its intrinsic antibacterial quality, the EO from *E. globulus* leaves may find usage in medicaments such as mouthwash and toothpaste [110, 120]. EOs, including cinnamon oil, are being utilized in animals as an alternative to antibiotics. The action, however, is nonspecific to microbes, parasites, and fungi [121, 122]. The effectiveness of the EO in inhibiting the development of 11 bacterial strains and 1 fungus was studied. In addition to antifungal action against *C. albicans*, the EOs showed antibacterial activity against both Gram-positive and Gram-negative microorganisms [123].

A study was conducted to assess the resoluteness of the MIC for the antimicrobial activity of EOs and pure chemicals. Thymol (38.99-52.92%), p-cymene (14.38-26.58%), terpinene (10.43-19.09%), linalool (2.39-3.56%), and carvacrol (1.87-3.3%) were the main constituents of all analysed samples. The EOs has shown the most antibacterial and antioxidant activity against *S. aureus*, *E. coli*, and *S. typhimurium* (MIC = 20 g/mL, 50 g/mL, and 500 g/mL, respectively). When compared to the analyses of virgin compounds, only thymol and carvacrol have shown strong antibacterial activity, free radical scavenging ability, and potency against *S. aureus, E. coli, and S. typhimurium* (MICs of 250 g/mL, 120 g/mL, and 60 g/mL, respectively). Data indicated that the best time to extract thyme EO is in the spring (20°C in Brazil) [124]. Several EOs exhibited antibacterial effectiveness against a variety of resistant bacteria [125]. Combining bactericidal medicines with EOs is one way to improve their efficacy [126, 127]. According to a recent study, certain phytochemicals can effectively inhibit the ion as efflux pumps responsible for the evolution of antibiotic resistance [128]. Thyme is one of the most often used medicinal plants in traditional treatments. It possesses exceptional antibacterial and antifungal activities due to phenolics such as quercetin, linalool, terpinene, and p-cymene [129 - 132]. Conventional antibiotics and Moroccan regional thyme EOs work together against MDR bacteria. Using these cumulations may curtail the lowest effective dose of drugs, reducing the risk of adverse side effects and the cost of therapy. More study is needed, however, to analyze the mechanism of action of EOs and appreciate the molecular pathways of their association with other chemically related antibacterial drugs to assess the therapeutic potential of these cumulations [133].

M. tuberculosis, the usual cause of tuberculosis (TB), was discovered by Robert Koch in 1882. It usually affects the lungs, although it can also affect other organs.

Furthermore, the ongoing pandemic and the emergence of MDR bacteria exacerbate the symptoms of this condition. Indeed, Koch's bacillus and HIV interact dangerously with one infectious agent taking advantage of the magnifying potential of the other [134]. For *T. satureioides*, the principal compounds were borneol (34.26%), carvacrol (31.21%), and thymol (3.71%), but for *M. pulegium*, the important compounds were R(+)- pulegone (75.48%), carvone (6.66%), and dihydrocarvone (4.64%). Following that, the micro-dilution technique employed to test their antimycobacterial action revealed that the MIC of *T. satureioides* EO against *M. aurum* and *M. smegmatis* was 0.062-0.015% and 0.125-0.031% (v/v) for *M. pulegium*. The data demonstrate unequivocally that Moroccan herbal herbs hold great promise for application as anti-tuberculosis treatments. These findings may enable researchers to launch several attempts to identify natural compounds that can be employed as early-stage anti-tuberculosis treatments [135]. The results demonstrated that *P. graveolens* EO and norfloxacin had a notable synergistic impact on three of the five bacterial species under investigation, with MIC values ranging from 0.37 to 0.50. These antibacterial characteristics were also shown to improve, albeit to a lesser level, when norfloxacin was combined with the main components of *P. graveolens* EO. The lowest effective dose of norfloxacin can be decreased to treat infections caused by certain bacterial species by combining it with *P. graveolens* EO or any of its constituent components. This will lessen the negative effects of the antibiotic [136]. In response to this revitalized interest, the current work expands on the chemical composition and antibacterial properties of EOs derived from Moroccan aromatic herbs *M. pulegium* and *J. phoenicea*. It first reports on the EO of *C. longus* during inclusion. Certain EOs, most notably *M. pulegium* EO, appear to be potential natural food preservation agents. Despite *J. phoenicea* and *C. longus* low activity, the findings in this study are particularly intriguing because the antibacterial activity of these EOs against the tested bacterial strains has never been examined or reported [137].

3.3. Antiviral Activity

EOs also partake antiviral properties. Natural materials provide limitless prospects for antiviral medication development due to their chemical variety and unrivalled availability, whether they are pure compounds or standardised plant extracts [138]. Natural products, as well as tiny chemicals from the biomedical area, continue to be important sources of novel therapeutic agents for a variety of maladies, including infectious disorders. Infectious viral infections continue to be a major medical concern since many viruses have demonstrated to be more resistant to prophylactic or treatment approaches than other pathogens. There are currently relatively few antiviral medications available to aid in the treatment of infections [139]. Human fibroblasts and tumor cell lines were used in most *in vitro* studies. Others choose monkey kidney cells since they may be used in antiviral research as well. Depending on the time of incubation, EOs have *in vitro* cytotoxic doses (CC_{50}) ranging from 5.0 to 1,950 g/ml. *In vitro*, EO doses of roughly 20-20,000 g/ml are necessary to induce bactericidal effects. This implies that EOs can be lethal to the tissue even when no antibacterial activity is evident. EOs, on the other hand, have antiviral activity at inhibitory concentrations (IC_{50}) ranging from 1 to 200 g/ml. The various components of EOs determine their cytotoxic action. In bacterial cells, EOs and their components have been found to cause cell cycle arrest, depolarization, and a decrease in the activity of cell membrane-associated enzymes [140]. The antiviral properties of EOs from different aromatic plants on different virus are summarized in Table **5** [141].

Table 5. Antiviral activity of different plant-derived essential oils. Adapted from Ma and Yao [141].

S. No.	Source of Essential Oils	Viruses	IC50	SI	Intercellular or Intracellular Mechanisms	References
1	Star Anise	HSV-1	1 µg/mL	160	Intercellular	Astani *et al.* [142]
2	*Mentha suaveolens*	HSV-1	5.1 µg/mL	67	Intracellular	Civitelli *et al.* [143]
3	Australian tea tree	HSV-1	13.2 µg/mL	43	Intracellular	Civitelli *et al.* [143]
4	*Sinapis arvensis*	HSV-1	0.035%	1.5	Intercellular	Sharifi-Rad *et al.* [144]
5	*Lallemantia royleana*	HSV-1	0.011%	6.4	Intercellular	Sharifi-Rad *et al.* [144]
6	*Pulicaria vulgaris*	HSV-1	0.001%	1	Intercellular	Sharifi-Rad *et al.* [144]
7	Mexican oregano (*Lippia graveolens*)	HSV-1	99.6 µg/mL	7.4	Intercellular	Pilau *et al.* [145]
8	*Zataria multiflora*	HSV-1	0.003%	55.4	ND	Gavanji *et al.* [146]
9	*Eucalyptus caesia*	HSV-1	0.007%	38.8	ND	Gavanji *et al.* [146]
10	*Artemisia kermanensis*	HSV-1	0.004%	66.4	ND	Gavanji *et al.* [146]
11	*Satureja hotensis*	HSV-1	0.008%	32.2	ND	Gavanji *et al.* [146]
12	*Rosmarinus officinalis*	HSV-1	0.006%	46.1	ND	Gavanji *et al.* [146]

(Table 5) cont.....

S. No.	Source of Essential Oils	Viruses	IC50	SI	Intercellular or Intracellular Mechanisms	References
13	*Thymus capitatus*	HSV-1	17.6 µg/mL	6.9	Intercellular	Toujani *et al.* [147]
14	*Thymus capitatus*	HSV-2	18.6 µg/mL	6.0	Intercellular	Toujani *et al.* [147]
15	*Salvia desoleana*	Acyclovir-resistant HSV-2	28.6 µg/mL	55.2	Intercellular and intracellular a	Cagno *et al.* [148]
16	Mexican oregano (*Lippia graveolens*)	Acyclovir-resistant HSV-1	55.9 µg/mL	13.1	Intercellular	Pilau *et al.* [145]
17	Patchouli	IFV-A (H1N1)	0.088 mg/mL	1.15	ND	Wei *et al.* [149]
18	*Cinnamomum zeylanicum*	IFV-A (H1N1)	<3.1 µL/mL	>4	Intercellular	Vimalanathan and Hudson [150]
19	*Citrus bergamia*	IFV-A (H1N1)	<3.1 µL/mL	>5	Intercellular	Vimalanathan and Hudson [150]
20	*Cymbopogon flexuosus*	IFV-A (H1N1)	<3.1 µL/mL	>4	ND	Vimalanathan and Hudson [150]
21	*Thymus vulgaris*	IFV-A (H1N1)	<3.1 µL/mL	>4	Intercellular	Vimalanathan and Hudson [150]
22	*Lavandula officinalis*	IFV-A (H1N1)	<3.1 µL/mL	>8	Intercellular	Vimalanathan and Hudson [150]
23	*Eucalyptus globulus*	IFV-A (H1N1)	<50 µL/mL	>0.5	Intercellular	Vimalanathan and Hudson [150]
24	*Pelargonium graveolens*	IFV-A (H1N1)	<3.1 µL/mL	>21	Intercellular	Vimalanathan and Hudson [150]
25	*Citrus reshni* ripe fruit peel	Avian influenza virus A (H5N1)	2.5 µg/mL	8.7	ND	Negy *et al.* [151]
26	*Fortunella margarita* fruit	Avian influenza virus A (H5N1)	6.8 µg/mL	ND	ND	Ibrahim *et al.* [152]

(Table 5) cont.....

S. No.	Source of Essential Oils	Viruses	IC50	SI	Intercellular or Intracellular Mechanisms	References
27	*Thymus vulgaris vulgaris, Cymbopogon citratus, Rosmarinus officinalis*	HIV-1	0.05–0.83 µg/mL	1.13–3.6	ND	Feriotto *et al.* [153]
28	*Cymbopogon nardus*	HIV-1	1.2 mg/mL	ND	ND	Mori *et al.* [154]
29	*Dysphania ambrosioides*	Coxsackie virus B4	21.7 µg/mL	74.3	ND	El Mokni *et al.* [155]
30	*Osmunda regalis* (Tunisian fern)	Coxsackie virus B4	2.2 µg/mL	789.8	ND	Bouazzi *et al.* [156]
31	Eucalyptus globulus bicostata	Coxsackie virus B3	0.7 mg/mL	22.8	Intercellular	Elaissi *et al.* [157]
32	Patchouli	Coxsackie virus B3	0.081 mg/mL	1.2	ND	Wei *et al.* [149]
33	Mexican oregano (*Lippia graveolens*)	Bovine viral diarrhoea virus	78 µg/mL	7.2	Intracellular	Pilau *et al.* [145]
34	*Ocimum basilicum*	Bovine viral diarrhoea virus	474.3 µg/mL	3.7	ND	Kubiça *et al.* [158]
35	Patchouli	Respiratory syncytial virus	0.092 mg/mL	1.1	ND	Wei *et al.* [149]
36	Mexican oregano (*Lippia graveolens*)	Respiratory syncytial virus	68 µg/mL	10.8	Intercellular	Pilau *et al.* [145]
37	*Lippia alba*	Yellow fever virus	4.3 µg/mL	30.6	Intercellular and intracellular	Gómez *et al.* [159]
38	Patchouli	Adenovirus-3	0.084 mg/mL	1.2	ND	Astani *et al.* [160]
39	Mexican oregano (*Lippia graveolens*)	Bovine herpes virus 2	58.4 µg/mL	9.7	Intercellular and intracellular	Pilau *et al.*, [145]
40	*Ayapana triplinervis*	Zika virus	38 µg/mL	12.5	Intercellular	Haddad *et al.* [161]
41	*Teucrium pseudochamaepitys*	Coxsackievirus B	589.6 µg/mL	1.11	ND	Hammami, [162]

Note: SI, selectivity index; HSV, human herpes viruses; HIV, human immunodeficiency virus; ND, not determined. "Intercellular" signifies mechanisms of action targeting virus surface during or before adsorption, while "intracellular" indicates action on intracellular events in viral lifecycle. a The late stage of viral lifecycle.

Virus adhere to, infiltrate, and invade the host cell, leading to the replication of their genetic material, culminating in the production and liberation of new virions [163]. Viral activity can be inhibited by the adverse actionon the related target involved in the infection phase (Fig. **1**).

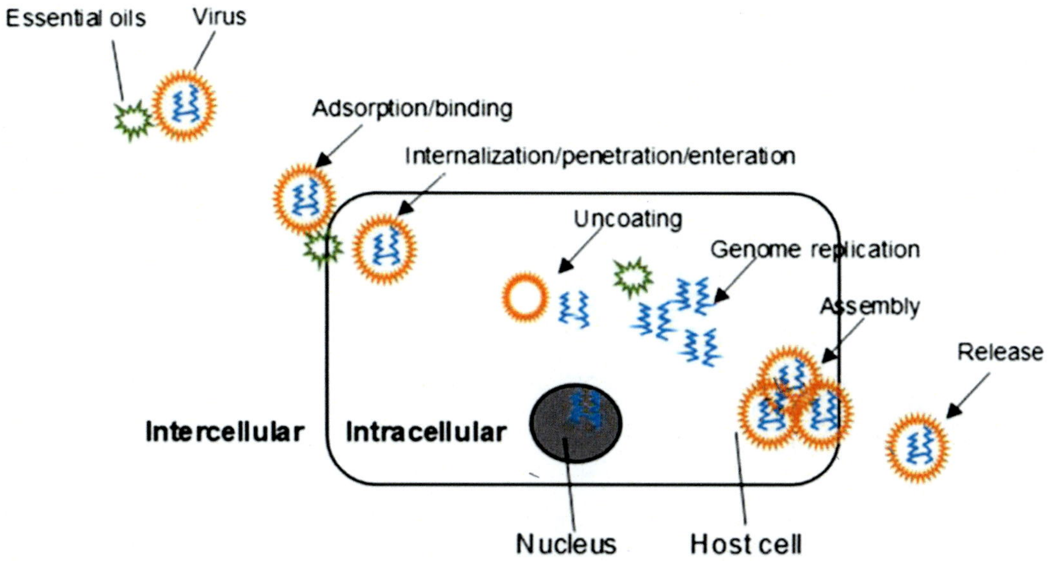

Fig. (1). Possible target sites of essential oil during viral lifecycle. Adapted from Ma and Yao [141].

Plant extracts, particularly EOs, may be a viable alternative to synthetic antiviral medications since they contain biocidal capabilities and are less hazardous than synthetic antiviral [164 - 166]. Herpes simplex virus (HSV-I, HSV-II) is a potentially lethal virus that is responsible for the vast majority of viral infections. *Artemisia arborescent* EO significantly improved the anti-intracellular HSV-1 activity of multilamellar lipid vesicles [81]. *Melissa officinalis* EO includes citral and citronellal, which can inhibit HSV-2 proliferation [167]. In viral suspension studies, *Mentha piperita* EO has shown excellent biocidal effectiveness against HSV-1, HSV-2, and an acyclovir-resistant version of HSV-1 [168]. *Lippia junelliana* and *Lippia turbinate* EOs successfully suppressed the Junin virus [169]. To a lesser extent, Australian eucalyptus and tea tree EOs had antiviral efficacy against HSV-1,2. *Santolina insularis* EO showed 100% antiviral efficacy against HSV-1,2 under *in vitro* conditions and was able to block virus replication from cell to cell in infected cells [170]. The oil reduced virion adsorption to host cells by directly inactivating virions. Isoborneol, a common monoterpenoid alcohol, demonstrated dual virucidal activity against HSV-1 and particularly decreased viral peptide glycosylation [171].

3.4. Antioxidant Activity

The phenolic components of EOs are highly powerful free radical scavengers [172, 173]. A variety of factors have been assessed to determine the antioxidant capabilities of foods, plant extracts, and EOs, including reducing power (RP), total phenolic content (TPC), carotene bleaching (BCB) activity [174 - 176], Trolox equipollent antioxidant capacity (TEAC), and 1,1-diphenyl-2 picrylhydrazyl (DPPH) [177, 178]. TPC, RP, BCB, TEAC, and DFRS activities were tested to measure the antioxidant levels of activity and major chemical components of 26 commonly used EOs. Across all tests, the clove bud EOs eugenol had the best results. The thymol and carvacrol in *Thyme borneol,* EO fared well in the RP, TPC, and BCB tests. A little amount of eugenol from jasmine absolute EO also displayed good DFRS proficiency. RP, TPC, BCB activity, TEAC, and DFRS competence were all substantially linked to chemical components with high phenol contents that displayed excellent antioxidant properties. These results indicate that clove bud, *Thyme, borneol,* and jasmine absolute EOs might be employed as antioxidants in functional cosmetics and foods [179].

Over the past ten years, there has been a surge in interest in herbal antioxidants, specifically polyphenolic compounds, owing to their health benefits in the treatment of several ailments, including carcinoma, cardiac, inflammation, and neurodegenerative problems, in addition to the prevention of aging [180 - 185]. Depending on the widely accepted action mechanism of such components, polyphenols' ability to absorb oxidizing agents aids in the mitigation of oxidative stress and the prevention of sickness [183, 186].

Numerous research investigated the antioxidant properties of EOs derived from eucalyptus species such as *E. polyanthemos, E. perriniana*, and *E. camaldulensis* [187 - 190]. *E. tereticornis* leaves, both decaying and fresh, exhibit strong antioxidant activity against DPPH, OH•, and O_2 radicals [118, 190]. The visual antioxidant activity of *E. citriodora* oil is supported by the long history of using eucalyptus oils in flavour, smell, aroma, and medicine. However, research confirming its antioxidant efficacy are few. On the other hand, it has been demonstrated that the oil extracted from the aerial portions of *E. radiata* and *E. camaldulensis* possesses significant DPPH• scavenging activity [189, 191].

Natural antioxidants have sparked a surge of innovation and technological advancement, with consequences for pharma industry. It has frequently been noticed that including these compounds in people's diets might assist them to avoid the harm caused by diseases characterized by reactive oxygen species (ROS). Indeed, the production of ROS such as superoxide ion ($O2^-$), hydroxyl radical (OH•), and hydrogen peroxide (H_2O_2) has been linked to several chronic health issues and ailments, including DNA damage, protein carbonylation, lipid peroxidation, Parkinson's disease, Vascular dementia, melanoma, cell cycle arrest, and heart conditions [192 - 194]. Thymoquinone (TQ), a significant component of VO from *Nigella sativa* seeds, has also been demonstrated to reduce lipid peroxidation in phospholipid liposomes in the encephalon, hence preventing the formation of eicosanoids in leukocytes [195, 196].

3.5. Anti-Inflammatory Activity

The composition of the EOs of 11 mentha plants revealed a prevalence of oxygenated monoterpenes, notably iso-menthone, menthol, menthofuran, D-neoisomenthol, 1,8-cineole, D-carvone, linalool, linalyl acetate, piperitenone oxide, and pulegone. The presence of increased piperitenone oxide, notably *M. longifolia* oil, is associated with the mentha species antioxidant action. According to the visual examination of *M. piperita* and *M. spicata*, both of which have anti-parkinsonian activity, the inhibitory action of this enzyme must occur *via* a synergistic mechanism between the major and minor components, with the major components being piperitenone oxide, menthofuran, 1,8-cineole, and limonene. The results of antioxidant and AChE inhibitory activities may expound the main utilization of plants of the genus *Mentha* in the treatment of gastrointestinal tract disorders, as oxidative stress is linked to inflammatory action in the gastric tract mucous membrane and AChE inhibitors may be useful in the treatment of intestinal motility disorders. Mentha EOs have been demonstrated to have minor antifungal properties. Pulegone's antifungal properties, which are highlighted in *M. spicata*, are directly connected to its presence in the oil composition [8]. Cinnamic acid, a chemical found in cinnamon and propolis and used by honeybees to seal their hives, has a variety of medicinal properties. Conti *et al.* [197] demonstrated that cinnamic acid inhibited the production of TNF- and IL-10 by inhibiting Toll-like receptors (TLR-4), a kind of pattern recognition receptor (PRR) located on immune cells that are implicated in the generation of inflammation in the intestinal mucosa [197, 198].

3.6. Cytotoxicity / Anticancer / Chemoprotective Activity

EOs and/or their constituent components are used to treat human ailments, including cancer. They have positive effects on chemoprevention and directly suppress the development of various human cancer cell lines due to their antioxidant, antiproliferative, and antimutagenic capabilities [199 - 202]. Furthermore, by activating various enzymes, EOs may reduce angiogenesis, enhance the immune system, and initiate the detoxification process [200]. Many EOs' active constituents have been demonstrated to alter gene expression, ion homeostasis, mitochondrial and plasma membrane activity, signaling, and metabolic pathways, resulting in cell cycle arrest [200 - 203].

Melanoma, one of the deadliest and most severe types of skin cancer, is mostly treated based on the time of diagnosis and becomes exceedingly resistant to existing treatments at the metastatic stage [204]. A surge in mammalian tumor cell resistance to chemotherapy and the severe side effects of this traditional treatment has fueled the hunt for novel, natural anticancer medicine. Terpenoids are responsible for the majority of plant EOs' anticancer properties [205]. The existence of diterpenoids with different skeletons, such as abietanes, labdanes, clerodanes, pimaranes, and icetexanes, is suggested to be responsible for the anticancer effects of *Salvia sp.* Many of these diterpenes, specifically tanshinones, have been shown to cause apoptosis and activate caspase-3 in the process [206]. Except for *Salvia viscose*, whose methanol extract has been researched for its cell magnification-inhibitory effect on human cervical adenocarcinoma (HeLa), skin carcinoma (A431), and breast adenocarcinoma (MCF7) cells, no other sal*via* species has been studied for anticancer activities. Many documentary evidences are avaliable on the anticancer properties of Sal*via* EOs and their constituents [207]. It might provide *in vitro* scientific evidence in favor of using *Salvia sp.* in traditional herbal cancer therapies utilized in Lebanon and other countries. The capacity of *S. aurea*, *S. judaica*, and *S. viscosa* EOs to target cancer cells while sparing healthy cells implies that these natural products might be interesting candidates for additional research into reducing the damaging side effects of chemotherapeutics in melanoma patients, as they include a lot of active ingredients that might operate together [208].

The EO extracted from the leaves of *Lippia gracilis* was found to be cytotoxic to a variety of tumor cell types [209]. However, the mechanisms behind these effects were not studied. The morphological changes were examined using hematoxylin and eosin staining in the presence of 5.0 g/ml EO cells demonstrated morphology consistent with apoptosis, such as cell volume loss, chromatin condensation, and nucleus fragmentation condensation. The proportions of viable, apoptotic, and necrotic cells were assessed using a cytotoxic drug screen and fluorescence microscopy. After 24 hours of exposure, EO-treated cells showed an increase in the number of apoptotic cells at a dose of 5 g/ml [210]. It is critical to emphasize that cytotoxicity is substantial as a result of legislation in the scent, cosmetic, tobacco, and aroma sectors [211]. Despite substantial studies on the use of EOs in sickness treatment, much more knowledge is needed on their potential to prevent disease. To address the bioactive components of EOs to specific targets, which may adopt the cytotoxicity property towards dysfunctioning loci, it remains preferable to develop and build preliminary procedures. Particles with bioactive components include toxins, agonists or antagonists, peptides, monoclonal antibodies, and other particles that target the receptors of either normal or malignant cells. Given their great chemical variety and broad spectrum of action, EOs and their constituents would very certainly be among the finest preventive care medicines once cytotoxicity is controlled [201].

Human umbilical vein endothelial cells (HUVEC), human ovarian carcinoma (A2780), cervical cancer (Hela), human colon adenocarcinoma (LS180), human breast adenocarcinoma (MCF-7), and HUVEC *in vitro* cytotoxicity tests revealed that nepeta oil had a significant anti-proliferative activity with the lowest IC_{50} value [123]. EOs and their constituents have also been shown to promote apoptosis and contribute to cellular metabolism [140, 212 - 214]. The 18 sage EOs were tested for their ability to inhibit enlargement and increase apoptosis in three human melanoma cell lines, A375, M14, and A2058 [215].

α—Bisabolol, a significant sesquiterpene alcohol discovered in *Matricaria chamomilla* EOs, can induce apoptosis in cells of particularly aggressive gliomas while remaining safe for animals and common astroglial cell survival [213]. Geraniol, a monoterpene alcohol, dramatically decreased thymidylate synthase (TS) and thymidine kinase (TK) production in colon cancer cells [216]. D-limonene inhibits tumor formation and spread by having anti-angiogenic and pro-apoptotic effects on human stomach cancer transplanted in unclad mice [217]. Furthermore, in a dose- and time-dependent fashion, d-limonene can stimulate the development of apoptotic bodies in BGC-823 gastric cancer cells [217]. Diallyl trisulfide (DATS), the major component of garlic EOs, has shown remarkable effectiveness in inhibiting human liver tumor cells at the G2/M phase of the cell cycle [218]. The mechanism of action is most likely the modulation of cyclin B1 and Cdk7 protein expression [219], 1,8-cineol is contained in large levels in *Elettaria cardamomum* and *Eucalyptus globulus* EO, ranging from 60% to 90% [220]. Human leukemia was treated after exposure to eucalyptol, HL-60 cells demonstrated morphological changes (DNA fragmentation) suggestive of apoptotic induction [221]. When delivered by hepatic arterial infusion, curcuma oil had a comparable consistently beneficial effect in treating primary liver cancer as a pharmacologic therapy [222].

3.7. Repellent and Insecticidal Activity

Bacterial resistance compositions derived from *Nepeta sp.* exhibit antibacterial and insecticidal properties due to the high flavonoid content [223, 224]. As a result, they have the potential to be employed as biocontrol agents and natural preservatives to prevent microbial degradation and extend food shelf life [225]. Insects, particularly mosquitos, carry serious human illnesses such as dengue, Japanese encephalitis, yellow pyrexia, hemorrhagic fever, and giardiasis. Due to the emergence of resistance, cross-resistance, and potential toxicity risks associated with synthetic insecticides, as well as their rising cost, interest in plant-based goods such as phytochemicals has recently been rekindled. *N. cataria* demonstrated strong insecticidal effectiveness against *Spodoptera littoralis* larvae with a median lethal dose (LC_{50}) value of 10.0 mL/m3 [226].

The major disease vector mosquitoes in a separate study that examined the repellent qualities of *N. cataria* EO and its components were *A. gambiae* and *C. quinquefasciatus*, the brown auditory perceiver tick *R. appendiculatus*, and the red poultry mite *Dermanyssus gallinae* [224]. This study's findings support the use of *N. cataria* derived materials as a prophylactic tool against sub-tropical and tropical mosquito disease vectors. Finally, *N. faassenii* is another nepeta species, utilized to repel mosquitoes [227]. It was recently reported that Pakistan natives were using *N. praetervisa* Rech. f. to treat children's geohelminth infections [228]. The larvicidal properties of *N. menthoides* EO and methanol extract killed *A. stephensi*, an important malaria vector. The LC_{50} and LC_{90} values for the EO and methanol extract, accordingly, were 243.3 and 69.5 ppm and 419.9 and 175.5 ppm, indicating that the methanol extracts had a greater impact than the EO [229, 230]. In Africa, it has been stated that burning the leaves of the *E. citriodora* plant is an effective and inexpensive approach to protecting dwellings against mosquitoes [231].

3.8. Hepatoprotective / Nephroprotective Activity

Several studies have found that herbal remedies can help heal liver problems [232]. Natural antioxidant-rich plants and herbs, such as carbolic acid, isoprene derivatives, carotene, terpenes, and polyphenols, may operate as hepatoprotective and nephroprotective agents [233]. According to the data, antioxidants from *Thymus algeriensis* essential oil (TEO) can protect cells from H_2O_2-induced damage. By restoring the cellular balance between oxidants and antioxidants [234]. TEO has been shown to protect rats from acute stomach injury, testicular toxicity, and H_2O_2-induced liver and kidney damage [234, 235]. TEO treatment partly or completely decreased H_2O_2-mediated oxidative stress and antioxidant capacity in kidney tissues. when measured in comparison to the control, the activities of GST, GPX, GSH, FELINE, and SOD were significantly curtailed by H_2O_2 delivery. TEO treatment, similar to the pattern reported in liver tissues, entirely recovered SOD and GPX activities while only partially restoring FELINE activity and GSH levels. TEO significantly boosted both GPX activity and GSH levels in renal tissues. TEO is a powerful antioxidant that has been proven to affect serum biochemical parameters, decrease lipid peroxidation, and restore antioxidant enzyme activity to mitigate the effects of H_2O_2-induced hepatorenal injury. According Fatma *et al.* [236], physiological changes are caused by several recognized chemotherapeutic agents, insecticides, and pharmaceuticals, the number of which has expanded dramatically in recent decades [236].

3.9. Analgaesia / Antinociceptive Activity

A constituent-based method, similar to generalizations about EOs toxicity to humans, can provide easy guidance in estimating EOs antimicrobial activity, but the true activity cannot be confirmed until a sample is tested, and even then, the findings can be surprising. This basic generalization offers the maximum activity to EOs components with a high lipophilic character on the hydrocarbon skeleton but a high hydrophilic character on its functional group, with the following ranking: phenol > aldehyde > ketone > alcohols > esters > hydrocarbons [41]. Analgesia is related to central nervous system activity, although it is referred to as antinociceptive activity in this context. When other ill states such as depression, solicitude, or hysteria are present, antinociceptive activity can be more closely linked with psychological consequences [40].

EOs' biological action is determined by their antinociceptive effect. The most commonly used methods for assessing these effects rely mostly on animal models that induce pain or intestinal writhing after intraperitoneal infusion. The goal of the therapy is to shorten these obvious consequences [40, 42]. Eugenol is a phenylpropanoid found in the plant known as "cravo da India," *Syzygium aromaticum* L. These usages include antibacterial and analgesic applications in dentistry, where the pure oil may be applied to the gums to relieve toothache [237].

3.10. Skin Care Activity

EOs have a long history of traditional usage and have recently gained popularity for skincare use. Nonetheless, research on the biological effects of EOs on human skin cells is scarce. Scientific investigations on EOs in human dermal fibroblasts found that these chemicals have a considerable influence on the proteins, genes, and metabolic pathways involved in inflammation and tissue remodeling [238, 239]. *Citrus aurantium* (petitgrain), *Coriandrum sativum* (cilantro), *Pelargonium graveolens* (geranium), *Helichrysum italicum* (helichrysum), *Pogostemon cablin* (patchouli), *Santalum album* (sandalwood), *Nardostachys jatamansi* (spikenard), and Cananga were used to study the biological functions of ten EOs. All 10 oils tested demonstrated considerable and potent antiproliferative effects on these cells. These oils have varied effects on protein molecules that are involved in tissue remodeling, immunological control, and inflammation. Helichrysum, ylang ylang, and Immortelle essential oils mostly showed tissue remodeling effects, whereas bergamot, cilantro, and spikenard EOs primarily demonstrated anti-inflammatory and tissue remodeling benefits. Given the results indicating therapeutic potential, these EOs might be a useful adjuvant treatment for a variety of disorders [39].

Excruciating pain is experienced by burn sufferers during operations such as dressing and debridement. Furthermore, there is a direct relationship between pain and solicitousness, with rising pain leading to increased dread. EOs may be the most effective alternative therapy for healing burn sufferers [240 - 242].

3.11. Memory Booster

The effects of rosemary EO on human quick visual and numerical recollection have been investigated. The research included 53 secondary school students from the Ukrainian capital (24 boys and 29 girls), aged 13 to 15. Participants were divided into two groups: the control group and the "Rosemary" group, which got a rosemary EO spray. While no gender disparities were found in the uniform groups, there were significant statistical differences in individuals' short-term memory productivity. As a consequence, compared to the control, rosemary EO significantly boosted visual recall. Inhaling rosemary EO increases one's capacity to memorize numbers. The findings add an overall understanding of the effects of EOs on human short-term memory and forward research into possible ways for boosting short-term memory for both pictures and numbers. There are statistically significant differences in the values of the quick recollection of the participants of different groups, as demonstrated by tests identifying the effect of the EO of rosemary on the cognitive features of students and the results obtained in the study, where the EO of rosemary has a statistically significant increase in the image and numeric recollection of the study participants when compared to the control [243].

In neurodegenerative diseases such as Alzheimer's, prominent immune cells in the encephalon known as microglial cells are activated. One of the proinflammatory chemicals released by activated microglia is nitric oxide (NO), a critical mediator of neuropathology and neuron cell death. The research found that geranium oil reduced NO generation as well as the expression of the proinflammatory enzymes cyclooxygenase-2 (COX-2) and induced nitric oxide synthase (iNOS), both of which are implicated in inflammation, in primary cultures of activated microglia. When examined in their natural relative levels in the oil, none of the key oil components could inhibit NO formation. Citronellol exhibited an inhibiting effect at higher doses. The data suggest that these components may have a synergistic connection. Geranium oil may be safe for use in the prevention or treatment of neurodegenerative disorders because neuroinflammation is a component of their development. EO of *P. graveolen* can reduce NO production as well as the expression of the inflammatory enzymes COX-2 and iNOS in initial cultures of excited microglia [244].

3.12. Respiratory Tract

Tonsillitis, sinusitis, bronchitis, and pneumonia are bacterial respiratory system disorders that typically originate from viral infections. The bacteria most commonly identified from the respiratory system include *S. pneumoniae, H. influenzae, M. catarrhalis*, and *S. pyogenes*. As a result, it is fascinating to investigate how these bacteria react to EOs. *In vitro* applications of, lemon balm (*M. officinalis*), thyme (*T. vulgaris*), cinnamon bark (*C. verum*), and lemongrass (*C. citratus*) oils were very effective, as were eucalyptus (*E. globulus*) and peppermin (*M. Piperita*) oils, which are commonly used to treat colds. Surprisingly, doses of 1.56-6.25 g/ml of the most active oils were enough to limit bacterial multiplication in the gaseous phase, indicating that an antibacterial effect of inhalation may be achievable [245, 246]. Cineole is used in conventional medicine to treat infections of the airways [247]. The gastroprotective effect of cineole was studied using a 100% ethanol gastric lesion model in rats [248].

3.13. Anxiety

EOs have a positive impact on mood and emotional well being. Fear disorders are among the most common mental illnesses [249]. Anxiety is characterized by a vague, unpleasant, blurry sense. Autonomic symptoms such as headache, sweating, palpitations, chest tightness, and mild stomach pain [250], The benzodiazepine family is the most often prescribed class of antianxiety drugs [251]. Thymus species are widespread, totaling over 150, and are largely found in Asia, Africa, and North America. With the majority of the species being indigenous, its distribution has lately been substantially expanded to the Iberian Peninsula [252]. According to one study, an oral dose of *T. vulgaris* extract may have an anxiolytic effect in rats. The presence of polyphenols, flavonoids, and EO in *T. vulgaris* plant extract enhances its anxiolytic activity. In addition to flavonoid content, it is likely that the anxiolytic impact visually observed in studies was connected to additional substances having antioxidant activity. More studies would be required to determine whether additional substances contributed to the reported activity because it is yet unknown which molecules created these effects [253].

The research was done to determine if taking *Satureja brevicalyx* or *Satureja boliviana* EOs in conjunction with mindful contemplation may lessen human solicitude levels. A randomized experimental study was undertaken with 108 participants divided into six groups, A control group and five experimental groups. Aromatherapy was conducted by inhaling EOs, but the mindfulness intervention program's focus was "flow meditation." The apprehensiveness index was calculated using the State-Trait Solicitousness Inventory (STAI). Measurements were obtained before and after the test. State and Trait solicitousness ratings dropped in all experimental groups during the post-test study period compared to the pre-test [254].

3.14. Anti Ulcer / Gastroprotective Activity

The current goals of ulcerative colitis treatment are to alleviate pain, revive the ulcer, and prevent ulcer recurrence [255]. As a result, some of the the common existing options for ulcerative colitis treatment include i) antacids *viz.* aluminum hydroxide and magnesium trisilicate; ii) chemopreventive medications *viz.* sucralfate and the prostaglandin analogue misoprostol; iii) muscarinic antagonists *viz.* pirenzepine; iv) *H. pylori* antibiotics *viz.* amoxicillin and metronidazole; v) H_2 receptor antagonists *viz.* cimetidine and ranitidine, and vi) proton pump inhibitors such as omepra [256, 257]. The usage of H_2 receptor blockers and proton pump inhibitors over an extended period has been related to several negative side effects, including intolerance, cardiomyopathy, infertility, hyperplasia, and hypomagnesemia [258]. Furthermore, some of these medicines are costly, and they may increase the risk of injury, asthma, and bowel cancer [259, 260]. As a result, early therapeutic pharmaceutical development for the treatment of stomach ulcers is crucial. It is well acknowledged in this context that medicinal herbs are the primary sources of bioactive compounds with anti-ulcerogenic potential [261, 262]. Many plants have anti-ulcerogenic effects and have been used in traditional medicine. Fragrant medicinal plant species have been employed since antiquity for their therapeutic benefits, which are often connected with the presence of EOs [199, 263, 264].

According to Rozza *et al.* [265] investigation, oral menthol therapy (50 mg/kg) had a strong protective effect on the stomach mucosa, 88% and 72% against ethanol and indomethacin, respectively. Isopulegol is a monoterpene found in the EOs of a variety of plants, including *Zanthoxylum schinifolium* Siebold & Zucc. and *Corymbia citriodora* Hill & Johnson [248, 266, 267]. Silva *et al.* [268] demonstrated that isopulegol (100 and 200 mg/kg) significantly reduced stomach ulcers in mice caused by 100% alcohol. Acute alcohol intake causes bleeding, edema, infiltration of inflammatory cells, and a reduction in internal sulfhydryl levels [269, 270]. Prostaglandins protect the stomach mucosa by encouraging mucus and bicarbonate formation [271]. Whereas, NO appears to be a critical regulator of blood flow and gastric vasculature [272]. In experiments utilizing pure limonene or EOs including R (+) limonene, animal models demonstrated hepatoprotective benefits [273]. Citrus lemon EOs (250 mg/kg) and limonene (177 mg/kg) protected the stomach mucosa and elevated the expression of the

HSP-70 protein, which is associated with cellular adaptive defense mechanisms in response to alcohol intake [274, 275]. *Citrus aurantium*, often known as caustic orange, has long been used to cure rheumatism and stomach problems [276]. Limonene is the major constituent of the EO extracted from the peel of the acerbic orange fruit [277]. *C. aurantium* EO and limonene were studied in a model of an ethanol-induced stomach injury, and the results demonstrated a rise in the quantity of mucus adhesion in animals treated with the chemicals, which supports their hepatoprotective effect Cineole (1,8-cineole, epoxy-p-menthane), or eucalyptol, is the primary monoterpene, found in EOs with other genera such as *Artemisia*, *Salvia*, and *Mentha* that accounts for 80% of the content of eucalyptus EO [278]. The oral LD_{50} in rodents was 2.48 g/kg weight, indicating that this monoterpene is highly safe.

Thymoquinone (TQ) capacity to restore normal proton pump function in parietal cells or antihistaminic effects were attributed to acid level decreases. TQ also decreased gastric secretion peptic action, which may have involved lowering gastric acidity, which delayed or blocked the activation of pepsinogens in gastric secretion and histamine release. TQ's metabolite, dihydro-thymoquinone, may be responsible for some of TQ's free radical scavenging and antioxidant activities [279]. TQ LD_{50} in mice after intravenous administration was 57.5 mg/kg and 794.3 mg/kg after oral ingestion, which explains the compound's low levels of gastroprotective activity [280].

Terpineol possesses gastroprotective effects against ethanol-induced ulcers [281]. Terpinen-4-ol is a cyclic monoterpene found in several aromatic plants, including *Zingiber montanum* [282], *Zingiber cassumunar* [283], *Melaleuca alternifolia Cheel* [284], and *Origanum majorana* [285]. Epoxycarvone (EC) is a monocyclic monoterpene found in the EOs of several plants, including *Carum carvi* and *Kaempferia galangal* [286]. Epoxycarvone (10 to 50 mg/kg) indicated gastroprotective effects in all ulcer models. However, no enhanced nitric oxide, prostaglandin, or anti-secretory activity was observed in such actions. Cyclohexanemethanol is a nontoxic sesquiterpene that is utilised as a fragrance component in cosmetics, high-end perfumes, shampoos, and soaps, as well as non-cosmetic goods such as household cleaners and detergents [287, 288]. EO from the leaves of *Cryptomeria japonica* has anti-ulcer action and dramatically decreases stomach lesions in the HCl/ethanol, HCl/aspirin, water-immersion stress, and pylorus ligation models [289]. Natural aliphatic nerolidol (3,7,11-trimethyl-1,6,10-dodecatrien-3-ol) is a key component of plant EOs [290, 291]. The anti-ulcer activity of *Baccharis dracunculifolia* EO and its major component nerolidol was evaluated using an ethanol-induced model of acute gastric ulcers [292]. According to the phytochemical analyses of the oil, the anti-ulcer effect of *B. dracunculifolia* EO can be attributed mostly to nerolidol (23.58%). Anethole

(300 mg/kg) had a hepatoprotective effect without altering mucus production by improving the quality of gastric mucus. Based on the study, the side chains of anethole's double bond and polar group improved its hepatoprotective function while decreasing its mucus secretion-inducing properties [293].

Capasso *et al.* [294] demonstrated dose-dependent gastroprotection (10 to 100 mg/kg) using alcohol injury models. Eugenol is derived from platelet membranes, involved in the etiology of various pathophysiological conditions such as gastric ulcers [295], and associated with vicissitudes in the gastric epithelium of mice [296]. *Alpinia galanga* (galanga) is widely grown in China, India, and Southeast Asia. Galangal rhizomes are commonly employed in herbal medicine and as ginger or spice substitutes in cooking [297]. 1'S-1'-acetoxychavicol and a few related phenylpropanoids from the rhizomes of *A. galangal* had protective effects against gastric lesions caused by various necrotizing agents in their study on the protective effects of 1'S-1'-acetoxychavicol and a few related phenylpropanoids from the rhizomes of (2.0 mg) [298].

Cinnamon powder (100 mg daily for four weeks) effectively protected mice from ulcers caused by stress, alcohol, HCl, and oral aspirin medication, but not indomethacin ulceration [299]. Citral is a superseded vinyl aldehyde found in plants such as myrtle trees, African basil, lemons, limes, and oranges [300]. At the 3 hr time point, the stomach injury caused by naproxen (100 mg/kg, p.o.) might cause substantial harm. These findings indicate that naproxen and citral have systemic interactions, induce little stomach injury, and may have therapeutic benefits in the treatment of inflammatory pain [301]. Antihistamine activity is a good prophylactic therapy for alcohol-induced stomach discomfort [302].

3.15. Diabetes Remedy

Diabetes is a condition in which the body is unable to produce or utilize insulin properly. Few researches have been published evaluating the potential advantages of EOs as hypoglycemic agents. Some EOs may worsen diabetes. Diabetic rabbits treated with rosemary EO had hyperglycemic and insulin-release inhibitory action [303]. An oral dose of EOs, including cinnamon, cumin, fennel, oregano, and myrtle, increased insulin sensitivity in type 2 diabetes while also lowering circulating glucose in the thigh [304]. Lipophilic component of EOs has no antidiabetic properties. In diabetic mice, the *Satureja khuzestanica* EO resulted in comparable reductions in fasting blood glucose levels [305, 306]. More research is needed to show the reliability of other EOs' low blood sugar properties and to elucidate their process of action [199].

3.16. Antherosclerosis Remedy

Atherosclerosis develops when plaque deposits form in the intima, the innermost layer of the artery [307]. EOs high in phenolic components, such as eugenol and thymol, have the most antioxidative effect on LDL oxidation, which can also change the LDL receptor's affinity [308]. Terpinene is found in high concentrations in citrus peel EOs such as bergamot (14%), mandarin (17%), and lemon (10%). Terpinene (23.0%) is prevalent in tea tree EO [309, 310]. It has been proposed as a food and beverage component to prevent LDL oxidation and plaque development [311]. The EO of the native Iranian plant *Satureja khuzestanica* lowers the level of common blood lipid peroxidation [306].

3.17. Wound Rejuvenating and Remedy

Wound rejuvenation is a worldwide medical issue that confronts several challenges, including the increased incidence of obesity and type II diabetes, an aging population, and the need for more effective but also cheap bandages [312]. To achieve tissue and wound renewal, an involuntary process comprising several linked biological and molecular activities is required [313, 314]. The key physiological processes are clotting, irritation, and abstraction of injured matrix components, which are subsequently followed by cellular cell migration and proliferation, vasculature, matrix synthesis, layering, re-epithelization, and remodeling (Table **6**).

Table 6. Summary of the evidences for the use of EO in surgical patients. Adapted from Stea *et al.* [37].

Condition	Essential Oil	References
Anxiety	Lavender	Lehrner *et al.* [315]; Bradenet *et al.* [316]; Kim *et al.* [317]; Perry *et al.* [318]
	Citrus sinensis	Lehrner *et al.* [315]; Goes *et al.* [319]; Jafarzadeh *et al.* [320]
	Rosa damascene	Hongratanaworakit [321]
	Neroli	Hu *et al.* [322]
	Lavandula officinalis +Anthemis nobilis +Neroli	Cho *et al.* [323]
Pain	*Citrus reticulata*	Jong *et al.* [324]
-	Lavender	Kim *et al.* [325]; Soltani *et al.* [326]; Olapour *et al.* [327]
Nausea	*Menta × piperita*	Tate [328]; Hines *et al.* [329]; Lane *et al.* [330]; Lua and Zakaria [331]; Ferruggiari *et al.* [332]; Hunt *et al.* [333]; Hiki *et al.* [334]; Shavakhi *et al.* [335]
-	*Zingiber officinale + Mentha spicata + Menta × piperita*	Hunt *et al.* [333]

(Table 6) cont.....

Condition	Essential Oil	References
Infection	*Melaleuca alternifolia*	Halc´on and Milkus [336]; Chin and Cordell [337]; Edmondson *et al.* [338]; Blackwood *et al.* [339]
-	*Menta spicata + Thymus vulgaris + Eucalyptus globulus*	Cavalca Cortelli *et al.* [340]; Osso and Kanani [341]

Because of ecumenical's significant expense burden, novel techniques for fast wound regeneration are sought. Numerous research on the real situation of wound renewal and wound healing products have been undertaken, with an emphasis on the governing directive for more sophisticated forms of wound therapy, as well as a few of the current difficulties and driving forces behind this governing directive. The treatment of long-term wounds, such as amputees, diabetics, skin ulcers, bed sores, surgical wounds, and traumatic wounds (burns and accidents), is an essential area of attention when patient immunity is poor and the risk of infection and consequences is high. Initial dressings include medicated moist dressings, tissue-engineered substitutes, biological dressings based on biomaterials originating from natural sources, medicated sutures, and various coalescences of the previous groupings.Plant extracts from *Chamomilla recutita* [342], *Hamamelis virginiana* [343], *Polisiphonia lanose* seaweed [344], *Acacia arabica*, and *Moringa oleifera* are already being used to make advanced wound dressings [345]. A collagen sponge infused with *Macrotyloma uniflorum* extract, which is widely used in cow feeding [346]. The plant extract provides antimicrobial quality to the sponge while also increasing its strength properties and collagenase enzyme consistency. Table **7** is a list of herbal metabolites that can be used to heal wounds [347].

Table 7. Extracts from Different Plants Useful in Wound Healing. Adapted from Sharma *et al.* [347].

S. No.	Medicinal Plants	Part Used	Metabolites	Uses	References
1.	Turmeric (*Curcuma longa*)	Rhizomes	Curcumin, vitamin A, proteins	Chronic wound healing	Jain *et al.* [348]
2.	Liquorice (*Glycyrrhiza glabra*)	Roots	Glycyrrhizin, glycyrrhetinic	Acute/chronic wound healing	Ameri *et al.*[349]
3.	Centella (*Centella asiatica*)	Leaves	Asiatic acid, asiaticoside madecassoside, madecassic acid	Incision wound healing	Shukla *et al.*,Chen *et al.* [350, 351]
4.	Carbonal (*Mimosa tenuiflora*)	Stem	Mimosine (an alkaloid), sitosterol, amino acids, linoleic acid, tannins, polyphenols, and oleic acid	Chronic wound healing	Kumarasamyraja *et al.*[352]

(Table 7) cont.....

S. No.	Medicinal Plants	Part Used	Metabolites	Uses	References
5.	Honey (*Apis mellifera*)	Secretion from hive	5-Hydroxyimidacloprid, 4,5-dihydroxyimidacloprid, desnitroimidacloprid, 6-chloronicotinic acid, olefin	Acute wound healing	Gorgescu *et al.*[353]
6.	Theaceae (*Camellia pubipetala*)	Leaves	Flavonoids, theanine and caffeine	Excision wound healing	Yang *et al.* [354]
7.	Forest Champa (Spermadictyon suaveolens)	Roots	Triterpenes, sesquiterpenes, alkaloids	Chronic wound healing	Rani *et al.* [355]
8.	Neem (*Azadirachta indica*)	All portions	Azadirachtin, azadirone, nimbin, nimbidin, nimbinin	Open wound healing	Osunwokeemek *et al.* [356]
9.	Sesame (*Sesamum indicum* L.)	Seeds	Metronidazole, E and C vitamins, sesamolinol, sesamol, sesaminol, sesamolin	Acute/chronic wound healing	Kiran and Asad [357]
10.	Trumpet tree (*Cecropia peltata*)	Leaves	Flavanoids, terpenes phenols, alkaloids, sterols, waxes, fats, tannins, gums, resin acids	Closed wound healing	Sana *et al.* [358]
11.	Kencur (*Kaempferia galanga*)	Rhizomes	Amino acids, protein, carbohydrate, alkaloids, steroids, cholesterol, cardiac glycosides,	Incision wound healing	Himesh and Singhai [359]
12.	Druce (*Prosopis cineraria*)	Leaves	Patulitrin, diketones, spicigerin, β-sitosterol, stigmasterol, hentria- contane, octasanol, and prosogerin A, B, C, and D	Closed wound healing	Kumarasamyraja *et al.* [352]
13.	Maidenhair (*Ginkgo biloba*)	Leaves and seeds	Flavonoids, lactones, and ginkgolic acid	Closed wound healing	Muhammad *et al.* [360]
14.	Indian mulberry (*Morinda citrifolia*)	Leaves and fruit	Anthraquinones, steroid, phenol, tannin, and terpenoids	Closed wound healing	Nayak *et al.* [361]
15.	Club Moss (*Lycopodium serratum*)	Spores and whole fern	Alkaloids, steroids, tannins	Acute/chronic wound healing	Manjunatha *et al.* [362]
16.	Madagascar periwinkle (*Catharanthus roseus*)	Leaves	Monoterpenoids alkaloids, vinblastine, Vincristine	Acute/chronic wound healing	Nayak *et al.* [363]
17.	Asthma Weed (*Euphorbia hirta*)	Leaves	Saponins, tannins, flavonoids, alkaloids, glycosides	Chronic wound healing	Mittal *et al.* [364]

(*Table 7*) *cont.....*

S. No.	Medicinal Plants	Part Used	Metabolites	Uses	References
18.	Red sandalwood (*Pterocarpus santalinus*)	Bark wood	Santalin A and B, savinin, calocedrin, pterolinus K and L, and pterostilbenes	Acute/chronic wound healing	Yogesh and Jeyabalan [365]
19.	Lawsonia alba (*Lawsonia inermis*)	Leaves and roots	Coumarins, naphthoquinone, flavonoids, sterols, triterpene, and xanthones	Chronic wound healing	Chaudhary *et al.* [366]
20.	Jandi or Ghaf (*Prosopis cineraria*)	Leaves and pods	Patulitrin, diketones, spicigerin, β-sitosterol, stigmasterol, hentria- contane, octasanol, and prosogerin A, B, C, and D	Cutaneous wound healing	Asif *et al.* [367]
21.	Aloe (*Aloe vera*)	Leaves	Anthaquinone, C and E vitamins, amino acids	Open wound healing	Galehdsti *et al.*, Orue *et al.* [368,369]
22.	Bay (*Sphagneticola trilobata*)	Leaves	Flavonoids, terpenoids, alkaloid, and saponin	Incision wound healing	Balekar *et al.*, Govindapa. [370, 371]
23.	Adusa (*Adhatoda vasica*)	Leaves	Flavonoids, tannins	Excision wound healing	Vinothapooshan and Sundar [372]
24.	Humble plant (*Mimosa pudica*)	Whole plant	Mimosine (an alkaloid), sitosterol, amino acids, linoleic acid, tannins, polyphenols, and oleic acid	Excision wound healing	Kumarasamyraja *et al.*[352]
25.	Papaya (*Caricapapaya*)	Latex, fruit	Papain	Diabetic, burn, soft tissue wounds	Mahmood and Salmah [373]
26.	Jungle flame (*Ixora coccin ea*)	Roots, leaves	Sesquiterpenes, Triterpenes, geranyl acetate, ursolicacid	Cutaneous, excision	Selvaraj*et al.* [374]

4. MECHANISM OF THE BIOLOGICAL ACTIVITIES OF ESSENTIAL OILS

Many EOs contain active ingredients that can regulate the paradoxical replications caused by various genes and pathways. To develop early treatment options for a variety of diseases, it is necessary to understand the action mechanism of the bioactive components, whether inside or across distinct cell types.The focus should be on identifying how interactions between bioactive components might boost replication efficiency. Specificity and cytotoxicity must be addressed when using EOs and their active components for therapeutic and prevention purposes [201].

A wide range of volatile chemical ingredients make up essential oils. An innovative administrative approach based on nanotechnology has been created to aid in the adoption of EOs. Using this technique, EOs are encapsulated into nanoparticles to increase their absorption and effectiveness. Depending on their molecular size, EO molecules take distinct routes to enter the brain after inhalation. The respiratory and olfactory systems are included in the inhalation delivery pathway (Fig. **2**). The nasal cavity, which is the starting point of the olfactory system and is related to the olfactory bulb, is important for the transmission of odorant signals. The olfactory system is closely associated with other brain regions, such as the hippocampus and hypothalamus. A few extremely tiny chemical molecules have the ability to cross the olfactory mucosa or sensory neuron cells' axons and enter the central nervous system (CNS), where they can directly affect an individual's emotional reaction. On the other hand, gaseous exchange is principally managed by the respiratory system. Vapour molecules have the ability to spread throughout the respiratory system in different parts. For example, they diffuse to the alveoli, dissolve into the pulmonary epithelium, and ultimately reach the circulation, which carries them to the brain regenerate reaction [375].

Hydrophobicity of EOs is required for their antimicrobial properties. It indicates that the liquid stages of EOs will selectively partition into the cytoplasmic lipid bilayer membrane, where they will then accumulate. One or more of EOs' antimicrobial effects are considered directed from inside the phospholipid bilayer membrane by modulating penetrability, which interferes with ion conduction mechanisms, connecting with membrane proteins, and other subcellular components. This EO-mediated replication occurs either from within the plasma membrane or through diffusion into the cytosol. Because EOs are combinations of various SMs, they may have several types of action mechanisms [376]. Thymol and curcumin, two phenolic terpenoids found in oregano EO, have antibacterial activities [113, 377, 378]. They have been demonstrated to increase the permeability and solubility of cell membranes when combined with oregano EO, resulting in cell content loss and autolysis [379 - 381]. Microbes exposed to these phenolic terpenoids showed a greater ratio of saturated to unsaturated membrane fatty acids, perhaps due to thymol and curcumin's increased permeability of cell membranes [380, 382, 383]. According to studies, both thymol and curcumin diminish H^+ ion and K^+ ion gradients and thus proton motive potential, lowering intracellular ATP levels by slowing ATP synthesis or boosting the rates of ATP hydrolysis [75]. The hydroxy group of these phenolic monoterpenes functions as a transmembrane proton transporter [95], similar to coccdiostats [384].

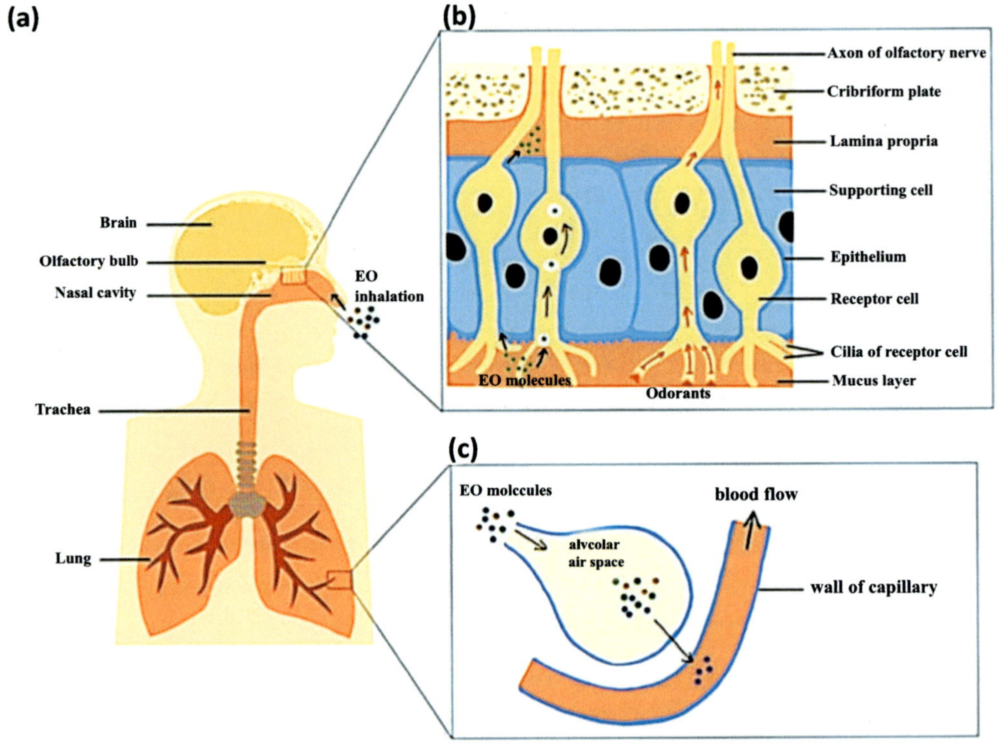

Fig. (2). Inhaled EO response delivery to brain through the respiratory and olfactory systems: (**a**) Inhaled EO passes through the nasal cavity and reaches the olfactory system or respiratory system (**b**) Overview of EO molecules' delivery pathway in the olfactory system (**c**) Overview of EO molecules crossing the air–blood barrier to reach the circulatory system. Adapted from Fung *et al.* [375].

SMs may have an important role in defending plants from herbivores, pathogens, and competitors [385]. They can also operate as an acid during seed disposal, as a barrier against external abiotic agents, or as a combination of these roles. Because of their unique features, the metabolites may be able to perform the aforesaid roles. Examples include smell, biological processes, and odour. SMs are naturally occurring substances that fall into three broad categories: alkaloids (12,000 different types), phenolic compounds (8,000 different types), and terpenes and terpenoids (25,000 different types) [386, 387].

Oxygenated monoterpenes are prevalent in the EO derived from the aerial portions of the bioactive natural product *N. sintenisii*, particularly 4a,7,7a-nepetalactone, which accounts for 51.74% of the total oil content. According to scientific investigations, the oil shows powerful antifungal and antimicrobial effects, along with dose-dependent cytotoxic activity against tumor cell lines, suggesting that it should be researched for possible therapeutic advantages in lab animals of infection and cancer [123]. Olive fruit and its related products, notably extra-virgin olive oil, are popular in Mediterranean countries due to their subtle flavor, pleasant perfume, and medical benefits [388 - 390]. The main scent components that pass from olive fruits to oil are trans-2-hexenal, hexanal, and cis-3-hexenal [391, 392]. Because the major purpose of aromatization is to supply clients with new flavors. Herbs and aromatic plants are frequently utilized in aromatization because of their powerful scents.

Rosmarinus officinalis is a common plant used in the aromatization of olive oil because of its good benefits to health and great nutritional potential with strong antibacterial, antidiabetic, and antioxidant activity [393, 394]. The main volatile compounds responsible for rosemary's strong aroma include -pinene, citronellol, eugenol, cinnamon, p-cymene, myrcene, limonene, and -caryophyllene [395, 396]. When the aromatic material is coupled to olive paste at the absorption stage rather than crushing or infusion in olive oil, the transfer of fragrance components from rosemary to olive oil is independent of the malaxation parameters studied. This provides an opportunity for producers, particularly if they manufacture aromatized olive oil under conditions comparable to those utilized in the study. The absence or limited effect of malaxation conditions on the aroma component transfer from rosemary to olive oil indicates a more controlled aromatization mechanism [397].

It has been reported that EOs derived from fragrant medicinal herbs such as thyme (*Thymus vulgaris*), fennel (*Foeniculum vulgare*), and peppermint (*Mentha piperita*) are efficient against microbes, fungi, and viruses along with Gram-positive and Gram-negative bacteria. They have a nice odour and are made up of a variety of volatile and lipophilic chemicals, including terpenoids, sesquiterpenes, and phenolics. They are also regarded to be a component of the higher plants' natural defensive mechanism [398, 399]. Despite intensive testing against a wide range of bacteria, yeasts, and fungi, the interaction between EOs and microorganisms that results in antimicrobial activity is not fully understood. the influence of various concentrations of *Cymbopogon densiflorus* EO on *Staphylococcus aureus* metabolism, magnification, and morphology, at low oil concentrations made metabolism inefficient owing to heat loss, whereas relatively high oil concentrations inhibited *staphylococcal* multiplication in a bacteriostatic way [400]. According to the electron microscopy studies, bacteriolysis is a topological shift generated by bactericidal medications. The antifungal efficacy of tea tree (*Melaleuca alternifolia*) oil and many of its constituents against *Candida albicans, Candida glabrata*, and *Saccharomyces cerevisiae* was investigated [401].

CONCLUSION

This chapter illustrates the potentials of EOs as expectorants and diuretics, antibacterial and antifungal actions, antiviral activity, antioxidant activity, anti-Inflammatory activity, chemoprotective activity, repellent and insecticidal activity, protective activity, analgaesia / antinociceptive activity, skin care activity, recollection booster respiratory tract, Solicitousness, gastroprotective activity, diabetes remedy, artherosclerosis remedy, wound rejuvenating and remedy and have explored the probable EOs that can be utilized in drug development. Different modes of application of EOs were discussed. An approach to exhibit enhanced efficacy *via* combinatorial effects of EO–EO or EO–antibiotics have additionally been reported.

There are adequate reports available on the correlation amid the structure of EO compounds and its cognition with its antimicrobial activity. However, the mechanisms by which the EO function are not plenarily understood in detail. Moreover, there have been reports of the negative impact of exorbitant doses of EO on human health. Although generally regarded as safe, natural products and EOs are not thoroughly safe due to the diversity of metabolites in them when utilized as antimicrobial agents. The substantial magnitude of secondary metabolites may have synergistic or antagonistic properties when utilized in non-standardized forms. Thus, there is a desideratum to optimize the analysis of a range of EOs and compounds more pellucidly for the efficacious yet safe utilization of EO for human beings. The formation of residues in biological systems and allergic reactions associated with the utilization of EOs are additionally among other challenges regarding their utilization as antimicrobial agents.

In the forthcoming days, research studies should be designed to determine the exact mechanism of action that is categorical for each EO and the synergistic mechanisms between its components. Further extensive studies might be designed to evaluate or prognosticate the adoptive comportment of microbes to the EO after chronic or subchronic use. However, with the evolving concept of green technology, probably the utilization of EO and medicinal plants will upsurge. The utilization of natural plant products-predicated drugs, herbs, EOs, and isolated pristine compounds is enormously incremented in medicine, cosmetics, neutraceuticals, and aliment sectors. With the utilization of modern analytical techniques evidence-predicated medicine can be developed with more efficiency and fortification. Consequently, incipient nanotechnology predicated approaches and synergistic research will provide utilizable information about its uptake mechanism and dosage.

Despite the fact that genomics, proteomics, and metabolomics have provided us with consequential prospects to understand the bio-drug targets, the problematic situation is engendered by microbial-mediated infections which is still an ecumenical health challenge. Emergence of resistant genes and the indiscriminate utilization of antimicrobial agents is one of the very consequential reasons abaft this. Another most paramount reason is that the pharma sector predicated industries are in a hurry to develop more and more drugs with only a few derivatives of the pristine drugs. There is inadequate fixate on the detection of novel compounds with incipient mechanisms of action. Hence, for the advancement in the development of efficacious therapeutic agents, expertise's from numerous disciplines are required; which constitute of genomics, structural biology, biotechnologist, chemist, and bioinformatics. These oils are efficacious and utilized in raw and processed aliment preservation, perfumery, and in alternative medicine due to their antimicrobial and antioxidant activities for burn rejuvenating, and malarial infection. EOs are withal shown to give synergistic activity when utilized with antibiotics and thought to be efficacious to treat antimicrobial resistance, and in the public perspective, it is more accepted due to its traditional use. Precedent revelations of EOs against antimicrobials still did not explicate precisely the EO mechanism of action and their chemical nature, and this makes the efficacy and action of EOs against antimicrobials obscure and in the desideratum of amendment. EO can be efficacious by either the absorption, ingestion, or inhalation through the lungs of its volatile compounds.

REFERENCES

[1] Schnaubelt K. Medical Aromatherapy: Healing with Essential Oils. 1st ed., Berkeley, Canada: Frog Books 1999.

[2] Buchbauer G, Jirovetz L, Jäger W, Plank C, Dietrich H. Fragrance compounds and essential oils with sedative effects upon inhalation. J Pharm Sci 1993; 82(6): 660-4. [http://dx.doi.org/10.1002/jps.2600820623] [PMID: 8331544]

[3] Adorjan B, Buchbauer G. Biological properties of essential oils: An updated review. Flavour Fragrance J 2010; 25(6): 407-26. [http://dx.doi.org/10.1002/ffj.2024]

[4] Franz CM. Essential oil research: Past, present and future. Flavour Fragrance J 2010; 25(3): 112-3. [http://dx.doi.org/10.1002/ffj.1983]

[5] Bilia AR, Guccione C, Isacchi B, Righeschi C, Firenzuoli F, Bergonzi MC. Essential oils loaded in nanosystems: A developing strategy for a successful therapeutic approach. Evid Based Complement Alternat Med 2014; 2014: 1-14. [http://dx.doi.org/10.1155/2014/651593] [PMID: 24971152]

[6] Ali B, Al-Wabel NA, Shams S, Ahamad A, Khan SA, Anwar F. Essential oils used in aromatherapy: A systemic review. Asian Pac J Trop Biomed 2015; 5(8): 601-11. [http://dx.doi.org/10.1016/j.apjtb.2015.05.007]

[7] Bakkali F, Averbeck S, Averbeck D, Idaomar M. Biological effects of essential oils – A review. Food Chem Toxicol 2008; 46(2): 446-75. [http://dx.doi.org/10.1016/j.fct.2007.09.106] [PMID: 17996351]

[8] de Sousa Barros A, de Morais SM, Ferreira PAT, *et al.* Chemical composition and functional properties of essential oils from Mentha species. Ind Crops Prod 2015; 76: 557-64. [http://dx.doi.org/10.1016/j.indcrop.2015.07.004]

[9] Hale AL, Reddivari L, Nzaramba MN, Bamberg JB, Miller JC Jr. Interspecific variability for antioxidant activity and phenolic content among *Solanum* species. Am J Potato Res 2008; 85(5): 332-41. [http://dx.doi.org/10.1007/s12230-008-9035-1]

[10] Benjilali B, Ayadi A. Methode d'étude des proprieties antiseptiques deshuiles essentielles par contact direct en milieu gelose [Thymus capitatus,Rosmarinus officinalis, Eucalyptus globulus, Artemisia herba alba]. Plantesmédicinal phototherapies 1986; 2: 155-67.

[11] Burt S. Essential oils: their antibacterial properties and potential applications in foods—a review. Int J Food Microbiol 2004; 94(3): 223-53. [http://dx.doi.org/10.1016/j.ijfoodmicro.2004.03.022] [PMID: 15246235]

[12] Kaloustian J, Chevalier J, Mikail C, Martino M, Abou L, Vergnes MF. Étude de six huiles essentielles : Composition chimique et activité antibactérienne. Phytotherapie 2008; 6(3): 160-4. [http://dx.doi.org/10.1007/s10298-008-0307-1]

[13] Stefanakis MK, Touloupakis E, Anastasopoulos E, Ghanotakis D, Katerinopoulos HE, Makridis P. Antibacterial activity of essential oils from plants of the genus *Origanum.* Food Control 2013; 34(2): 539-46. [http://dx.doi.org/10.1016/j.foodcont.2013.05.024]

[14] Djenane D, Yangüela J, Gómez D, Roncalés P. Perspectives on the use of essential oils as antimicrobials against *Campylobacter jejuni* CECT 7572 in retail chicken meats packaged in microaerobic atmosphere. J Food Saf 2012; 32(1): 37-47. [http://dx.doi.org/10.1111/j.1745-4565.2011.00342.x]

[15] Gutierrez J, Barry-Ryan C, Bourke P. The antimicrobial efficacy of plant essential oil combinations and interactions with food ingredients. Int J Food Microbiol 2008; 124(1): 91-7. [http://dx.doi.org/10.1016/j.ijfoodmicro.2008.02.028] [PMID: 18378032]

[16] Batish DR, Singh HP, Kohli RK, Kaur S. Eucalyptus essential oil as a natural pesticide. For Ecol Manage 2008; 256(12): 2166-74. [http://dx.doi.org/10.1016/j.foreco.2008.08.008]

[17] Wei A, Shibamoto T. Antioxidant activities and volatile constituents of various essential oils. J Agric Food Chem 2007; 55(5): 1737-42. [http://dx.doi.org/10.1021/jf062959x] [PMID: 17295511]

[18] Musthaba M, Baboota S, Athar TM, Thajudeen KY, Ahmed S, Ali J. Patented herbal formulations and their therapeutic applications. Recent Pat Drug Deliv Formul 2010; 4(3): 231-44. [http://dx.doi.org/10.2174/187221110793237538] [PMID: 20626333]

[19] Miladi H, Slama RB, Mili D, Zouari S, Bakhrouf A, Ammar E. Essential oil of *Thymus vulgaris L.* and *Rosmarinus officinalis* L.: Gas chromatography–mass spectrometry analysis, cytotoxicity and antioxidant properties and antibacterial activities against food borne pathogens. Nat Sci 2013; 5(6): 729-39.

[20] Al-Asmari AK, Athar MT, Al-Faraidy AA, Almuhaiza MS. Chemical composition of essential oil of *Thymus vulgaris* collected from Saudi Arabian market. Asian Pac J Trop Biomed 2017; 7(2): 147-50. [http://dx.doi.org/10.1016/j.apjtb.2016.11.023]

[21] Lawless J. The Illustrated Encyclopedia of Essential Oils. Shaftesbury, UK: Element Books Ltd. 1995.

[22] Mishra AK, Dubey NK. Evaluation of some essential oils for their toxicity against fungi causing deterioration of stored food commodities. Appl Environ Microbiol 1994; 60(4): 1101-5. [http://dx.doi.org/10.1128/aem.60.4.1101-1105.1994] [PMID: 8017906]

[23] Horváth G, Ács K. Essential oils in the treatment of respiratory tract diseases highlighting their role in bacterial infections and their anti-inflammatory action: A review. Flavour Fragrance J 2015; 30(5): 331-41.
[http://dx.doi.org/10.1002/ffj.3252] [PMID: 32313366]

[24] Shah AJ, Gilani AH, Abbas K, Rasheed M, Ahmed A, Ahmad VU. Studies on the chemical composition and possible mechanisms underlying the antispasmodic and bronchodilatory activities of the essential oil of Artemisia maritima L. Arch Pharm Res 2011; 34(8): 1227-38.
[http://dx.doi.org/10.1007/s12272-011-0801-0] [PMID: 21910043]

[25] Santos BA, Roman-Campos D, Carvalho MS, *et al.* Cardiodepressive effect elicited by the essential oil of Alpinia speciosa is related to L-type Ca^2+ current blockade. Phytomedicine 2011; 18(7): 539-43.
[http://dx.doi.org/10.1016/j.phymed.2010.10.015] [PMID: 21112750]

[26] Turina AV, Nolan MV, Zygadlo JA, Perillo MA. Natural terpenes: self-assembly and membrane partitioning. Biophysics Chem 2006; 122(2): 101-2.
[http://dx.doi.org/10.1016/j.bpc.2006.02.007]

[27] Huang L, Abuhamdah S, Howes MJ, *et al.* Pharmacological profile of essential oils derived from Lavandula angustifolia and Melissa officinal is with anti-agitation properties: focus on ligand-gated channels. J Pharm Pharmacol 2009; 60(11): 1515-22.
[http://dx.doi.org/10.1211/jpp/60.11.0013]

[28] Dunning T. Aromatherapy: Overview, safety and quality issues. OA Alternat Med 2013; 1(1): 6.
[http://dx.doi.org/10.13172/2052-7845-1-1-518]

[29] Reynolds JEF. Martindale – the Extra Pharmacopoeia. 31st ed., London: Royal Pharmaceutical Society of Great Britain 1996.

[30] Lis-Balchin M, Deans SG. Bioactivity of selected plant essential oils against *listeria monocytogenes.* J Appl Microbiol 1997; 82(6): 759-62.
[http://dx.doi.org/10.1046/j.1365-2672.1997.00153.x] [PMID: 9202441]

[31] Hammer KA, Carson CF, Riley TV. Antimicrobial activity of essential oils and other plant extracts. J Appl Microbiol 1999; 86(6): 985-90.
[http://dx.doi.org/10.1046/j.1365-2672.1999.00780.x] [PMID: 10438227]

[32] Svoboda KP, Deans SG. Biological activities of essential oils from selected aromatic plants. Acta Hortic 1995; (390): 203-9.
[http://dx.doi.org/10.17660/ActaHortic.1995.390.28]

[33] Evans WC. Trease and Evans pharmacognosy. 4th ed., London: WB Saunders Co. 2000.

[34] Schiller C, Schiller D. 500 formulas for aromatherapy: mixing essential oils for every use. USA: Sterling Publications 1994.

[35] Wildwood C. The encyclopedia of aromatherapy. Rochester: Healing Arts Press 1996.

[36] Fayazi S, Babashahi M, Rezaei M. The effect of inhalation aromatherapy on anxiety level of the patients in preoperative period. Iran J Nurs Midwifery Res 2011; 16(4): 278-83.
[PMID: 23449862]

[37] Stea S, Beraudi A, Pasquale DD. Essential oils for complementary treatment of surgical patients: state of the art. Evid Based Complement Alternat Med 2014; 2014: 726341.
[http://dx.doi.org/10.1155/2014/726341]

[38] Filiptsova OV, Gazzavi-Rogozina LV, Timoshyna IA, Naboka OI, Dyomina YV, Ochkur AV. The effect of the essential oils of lavender and rosemary on the human short-term memory. Alex J Med 2018; 54(1): 41-4.
[http://dx.doi.org/10.1016/j.ajme.2017.05.004]

[39] Han X, Beaumont C, Stevens N. Chemical composition analysis and *in vitro* biological activities of ten essential oils in human skin cells. Biochim Open 2017; 5: 1-7.

[http://dx.doi.org/10.1016/j.biopen.2017.04.001] [PMID: 29450150]

[40] Buchbauer G. Biological activities of essential oils. Science, Technology and Applications. CRC Press, Taylor and Francis Group 2010.

[41] Koroch AR, Juliani HR, Zygadlo JA. Bioactivity of essential oils and their components. In: Berger RG, Ed. Fragrance and Flavours: Chemistr, Bioprocessing and Sustainability. 1st ed., Leipzig, Germany: Springer 2007.
[http://dx.doi.org/10.1007/978-3-540-49339-6_5]

[42] Sadgrove N, Jones G. A contemporary introduction to essential oils: Chemistry, bioactivity and prospects for australian agriculture. Agriculture 2015; 5(1): 48-102.
[http://dx.doi.org/10.3390/agriculture5010048]

[43] van Vuuren SF, du Toit LC, Parry A, Pillay V, Choonara YE. Encapsulation of essential oils within a polymeric liposomal formulation for enhancement of antimicrobial efficacy. Nat Prod Commun 2010; 5(9): 1934578X1000500.
[http://dx.doi.org/10.1177/1934578X1000500912] [PMID: 20922998]

[44] Karlsen J. Encapsulation and other programmed release techniques for essential oils and volatile terpenes. Handbook of Essential Oils: Science, Technology and Applications. CRC Press 2011.

[45] Lee M, Lim S, Song JA, Kim M-E, Hur M-H. The effects of aromatherapy essential oil inhalation on stress, sleep quality and immunity in healthy adults: Randomized controlled trial. Eur J Integr Med 2017; 12: 79-86.
[http://dx.doi.org/10.1016/j.eujim.2017.04.009]

[46] Baba Shahi F. The effect of aromatherapy massage and massage therapy on anxiety of patients before surgery: A clinical trial. J Evid-Based Care 2012; 2: 20-7.

[47] Bahraini S, Naji S, Mannani R. Effects of aromatherapy and its application. J Urmia Nurs Midwifery Faculty 2011; 9: 1-8.

[48] Kanani M, Mazloum SR, Emami A, Mokhber N. The effect of aromatherapy with orange essential oils on anxiety in patients undergoing hemodialysis. J Sabzevar Univ Med Sci 2012; 19: 249-57.

[49] Gaware V, Nagare R, Dhamak KB, *et al.* Aromatherapy: Art or science. Int J Biomed Res 2013; 4(2): 74-83.
[http://dx.doi.org/10.7439/ijbr.v4i2.231]

[50] Cooke B, Ernst E. Aromatherapy: A systematic review. Br J Gen Pract 2000; 50(455): 493-6.
[PMID: 10962794]

[51] Liakos I, Rizzello L, Scurr DJ, Pompa PP, Bayer IS, Athanassiou A. All-natural composite wound dressing films of essential oils encapsulated in sodium alginate with antimicrobial properties. Int J Pharm 2014; 463(2): 137-45.
[http://dx.doi.org/10.1016/j.ijpharm.2013.10.046] [PMID: 24211443]

[52] Altiok D, Altiok E, Tihminlioglu F. Physical, antibacterial and antioxidant properties of chitosan films incorporated with thyme oil for potential wound healing applications. J Mater Sci Mater Med 2010; 21(7): 2227-36.
[http://dx.doi.org/10.1007/s10856-010-4065-x] [PMID: 20372985]

[53] Kavoosi G, Dadfar SMM, Purfard AM. Mechanical, physical, antioxidant, and antimicrobial properties of gelatin films incorporated with thymol for potential use as nano wound dressing. J Food Sci 2013; 78(2): E244-50.
[http://dx.doi.org/10.1111/1750-3841.12015] [PMID: 23317304]

[54] Dias AMA, Braga MEM, Seabra IJ, Ferreira P, Gil MH, de Sousa HC. Development of natural-based wound dressings impregnated with bioactive compounds and using supercritical carbon dioxide. Int J Pharm 2011; 408(1-2): 9-19.
[http://dx.doi.org/10.1016/j.ijpharm.2011.01.063] [PMID: 21316432]

[55] Anghel I, Holban AM, Grumezescu AM, *et al.* Modified wound dressing with phyto-nanostructured coating to prevent staphylococcal and pseudomonal biofilm development. Nanoscale Res Lett 2012; 7(1): 690.
[http://dx.doi.org/10.1186/1556-276X-7-690] [PMID: 23272823]

[56] Charernsriwilaiwat N, Rojanarata T, Ngawhirunpat T, Sukma M, Opanasopit P. Electrospun chitosan-based nanofiber mats loaded with *Garcinia mangostana* extracts. Int J Pharm 2013; 452(1-2): 333-43.
[http://dx.doi.org/10.1016/j.ijpharm.2013.05.012] [PMID: 23680732]

[57] Catanzano O, Straccia MC, Miro A, *et al.* Spray-by-spray in situ cross-linking alginate hydrogels delivering a tea tree oil microemulsion. Eur J Pharm Sci 2015; 66: 20-8.
[http://dx.doi.org/10.1016/j.ejps.2014.09.018] [PMID: 25277680]

[58] Chung KF. Drugs to suppress cough. Expert Opin Investig Drugs 2005; 14: 19-27.
[http://dx.doi.org/10.1517/13543784.14.1.19]

[59] Dapaah G, Koffuor GA, Mante PK, Ben IO. Antitussive, expectorant and analgesic effects of the ethanol seed extract of Picralima nitida (Stapf) Th. & H. Durand. Res Pharm Sci 2016; 11(2): 100-12.
[PMID: 27168749]

[60] Eccles R. Placebo effects of antitussive treatments on cough associated with acute upper respiratory tract infection. In: Chung KF, Widdicombe JG, Boushey HA, Eds. Cough: Causes, Mechanisms and Therapy. Massachusetts: Blackwell Publishing 2003; pp. 259-68.
[http://dx.doi.org/10.1002/9780470755846.ch25]

[61] Eccles R. Central mechanisms IV: Conscious control of cough and the placebo effect. In: Chung KF, Widdicombe JG, Eds. Pharmacology and Therapeutics of Cough-handbook of Experimental Pharmacology. Berlin, Heidelberg: Springer 2009; Vol. 187: pp. 242-62.
[http://dx.doi.org/10.1007/978-3-540-79842-2_12]

[62] Dapaah G, Koffuor GA, Mante PK, Ben IO. The possible mode of antitussive and expectorant activity of the ethanol seed extracts of Picralima nitida ((Stapf) Th. & H. Durand). J Tradit Complement Med 2017; 7(1): 133-40.
[http://dx.doi.org/10.1016/j.jtcme.2016.05.003] [PMID: 28053900]

[63] Bassler BL. Small Talk. Cell 2002; 109(4): 421-4.
[http://dx.doi.org/10.1016/S0092-8674(02)00749-3] [PMID: 12086599]

[64] Fuqua WC, Winans SC, Greenberg EP. Quorum sensing in bacteria: The LuxR-LuxI family of cell density-responsive transcriptional regulators. J Bacteriol 1994; 176(2): 269-75.
[http://dx.doi.org/10.1128/jb.176.2.269-275.1994] [PMID: 8288518]

[65] Joint I, Allan Downie J, Williams P. Bacterial conversations: Talking, listening and eavesdropping. An introduction. Philos Trans R Soc Lond B Biol Sci 2007; 362(1483): 1115-7.
[http://dx.doi.org/10.1098/rstb.2007.2038] [PMID: 17360281]

[66] Waters C M, Bassler B L. Quorum sensing: Cell-to-cell communication in bacteria. Annual Rev Cell Develop Biol 2005; 319-46.
[http://dx.doi.org/10.1146/annurev.cellbio.21.012704.131001]

[67] Williams P. Quorum sensing: An emerging target for antibacterial chemotherapy? Expert Opin Ther Targets 2002; 6(3): 257-74.
[http://dx.doi.org/10.1517/14728222.6.3.257] [PMID: 12223068]

[68] Budzyńska A, Więckowska-Szakiel M, Sadowska B, Kalemba D, Różalska B. Antibiofilm activity of selected plant essential oils and their major components. Pol J Microbiol 2011; 60(1): 35-41.
[http://dx.doi.org/10.33073/pjm-2011-005] [PMID: 21630572]

[69] Schillaci D, Arizza V, Dayton T, Camarda L, Stefano VD. *In vitro* anti-biofilm activity of *Boswellia* spp. oleogum resin essential oils. Lett Appl Microbiol 2008; 47(5): 433-8.
[http://dx.doi.org/10.1111/j.1472-765X.2008.02469.x] [PMID: 19146534]

[70] Saharkhiz M J, Motamedi M, Zomorodian K, Pakshir K, Miri R, Hemyari K. Chemical composition, antifungal and antibiofilm activities of the essential oil of Mentha piperita L. ISRN Pharmaceut 2012. [http://dx.doi.org/10.5402/2012/718645]

[71] Adukwu EC, Allen SCH, Phillips CA. The anti-biofilm activity of lemongrass (*Cymbopogon flexuosus*) and grapefruit (*Citrus paradisi*) essential oils against five strains of *Staphylococcus aureus*. J Appl Microbiol 2012; 113(5): 1217-27. [http://dx.doi.org/10.1111/j.1365-2672.2012.05418.x] [PMID: 22862808]

[72] Mukherji R, Prabhune A. Novel glycolipids synthesized using plant essential oils and their application in quorum sensing inhibition and as antibio film agents. The Scientific World J 2014. [http://dx.doi.org/10.1155/2014/890709]

[73] Akthar MS, Birhanu DTA. Antimicrobial activity of essential oils extracted from medicinal plants against the pathogenic microorganisms: A review. Issues Biol Sci Pharmaceut Res 2014; 2(1): 001-7.

[74] Grohs BM, Kunz B. Use of spice mixtures for the stabilisation of fresh portioned pork. Food Control 2000; 11(6): 433-6. [http://dx.doi.org/10.1016/S0956-7135(00)00005-0]

[75] Lambert RJW, Skandamis PN, Coote PJ, Nychas GJE. A study of the minimum inhibitory concentration and mode of action of oregano essential oil, thymol and carvacrol. J Appl Microbiol 2001; 91(3): 453-62. [http://dx.doi.org/10.1046/j.1365-2672.2001.01428.x] [PMID: 11556910]

[76] Elgayyar M, Draughon FA, Golden DA, Mount JR. Antimicrobial activity of essential oils from plants against selected pathogenic and saprophytic microorganisms. J Food Prot 2001; 64(7): 1019-24. [http://dx.doi.org/10.4315/0362-028X-64.7.1019] [PMID: 11456186]

[77] Ultee A, Smid EJ. Influence of carvacrol on growth and toxin production by *Bacillus cereus*. Int J Food Microbiol 2001; 64(3): 373-8. [http://dx.doi.org/10.1016/S0168-1605(00)00480-3] [PMID: 11294360]

[78] Hammer KA, Carson CF, Riley TV. *in vitro* activity of *Melaleuca alternifolia* (tea tree) oil against dermatophytes and other filamentous fungi. J Antimicrob Chemother 2002; 50(2): 195-9. [http://dx.doi.org/10.1093/jac/dkf112] [PMID: 12161399]

[79] Hood JR, Wilkinson JM, Cavanagh HMA. Evaluation of common antibacterial screening methods utilized in essential oil research. J. Essen. J Essent Oil Res 2003; 15(6): 428-33. [http://dx.doi.org/10.1080/10412905.2003.9698631]

[80] Lanciotti R, Gianotti A, Patrignani F, Belletti N, Guerzoni ME, Gardini F. Use of natural aroma compounds to improve shelf-life and safety of minimally processed fruits. Trends Food Sci Technol 2004; 15(3-4): 201-8. [http://dx.doi.org/10.1016/j.tifs.2003.10.004]

[81] Sinico C, De Logu A, Lai F, *et al.* Liposomal incorporation of *Artemisia arborescens* L. essential oil and *in vitro* antiviral activity. Eur J Pharm Biopharm 2005; 59(1): 161-8. [http://dx.doi.org/10.1016/j.ejpb.2004.06.005] [PMID: 15567314]

[82] Oussalah M, Caillet S, Lacroix M. Mechanism of action of Spanish oregano, Chinese cinnamon, and savory essential oils against cell membranes and walls of *Escherichia coli* O157:H7 and *Listeria monocytogenes*. J Food Prot 2006; 69(5): 1046-55. [http://dx.doi.org/10.4315/0362-028X-69.5.1046] [PMID: 16715803]

[83] Soković M, Vukojević J, Marin P, Brkić D, Vajs V, Van Griensven L. Chemical composition of essential oils of *Thymus* and *Mentha* species and their antifungal activities. Molecules 2009; 14(1): 238-49. [http://dx.doi.org/10.3390/molecules14010238] [PMID: 19136911]

[84] Mulyaningsih S, Sporer F, Zimmermann S, Reichling J, Wink M. Synergistic properties of the terpenoids aromadendrene and 1,8-cineole from the essential oil of *Eucalyptus globulus* against

antibiotic-susceptible and antibiotic-resistant pathogens. Phytomedicine 2010; 17(13): 1061-6. [http://dx.doi.org/10.1016/j.phymed.2010.06.018] [PMID: 20727725]

[85] Shan B, Cai YZ, Brooks JD, Corke H. Potential application of spice and herb extracts as natural preservatives in cheese. J Med Food 2011; 14(3): 284-90. [http://dx.doi.org/10.1089/jmf.2010.0009] [PMID: 21142945]

[86] Jafri H, Husain FM, Ahmad I. Antibacterial and antibiofilm activity of some essential oils and compounds against clinical strains of *Staphylococcus aureus*. Journal of Biomedical & Therapeutic Sciences 2014; 1(1): 65-71.

[87] Sfeir J, Lefrançois C, Baudoux D, Derbré S, Licznar P. *in vitro* Antibacterial Activity of Essential Oils against Streptococcus pyogenes. Evid-Based Complement Alternat Med 2013; 9. [http://dx.doi.org/10.1155/2013/269161]

[88] Bey-Ould Si Said Z, Haddadi-Guemghar H, Boulekbache-Makhlouf L, *et al.* Essential oils composition, antibacterial and antioxidant activities of hydrodistillated extract of *Eucalyptus globulus* fruits. Ind Crops Prod 2016; 89: 167-75. [http://dx.doi.org/10.1016/j.indcrop.2016.05.018]

[89] Oh HK, Sakai T, Jones MB, Longhurst WM. Effect of various essential oils isolated from Douglas fir needles upon sheep and deer rumen microbial activity. Appl Microbiol 1967; 15(4): 777-84. [http://dx.doi.org/10.1128/am.15.4.777-784.1967] [PMID: 6049303]

[90] Cosentino S, Tuberoso CIG, Pisano B, *et al.* In-vitro antimicrobial activity and chemical composition of Sardinian Thymus essential oils. Lett Appl Microbiol 1999; 29(2): 130-5. [http://dx.doi.org/10.1046/j.1472-765X.1999.00605.x] [PMID: 10499301]

[91] Dorman HJD, Deans SG. Antimicrobial agents from plants: Antibacterial activity of plant volatile oils. J Appl Microbiol 2000; 88(2): 308-16. [http://dx.doi.org/10.1046/j.1365-2672.2000.00969.x] [PMID: 10736000]

[92] Cristani M, D'Arrigo M, Mandalari G, *et al.* Interaction of four monoterpenes contained in essential oils with model membranes: implications for their antibacterial activity. J Agric Food Chem 2007; 55(15): 6300-8. [http://dx.doi.org/10.1021/jf070094x] [PMID: 17602646]

[93] Ross ZM, O'Gara EA, Hill DJ, Sleightholme HV, Maslin DJ. Antimicrobial properties of garlic oil against human enteric bacteria: evaluation of methodologies and comparisons with garlic oil sulfides and garlic powder. Appl Environ Microbiol 2001; 67(1): 475-80. [http://dx.doi.org/10.1128/AEM.67.1.475-480.2001] [PMID: 11133485]

[94] Corzomartinez M, Corzo N, Villamiel M. Biological properties of onions and garlic. Trends Food Sci Technol 2007; 18(12): 609-25. [http://dx.doi.org/10.1016/j.tifs.2007.07.011]

[95] Ultee A, Bennik MHJ, Moezelaar R. The phenolic hydroxyl group of carvacrol is essential for action against the food-borne pathogen Bacillus cereus. Appl Environ Microbiol 2002; 68(4): 1561-8. [http://dx.doi.org/10.1128/AEM.68.4.1561-1568.2002] [PMID: 11916669]

[96] Bassolé IHN, Juliani HR. Essential oils in combination and their antimicrobial properties. Molecules 2012; 17(4): 3989-4006. [http://dx.doi.org/10.3390/molecules17043989] [PMID: 22469594]

[97] Pei R, Zhou F, Ji B, Xu J. Evaluation of combined antibacterial effects of eugenol, cinnamaldehyde, thymol, and carvacrol against *E. coli* with an improved method. J Food Sci 2009; 74(7): M379-83. [http://dx.doi.org/10.1111/j.1750-3841.2009.01287.x] [PMID: 19895484]

[98] Gallucci MN, Oliva M, Casero C, *et al.* Antimicrobial combined action of terpenes against the food-borne microorganisms *Escherichia coli, Staphylococcus aureus* and *Bacillus cereus*. Flavour Fragrance J 2009; 24(6): 348-54. [http://dx.doi.org/10.1002/ffj.1948]

[99] Rivas L, McDonnell MJ, Burgess CM, *et al.* Inhibition of verocytotoxigenic Escherichia coli in model broth and rumen systems by carvacrol and thymol. Int J Food Microbiol 2010; 139(1-2): 70-8. [http://dx.doi.org/10.1016/j.ijfoodmicro.2010.01.029] [PMID: 20153068]

[100] Zhou F, Ji B, Zhang H, *et al.* The antibacterial effect of cinnamaldehyde, thymol, carvacrol and their combinations against the food-borne pathogen Salmonella typhimurium. J Food Saf 2007; 27(2): 124-33. [http://dx.doi.org/10.1111/j.1745-4565.2007.00064.x]

[101] Ultee A, Slump RA, Steging G, Smid EJ. Antimicrobial activity of carvacrol toward Bacillus cereus on rice. J Food Prot 2000; 63(5): 620-4. [http://dx.doi.org/10.4315/0362-028X-63.5.620] [PMID: 10826719]

[102] Bassolé IHN, Lamien-Meda A, Bayala B, *et al.* Composition and antimicrobial activities of *Lippia multiflora* Moldenke, *Mentha* x *piperita* L. and *Ocimum basilicum* L. essential oils and their major monoterpene alcohols alone and in combination. Molecules 2010; 15(11): 7825-39. [http://dx.doi.org/10.3390/molecules15117825] [PMID: 21060291]

[103] Moleyar V, Narasimham P. Antibacterial activity of essential oil components. Int J Food Microbiol 1992; 16(4): 337-42. [http://dx.doi.org/10.1016/0168-1605(92)90035-2] [PMID: 1457292]

[104] Vuuren SF, Viljoen AM. Antimicrobial activity of limonene enantiomers and 1,8-cineole alone and in combination. Flavour Fragrance J 2007; 22(6): 540-4. [http://dx.doi.org/10.1002/ffj.1843]

[105] Tserennadmid R, Takó M, Galgóczy L, *et al.* Anti yeast activities of some essential oils in growth medium, fruit juices and milk. Int J Food Microbiol 2011; 144(3): 480-6. [http://dx.doi.org/10.1016/j.ijfoodmicro.2010.11.004] [PMID: 21131081]

[106] de Azeredo GA, Stamford TLM, Nunes PC, Gomes Neto NJ, de Oliveira MEG, de Souza EL. Combined application of essential oils from *Origanum vulgare* L. and *Rosmarinus officinalis* L. to inhibit bacteria and autochthonous microflora associated with minimally processed vegetables. Food Res Int 2011; 44(5): 1541-8. [http://dx.doi.org/10.1016/j.foodres.2011.04.012]

[107] Fu Y, Zu Y, Chen L, *et al.* Antimicrobial activity of clove and rosemary essential oils alone and in combination. Phytother Res 2007; 21(10): 989-94. [http://dx.doi.org/10.1002/ptr.2179] [PMID: 17562569]

[108] Goñi P, López P, Sánchez C, Gómez-Lus R, Becerril R, Nerín C. Antimicrobial activity in the vapour phase of a combination of cinnamon and clove essential oils. Food Chem 2009; 116(4): 982-9. [http://dx.doi.org/10.1016/j.foodchem.2009.03.058]

[109] Bassolé IHN, Lamien-Meda A, Bayala B, *et al.* Chemical composition and antimicrobial activity of *Cymbopogon citratus* and *Cymbopogon giganteus* essential oils alone and in combination. Phytomedicine 2011; 18(12): 1070-4. [http://dx.doi.org/10.1016/j.phymed.2011.05.009] [PMID: 21665450]

[110] Gill AO, Holley RA. Mechanisms of Bactericidal Action of Cinnamaldehyde against *Listeria monocytogenes* and of Eugenol against *L. monocytogenes* and *Lactobacillus sakei.* Appl Environ Microbiol 2004; 70(10): 5750-5. [http://dx.doi.org/10.1128/AEM.70.10.5750-5755.2004] [PMID: 15466510]

[111] Walsh SE, Maillard JY, Russell AD, Catrenich CE, Charbonneau DL, Bartolo RG. Activity and mechanisms of action of selected biocidal agents on Gram-positive and -negative bacteria. J Appl Microbiol 2003; 94(2): 240-7. [http://dx.doi.org/10.1046/j.1365-2672.2003.01825.x] [PMID: 12534815]

[112] Ouwehand AC, Tiihonen K, Kettunen H, Peuranen S, Schulze H, Rautonen N. *in vitro* effects of essential oils on potential pathogens and beneficial members of the normal microbiota. Vet Med

(Praha) 2010; 55(2): 71-8.
[http://dx.doi.org/10.17221/152/2009-VETMED]

[113] Helander IM, Alakomi HL, Latva-Kala K, *et al.* Characterization of the action of selected essential oil components on Gram negative bacteria. J Agric Food Chem 1998; 46(9): 3590-5.
[http://dx.doi.org/10.1021/jf980154m]

[114] Fujisawa H, Watanabe K, Suma K, *et al.* Antibacterial potential of garlic-derived allicin and its cancellation by sulfhydryl compounds. Biosci Biotechnol Biochem 2009; 73(9): 1948-55.
[http://dx.doi.org/10.1271/bbb.90096] [PMID: 19734685]

[115] Münchberg U, Anwar A, Mecklenburg S, Jacob C. Polysulfides as biologically active ingredients of garlic. Org Biomol Chem 2007; 5(10): 1505-18.
[http://dx.doi.org/10.1039/B703832A] [PMID: 17571177]

[116] Riahi L, Elferchichi M, Ghazghazi H, *et al.* Phytochemistry, antioxidant and antimicrobial activities of the essential oils of *Mentha rotundifolia* L. in Tunisia. Ind Crops Prod 2013; 49: 883-9.
[http://dx.doi.org/10.1016/j.indcrop.2013.06.032]

[117] Singh BN, Singh BR, Singh RL, Prakash D, Sarma BK, Singh HB. Antioxidant and anti-quorum sensing activities of green pod of *Acacia nilotica* L. Food Chem Toxicol 2009; 47(4): 778-86.
[http://dx.doi.org/10.1016/j.fct.2009.01.009] [PMID: 19168114]

[118] Singh HP, Mittal S, Kaur S, Batish DR, Kohli RK. Characterization and antioxidant activity of essential oils from fresh and decaying leaves of *Eucalyptus tereticornis.* J Agric Food Chem 2009; 57(15): 6962-6.
[http://dx.doi.org/10.1021/jf9012407] [PMID: 19722579]

[119] Luís Â, Duarte A, Gominho J, Domingues F, Duarte AP. Chemical composition, antioxidant, antibacterial and anti-quorum sensing activities of *Eucalyptus globulus* and *Eucalyptus radiata* essential oils. Ind Crops Prod 2016; 79: 274-82.
[http://dx.doi.org/10.1016/j.indcrop.2015.10.055]

[120] Harkat-Madouri L, Asma B, Madani K, *et al.* Chemical composition, antibacterial and antioxidant activities of essential oil of Eucalyptus globulus from Algeria. Ind Crops Prod 2015; 78: 148-53.
[http://dx.doi.org/10.1016/j.indcrop.2015.10.015]

[121] Cobellis G, Trabalza-Marinucci M, Yu Z. Critical evaluation of essential oils as rumen modifiers in ruminant nutrition: A review. Sci Total Environ 2016; 545-546: 556-68.
[http://dx.doi.org/10.1016/j.scitotenv.2015.12.103] [PMID: 26760275]

[122] Ye D, Karnati SKR, Wagner B, Firkins JL, Eastridge ML, Aldrich JM. Essential oil and monensin affect ruminal fermentation and the protozoal population in continuous culture. J Dairy Sci 2018; 101(6): 5069-81.
[http://dx.doi.org/10.3168/jds.2017-13646] [PMID: 29605331]

[123] Shakeri A, Khakdan F, Soheili V, Sahebkar A, Shaddel R, Asili J. Volatile composition, antimicrobial, cytotoxic and antioxidant evaluation of the essential oil from *Nepeta sintenisii* Bornm. Ind Crops Prod 2016; 84: 224-9.
[http://dx.doi.org/10.1016/j.indcrop.2015.12.030]

[124] Lemos MF, Lemos MF, Pacheco HP, *et al.* Seasonal variation affects the composition and antibacterial and antioxidant activities of *Thymus vulgaris.* Ind Crops Prod 2017; 95: 543-8.
[http://dx.doi.org/10.1016/j.indcrop.2016.11.008]

[125] Bozin B, Mimica-Dukic N, Simin N, Anackov G. Characterization of the volatile composition of essential oils of some lamiaceae spices and the antimicrobial and antioxidant activities of the entire oils. J Agric Food Chem 2006; 54(5): 1822-8.
[http://dx.doi.org/10.1021/jf051922u] [PMID: 16506839]

[126] Hemaiswarya S, Kruthiventi AK, Doble M. Synergism between natural products and antibiotics against infectious diseases. Phytomedicine 2008; 15(8): 639-52.

[http://dx.doi.org/10.1016/j.phymed.2008.06.008] [PMID: 18599280]

[127] Rosato A, Vitali C, Gallo D, Balenzano L, Mallamaci R. The inhibition of Candida species by selected essential oils and their synergism with amphotericin B. Phytomedicine 2008; 15(8): 635-8. [http://dx.doi.org/10.1016/j.phymed.2008.05.001] [PMID: 18579358]

[128] Smith ECJ, Kaatz GW, Seo SM, Wareham N, Williamson EM, Gibbons S. The phenolic diterpene totarol inhibits multidrug efflux pump activity in *Staphylococcus aureus*. Antimicrob Agents Chemother 2007; 51(12): 4480-3. [http://dx.doi.org/10.1128/AAC.00216-07] [PMID: 17664318]

[129] Sakagami Y, Iinuma M, Piyasena KGNP, Dharmaratne HRW. Antibacterial activity of α-mangostin against vancomycin resistant Enterococci (VRE) and synergism with antibiotics. Phytomedicine 2005; 12(3): 203-8. [http://dx.doi.org/10.1016/j.phymed.2003.09.012] [PMID: 15830842]

[130] Kizil S, Uyart F. Antimicrobial activities of some Thyme (Thymus, Staureja, Origanum and Thymbra) species against important plant pathogens. Asian J Chem 2006; 18: 1455-61.

[131] Nedorostova L, Kloucek P, Kokoska L, Stolcova M, Pulkrabek J. Antimicrobial properties of selected essential oils in vapour phase against foodborne bacteria. Food Control 2009; 20(2): 157-60. [http://dx.doi.org/10.1016/j.foodcont.2008.03.007]

[132] Saad A, Fadli M, Bouaziz M, Benharref A, Mezrioui NE, Hassani L. Anticandidal activity of the essential oils of *Thymus maroccanus* and *Thymus broussonetii* and their synergism with amphotericin B and fluconazol. Phytomedicine 2010; 17(13): 1057-60. [http://dx.doi.org/10.1016/j.phymed.2010.03.020] [PMID: 20554185]

[133] Fadli M, Saad A, Sayadi S, *et al.* Antibacterial activity of *Thymus maroccanus* and *Thymus broussonetii* essential oils against nosocomial infection – bacteria and their synergistic potential with antibiotics. Phytomedicine 2012; 19(5): 464-71. [http://dx.doi.org/10.1016/j.phymed.2011.12.003] [PMID: 22257599]

[134] Naidoo K, Grobler AC, Deghaye N, Reddy T, Gengiah S, Gray A, *et al.* Cost-effectiveness of initiating antiretroviral therapy at different points in TB treatment in HIV-TB coinfected ambulatory patients in South Africa. J Acquir Immune Deficy Syndrom 2015; 69(5): 576-84.

[135] Chraibi M, Farah A, Lebrazi S, El Amine O, Iraqui Houssaini M, Fikri-Benbrahim K. Antimycobacterial natural products from Moroccan medicinal plants: Chemical composition, bacteriostatic and bactericidal profile of *Thymus satureioides* and *Mentha pulegium* essential oils. Asian Pac J Trop Biomed 2016; 6(10): 836-40. [http://dx.doi.org/10.1016/j.apjtb.2016.08.002]

[136] Rosato A, Vitali C, De Laurentis N, Armenise D, Antonietta Milillo M. Antibacterial effect of some essential oils administered alone or in combination with Norfloxacin. Phytomedicine 2007; 14(11): 727-32. [http://dx.doi.org/10.1016/j.phymed.2007.01.005] [PMID: 17303397]

[137] Ait-Ouazzou A, Lorán S, Arakrak A, *et al.* Evaluation of the chemical composition and antimicrobial activity of *Mentha pulegium, Juniperus phoenicea*, and *Cyperus longus* essential oils from Morocco. Food Res Int 2012; 45(1): 313-9. [http://dx.doi.org/10.1016/j.foodres.2011.09.004]

[138] Jassim SAA, Naji MA. Novel antiviral agents: A medicinal plant perspective. J Appl Microbiol 2003; 95(3): 412-27. [http://dx.doi.org/10.1046/j.1365-2672.2003.02026.x] [PMID: 12911688]

[139] Reichling J, Schnitzler P, Suschke U, Saller R. Essential oils of aromatic plants with antibacterial, antifungal, antiviral, and cytotoxic properties--an overview. Forsch Komplement Med 2009; 16(2): 79-90. [PMID: 19420953]

[140] Carnesecchi S, Schneider Y, Ceraline J, *et al.* Geraniol, a component of plant essential oils, inhibits growth and polyamine biosynthesis in human colon cancer cells. J Pharmacol Exp Ther 2001; 298(1): 197-200.
[PMID: 11408542]

[141] Ma L, Yao L. Antiviral effects of plant-derived essential oils and their components: An Updated review. Molecules 2020; 25(11): 2627.
[http://dx.doi.org/10.3390/molecules25112627]

[142] Astani A, Reichling J, Schnitzler P. For antiviral activities of isolated compounds from essential oils. Evid Based Complement Altern Med 2011; 1-8.
[http://dx.doi.org/10.1093/ecam/nep187]

[143] Civitelli L, Panella S, Marcocci ME, *et al. In vitro* inhibition of herpes simplex virus type 1 replication by *Mentha suaveolens* essential oil and its main component piperitenone oxide. Phytomedicine 2014; 21(6): 857-65.
[http://dx.doi.org/10.1016/j.phymed.2014.01.013] [PMID: 24629600]

[144] Sharifi-Rad J, Salehi B, Schnitzler P, *et al.* Susceptibility of herpes simplex virus type 1 to monoterpenes thymol, carvacrol, p-cymene and essential oils of *Sinapis arvensis* L., *Lallemantia royleana* Benth. and *Pulicaria vulgaris* Gaertn. Cell Mol Biol 2017; 63(8): 42-7.
[http://dx.doi.org/10.14715/cmb/2017.63.8.10] [PMID: 28886313]

[145] Pilau MR, Alves SH, Weiblen R, Arenhart S, Cueto AP, Lovato LT. Antiviral activity of the *Lippia graveolens* (Mexican oregano) essential oil and its main compound carvacrol against human and animal viruses. Braz J Microbiol 2011; 42(4): 1616-24.
[http://dx.doi.org/10.1590/S1517-83822011000400049] [PMID: 24031796]

[146] Gavanji S, Sayedipour SS, Larki B, Bakhtari A. Antiviral activity of some plant oils against herpes simplex virus type 1 in Vero cell culture. Journal of Acute Medicine 2015; 5(3): 62-8.
[http://dx.doi.org/10.1016/j.jacme.2015.07.001]

[147] Toujani MM, Rittà M, Civra A, *et al.* Inhibition of HSV-2 infection by pure compounds from *Thymus capitatus* extract *in vitro*. Phytother Res 2018; 32(8): 1555-63.
[http://dx.doi.org/10.1002/ptr.6084] [PMID: 29673001]

[148] Cagno V, Sgorbini B, Sanna C, *et al. in vitro* anti-herpes simplex virus-2 activity of *Salvia desoleana* Atzei & V. Picci essential oil. PLoS One 2017; 12(2): e0172322.
[http://dx.doi.org/10.1371/journal.pone.0172322] [PMID: 28207861]

[149] Wei X, Cheng P, Feng W. Study on the effect of anti-respiratory viruses of Patchouli Oil *in vitro*. J Pharm Clin Chin Mater Med 2012; 6: 65-8.

[150] Vimalanathan S, Hudson J. Anti-influenza virus activity of essential oils and vapors. Am J Essent Oil 2014; 2: 47-53.

[151] Nagy MM, Al-Mahdy DA, Abd El Aziz OM, Kandil AM, Tantawy MA, El Alfy TSM. Chemical composition and antiviral activity of essential oils from *citrus reshni* hort. ex Tanaka (Cleopatra mandarin) Cultivated in Egypt. J Essent Oil-Bear Plants 2018; 21(1): 264-72.
[http://dx.doi.org/10.1080/0972060X.2018.1436986]

[152] Ibrahim NA, El-Hawary SS, Mohammed MM, *et al.* Chemical composition, antiviral against a*via*n influenza (H5N1) virus and antimicrobial activities of the essential oils of the leaves and fruits of *Fortunella margarita*, lour. swingle, growing in Egypt. J Pharm Sci 2015.

[153] Feriotto G, Marchetti N, Costa V, *et al.* Chemical Composition of Essential Oils from *Thymus vulgaris*, *Cymbopogon citratus*, and *Rosmarinus officinalis*, and Their Effects on the HIV-1 Tat Protein Function. Chem Biodivers 2018; 15(2): e1700436.
[http://dx.doi.org/10.1002/cbdv.201700436] [PMID: 29282856]

[154] Mori K, Obossou EK, Suwa S, *et al.* Human Immunodeficiency virus type 1 (hiv-1) reverse transcriptase inhibitory effect of Cymbopogon nardus essential oil. Int J Adv Res 2016; 2: 7-13.

[155] Mokni RE, Youssef FS, Jmii H, *et al.* The essential oil of tunisian *dysphania ambrosioides* and its antimicrobial and antiviral properties. J Essent Oil-Bear Plants 2019; 22(1): 282-94. [http://dx.doi.org/10.1080/0972060X.2019.1588171]

[156] Bouazzi S, Jmii H, El Mokni R, *et al.* Cytotoxic and antiviral activities of the essential oils from Tunisian Fern, *Osmunda regalis.* S Afr J Bot 2018; 118: 52-7. [http://dx.doi.org/10.1016/j.sajb.2018.06.015]

[157] Elaissi A, Rouis Z, Ben Salem NA, *et al.* Chemical composition of 8 eucalyptus species' essential oils and the evaluation of their antibacterial, antifungal and antiviral activities. BMC Complement Altern Med 2012; 12: 81.

[158] Kubiça TF, Alves SH, Weiblen R, Lovato LT. *In vitro* inhibition of the bovine viral diarrhoea virus by the essential oil of *Ocimum basilicum* (basil) and monoterpenes. Braz J Microbiol 2014; 45(1): 209-14. [http://dx.doi.org/10.1590/S1517-83822014005000030] [PMID: 24948933]

[159] Gómez LA, Stashenko E, Ocazionez RE. Comparative study on *In vitro* activities of citral, limonene and essential oils from *Lippia citriodora* and L. alba on yellow fever virus. Nat Prod Commun 2013; 8(2): 1934578X1300800. [http://dx.doi.org/10.1177/1934578X1300800230] [PMID: 23513741]

[160] Astani A, Reichling J, Schnitzler P. Comparative study on the antiviral activity of selected monoterpenes derived from essential oils. Phytother Res 2010; 24(5): 673-9. [http://dx.doi.org/10.1002/ptr.2955] [PMID: 19653195]

[161] Haddad JG, Picard M, Bénard S, *et al. Ayapana triplinervis* essential oil and its main component thymohydroquinone dimethyl ether inhibit zika virus at doses devoid of toxicity in zebrafish. Molecules 2019; 24(19): 3447. [http://dx.doi.org/10.3390/molecules24193447] [PMID: 31547527]

[162] Hammami S, Jmii H, Mokni R, *et al.* Essential oil composition, antioxidant, cytotoxic and antiviral activities of *teucrium pseudochamaepitys* growing spontaneously in tunisia. Molecules 2015; 20(11): 20426-33. [http://dx.doi.org/10.3390/molecules201119707] [PMID: 26580590]

[163] Schnitzler P, Astani A, Reichling J. Lipids and Essential Oils as Antimicrobial Agents. John Wiley and Sons 2010.

[164] Baqui AAMA, Kelley JI, Jabra-Rizk MA, DePaola LG, Falkler WA, Meiller TF. *In vitro* effect of oral antiseptics on human immunodeficiency virus-1 and herpes simplex virus type 1. J Clin Periodontol 2001; 28(7): 610-6. [http://dx.doi.org/10.1034/j.1600-051x.2001.028007610.x] [PMID: 11422581]

[165] Primo V, Rovera M, Zanon S, *et al.* [Determination of the antibacterial and antiviral activity of the essential oil from *Minthostachys verticillata* (Griseb.) Epling]. Rev Argent Microbiol 2001; 33(2): 113-7. [PMID: 11494754]

[166] Schnitzler P, Schön K, Reichling J. Antiviral activity of Australian tea tree oil and eucalyptus oil against herpes simplex virus in cell culture. Pharmazie 2001; 56(4): 343-7. [PMID: 11338678]

[167] Allahverdiyev A, Duran N, Ozguven M, Koltas S. Antiviral activity of the volatile oils of *Melissa officinalis* L. against Herpes simplex virus type-2. Phytomedicine 2004; 11(7-8): 657-61. [http://dx.doi.org/10.1016/j.phymed.2003.07.014] [PMID: 15636181]

[168] Schuhmacher A, Reichling J, Schnitzler P. Virucidal effect of peppermint oil on the enveloped viruses herpes simplex virus type 1 and type 2 *in vitro*. Phytomedicine 2003; 10(6-7): 504-10. [http://dx.doi.org/10.1078/094471103322331467] [PMID: 13678235]

[169] García CC, Talarico L, Almeida N, Colombres S, Duschatzky C, Damonte EB. Virucidal activity of essential oils from aromatic plants of San Luis, Argentina. Phytother Res 2003; 17(9): 1073-5.

[http://dx.doi.org/10.1002/ptr.1305] [PMID: 14595590]

[170] De Logu A, Loy G, Pellerano ML, Bonsignore L, Schivo ML. Inactivation of HSV-1 and HSV-2 and prevention of cell-to-cell virus spread by *Santolina insularis* essential oil. Antiviral Res 2000; 48(3): 177-85.
[http://dx.doi.org/10.1016/S0166-3542(00)00127-3] [PMID: 11164504]

[171] Armaka M, Papanikolaou E, Sivropoulou A, Arsenakis M. Antiviral properties of isoborneol, a potent inhibitor of herpes simplex virus type 1. Antiviral Res 1999; 43(2): 79-92.
[http://dx.doi.org/10.1016/S0166-3542(99)00036-4] [PMID: 10517310]

[172] Ozcan M, Ere O, Herken E. Antioxidant activity, phenolic content, and peroxide value of essential oil and extracts of some medicinal and aromatic plants used as condiments and herbal teas in Turkey. J Med Food 2009; 12: 198-202.

[173] Zheng W, Wang SY. Antioxidant activity and phenolic compounds in selected herbs. J Agric Food Chem 2001; 49: 516-70.

[174] Fukumoto LR, Mazza G J. Assessing antioxidant and prooxidant activities of phenolic compounds. Agric Food Chem 2000; 48: 3597-604.
[http://dx.doi.org/10.1021/jf000220w]

[175] Tura D, Gigliotti C, Pedò S, Failla O, Bassi D, Serraiocco A. Influence of cultivar and site of cultivation on levels of lipophilic and hydrophilic antioxidants in virgin olive oils (*Olea Europea* L.) and correlations with oxidative stability. Sci Hortic (Amsterdam) 2007; 112(1): 108-19.
[http://dx.doi.org/10.1016/j.scienta.2006.12.036]

[176] Gulcin I. Antioxidant properties of resveratrol: A structure activity insight. Innov Food Sci Emerg Technol 2009; 11: 2108.

[177] Yamaguchi T, Takamura H, Matoba T, Terao J. HPLC method for evaluation of the free radical-scavenging activity of foods by using 1,1-diphenyl-2-picrylhydrazyl. Biosci Biotechnol Biochem 1998; 62(6): 1201-4.
[http://dx.doi.org/10.1271/bbb.62.1201] [PMID: 9692204]

[178] Gyamfi MA, Yonamine M, Aniya Y. Free-radical scavenging action of medicinal herbs from Ghana. Gen Pharmacol 1999; 32(6): 661-7.
[http://dx.doi.org/10.1016/S0306-3623(98)00238-9] [PMID: 10401991]

[179] Wang H. Anti-oxidant activity and major chemical component analyses of twenty-six commercially available essential oils. J Food Drug Analy 2017; 25: 881-9.

[180] Lu Y, Foo LY. Identification and quantification of major polyphenols in apple pomace. Food Chem 1997; 59(2): 187-94.
[http://dx.doi.org/10.1016/S0308-8146(96)00287-7]

[181] Bastianetto S, Quirion R. Natural extracts as possible protective agents of brain aging. Neurobiol Aging 2002; 23(5): 891-7.
[http://dx.doi.org/10.1016/S0197-4580(02)00024-6] [PMID: 12392793]

[182] Scalbert A, Johnson IT, Saltmarsh M. Polyphenols: Antioxidants and beyond. Am J Clin Nutr 2005; 81(1): 215S-7S.
[http://dx.doi.org/10.1093/ajcn/81.1.215S] [PMID: 15640483]

[183] Wang H, Zhao M, Yang B, Jiang Y, Rao G. Identification of polyphenols in tobacco leaf and their antioxidant and antimicrobial activities. Food Chem 2008; 107(4): 1399-406.
[http://dx.doi.org/10.1016/j.foodchem.2007.09.068]

[184] Ben Hassine D, Abderrabba M, Yvon Y, *et al.* Chemical composition and *in vitro* evaluation of the antioxidant and antimicrobial activities of *Eucalyptus gillii* essential oil and extracts. Molecules 2012; 17(8): 9540-58.
[http://dx.doi.org/10.3390/molecules17089540] [PMID: 22878228]

[185] Asgary S, Sahebkar A, Afshani MR, Keshvari M, Haghjooyjavanmard S, Rafieian-Kopaei M. Clinical evaluation of blood pressure lowering, endothelial function improving, hypolipidemic and anti-inflammatory effects of pomegranate juice in hypertensive subjects. Phytother Res 2014; 28(2): 193-9. [http://dx.doi.org/10.1002/ptr.4977] [PMID: 23519910]

[186] Huang YL, Chen CC, Chen Y. Identification and quantification of majorpolyphenols in grape seed. J Nat Prod 2001; 64: 903-6. [http://dx.doi.org/10.1021/np000583q] [PMID: 11473420]

[187] Lee KG, Shibamoto T. Antioxidant activities of volatile components isolated from *Eucalyptus* species. J Sci Food Agric 2001; 81(15): 1573-9. [http://dx.doi.org/10.1002/jsfa.980]

[188] Sacchetti G, Maietti S, Muzzoli M, *et al.* Comparative evaluation of 11 essential oils of different origin as functional antioxidants, antiradicals and antimicrobials in foods. Food Chem 2005; 91(4): 621-32. [http://dx.doi.org/10.1016/j.foodchem.2004.06.031]

[189] Barra A, Coroneo V, Dessi S, Cabras P, Angioni A. Chemical variability, antifungal and antioxidant activity of Eucalyptus camaldulensis essential oil from Sardinia. Nat Prod Commun 2010; 5(2): 1934578X1000500. [http://dx.doi.org/10.1177/1934578X1000500232] [PMID: 20334153]

[190] Singh HP, Kaur S, Negi K, *et al.* Assessment of *in vitro* antioxidant activity of essential oil of *Eucalyptus citriodora* (lemon-scented Eucalypt; Myrtaceae) and its major constituents. Lebensm Wiss Technol 2012; 48(2): 237-41. [http://dx.doi.org/10.1016/j.lwt.2012.03.019]

[191] Bendaoud H, Bouajila J, Rhouma A, Savagnac A, Romdhane M. GC/MS analysis and antimicrobial and antioxidant activities of essential oil of *Eucalyptus radiata*. J Sci Food Agric 2009; 89(8): 1292-7. [http://dx.doi.org/10.1002/jsfa.3585]

[192] Zhang J, Perry G, Smith MA, *et al.* Parkinson's disease is associated with oxidative damage to cytoplasmic DNA and RNA in substantia nigra neurons. Am J Pathol 1999; 154(5): 1423-9. [http://dx.doi.org/10.1016/S0002-9440(10)65396-5] [PMID: 10329595]

[193] Chaitanya KV, Pathan AAK, Mazumdar SS, Chakravarthi GP, Parine N. Bobbarala, Role of oxidative stress in human health: An overview. J Pharm Res 2010; 3: 1330-3.

[194] Hajlaoui H, Mighri H, Aouni M, Gharsallah N, Kadri A. Chemical composition and *in vitro* evaluation of antioxidant, antimicrobial, cytotoxicity and anti-acetylcholinesterase properties of Tunisian *Origanum majorana* L. essential oil. Microb Pathog 2016; 95: 86-94. [http://dx.doi.org/10.1016/j.micpath.2016.03.003] [PMID: 26997648]

[195] Houghton P, Zarka R, de las Heras B, Hoult J. Fixed oil of Nigella sativa and derived thymoquinone inhibit eicosanoid generation in leukocytes and membrane lipid peroxidation. Planta Med 1995; 61(1): 33-6. [http://dx.doi.org/10.1055/s-2006-957994] [PMID: 7700988]

[196] Kruk I, Michalska T, Lichszteld K, Kładna A, Aboul-Enein HY. The effect of thymol and its derivatives on reactions generating reactive oxygen species. Chemosphere 2000; 41(7): 1059-64. [http://dx.doi.org/10.1016/S0045-6535(99)00454-3] [PMID: 10879823]

[197] Conti BJ, Búfalo MC, Golim MA, Bankova V, Sforcin JM. Cinnamic Acid is partially involved in propolis immunomodulatory action on human monocytes. Evid Based Complement Alternat Med 2013; 2013: 1-7. [http://dx.doi.org/10.1155/2013/109864] [PMID: 23762102]

[198] Villena J, Kitazawa H. Modulation of intestinal TLR4-inflammatory signaling pathways by probiotic microorganisms: Lessons learned from *Lactobacillus Jessenia* TL2937. Front Immunol 2014; 4: 512. [http://dx.doi.org/10.3389/fimmu.2013.00512] [PMID: 24459463]

[199] Edris AE. Pharmaceutical and therapeutic Potentials of essential oils and their individual volatile

constituents: A review. Phytother Res 2007; 21(4): 308-23.
[http://dx.doi.org/10.1002/ptr.2072] [PMID: 17199238]

[200] Bhalla Y, Gupta VK, Jaitak V. Anticancer activity of essential oils: A review. J Sci Food Agric 2013; 93(15): 3643-53.
[http://dx.doi.org/10.1002/jsfa.6267] [PMID: 23765679]

[201] Saad NY, Muller CD, Lobstein A. Major bioactivities and mechanism ofaction of essential oils and their components. Flavour Frag J 2013; 28(5): 269-79.

[202] Raut JS, Karuppayil SM. A status review on the medicinal properties of essential oils. Ind Crops Prod 2014; 62: 250-64.
[http://dx.doi.org/10.1016/j.indcrop.2014.05.055]

[203] Greay SJ, Hammer KA. Recent developments in the bioactivity of mono- and diterpenes: Anticancer and antimicrobial activity. Phytochem Rev 2015; 14(1): 1-6.
[http://dx.doi.org/10.1007/s11101-011-9212-6]

[204] Smalley KSM. Understanding melanoma signaling networks as the basis for molecular targeted therapy. J Invest Dermatol 2010; 130(1): 28-37.
[http://dx.doi.org/10.1038/jid.2009.177] [PMID: 19571822]

[205] Langhasova L, Hanusova V, Rezek J, *et al.* Essential oil from *Myrica rubra leaves* inhibits cancer cell proliferation and induces apoptosis in several human intestinal lines. Ind Crops Prod 2014; 59: 20-6.
[http://dx.doi.org/10.1016/j.indcrop.2014.04.018]

[206] Akaberi M, Mehri S, Iranshahi M. Multiple pro-apoptotic targets of abietane diterpenoids from Sal*via* species. Fitoterapia 2015; 100: 118-32.
[http://dx.doi.org/10.1016/j.fitote.2014.11.008] [PMID: 25447154]

[207] Janicsák G, Zupkó I, Nikolova MT, *et al.* Bioactivity-guided study of antiproliferative activities of Sal*via* extracts. Nat Prod Commun 2011; 6(5): 1934578X1100600.
[http://dx.doi.org/10.1177/1934578X1100600501] [PMID: 21615011]

[208] Russo A, Formisano C, Rigano D, Cardile V, Arnold NA, Senatore F. Comparative phytochemical profile and antiproliferative activity on human melanoma cells of essential oils of three lebanese Sal*via* species. Ind Crops Prod 2016; 83: 492-9.
[http://dx.doi.org/10.1016/j.indcrop.2015.12.080]

[209] Ribeiro S, de Jesus A, dos Anjos C, *et al.* Evaluation of the cytotoxic activity of some Brazilian medicinal plants. Planta Med 2012; 78(14): 1601-6.
[http://dx.doi.org/10.1055/s-0032-1315043] [PMID: 22814822]

[210] Ferraz RPC, Bomfim DS, Carvalho NC, *et al.* Cytotoxic effect of leaf essential oil of Lippia gracilis Schauer (Verbenaceae). Phytomedicine 2013; 20(7): 615-21.
[http://dx.doi.org/10.1016/j.phymed.2013.01.015] [PMID: 23453306]

[211] Vigan M. Essential oils: renewal of interest and toxicity. Eur J Dermatol 2010; 20(6): 685-92.

[212] Yu SG, Hildebrandt LA, Elson CE. Geraniol, an inhibitor of mevalonate biosynthesis, suppresses the growth of hepatomas and melanomas transplanted to rats and mice. J Nutr 1995; 125(11): 2763-7.
[PMID: 7472655]

[213] Cavalieri E, Mariotto S, Fabrizi C, *et al.* α-Bisabolol, a nontoxic natural compound, strongly induces apoptosis in glioma cells. Biochem Biophys Res Commun 2004; 315(3): 589-94.
[http://dx.doi.org/10.1016/j.bbrc.2004.01.088] [PMID: 14975741]

[214] Kumar A, Malik F, Bhushan S, *et al.* An essential oil and its major constituent isointermedeol induce apoptosis by increased expression of mitochondrial cytochrome c and apical death receptors in human leukaemia HL-60 cells. Chem Biol Interact 2008; 171(3): 332-47.
[http://dx.doi.org/10.1016/j.cbi.2007.10.003] [PMID: 18070620]

[215] Russo A, Formisano C, Rigano D, *et al.* Chemical composition and anticancer activity of essential oils

of Mediterranean sage (*Salvia officinalis* L.) grown in different environmental conditions. Food Chem Toxicol 2013; 55: 42-7.
[http://dx.doi.org/10.1016/j.fct.2012.12.036] [PMID: 23291326]

[216] Carnesecchi S, Bras-Gonçalves R, Bradaia A, *et al.* Geraniol, a component of plant essential oils, modulates DNA synthesis and potentiates 5-fluorouracil efficacy on human colon tumor xenografts. Cancer Lett 2004; 215(1): 53-9.
[http://dx.doi.org/10.1016/j.canlet.2004.06.019] [PMID: 15374632]

[217] Lu XG, Feng BA, Zhan LB, Yu ZH. [D-limonene induces apoptosis of gastric cancer cells]. Zhonghua Zhong Liu Za Zhi 2003; 25(4): 325-7.
[PMID: 12921557]

[218] Wu CC, Chung JG, Tsai SJ, Yang JH, Sheen LY. Differential effects of allyl sulfides from garlic essential oil on cell cycle regulation in human liver tumor cells. Food Chem Toxicol 2004; 42(12): 1937-47.
[http://dx.doi.org/10.1016/j.fct.2004.07.008] [PMID: 15500931]

[219] Juergens UR, Stöber M, Vetter H. Inhibition of cytokine production and arachidonic acid metabolism by eucalyptol (1.8-cineole) in human blood monocytes *in vitro*. Eur J Med Res 1998; 3(11): 508-10.
[PMID: 9810029]

[220] Huang YB, Fang JY, Hung CH, Wu PC, Tsai YH. Cyclic monoterpene extract from cardamom oil as a skin permeation enhancer for indomethacin: *in vitro* and *in vivo* studies. Biol Pharm Bull 1999; 22(6): 642-6.
[http://dx.doi.org/10.1248/bpb.22.642] [PMID: 10408241]

[221] Moteki H, Hibasami H, Yamada Y, Katsuzaki H, Imai K, Komiya T. Specific induction of apoptosis by 1,8-cineole in two human leukemia cell lines, but not a in human stomach cancer cell line. Oncol Rep 2002; 9(4): 757-60.
[http://dx.doi.org/10.3892/or.9.4.757] [PMID: 12066204]

[222] Cheng J, Chang G, Wu W. A controlled clinical study between hepatic arterial infusion with embolized Curcuma aromatic oil and chemical drugs in treating primary livercancer. Chin J Integr Trad Western Med 2001; 21: 165-7.

[223] Adiguzel A, Ozer H, Sokmen M, *et al.* Antimicrobial and antioxidant activity of the essential oil and methanol extract of *Nepeta cataria.* Pol J Microbiol 2009; 58(1): 69-76.
[PMID: 19469289]

[224] Birkett MA, Hassanali A, Hoglund S, Pettersson J, Pickett JA. Repellent activity of catmint, Nepeta cataria, and iridoid nepetalactone isomers against Afro-tropical mosquitoes, ixodid ticks and red poultry mites. Phytochemistry 2011; 72(1): 109-14.
[http://dx.doi.org/10.1016/j.phytochem.2010.09.016] [PMID: 21056438]

[225] Zomorodian K, Saharkhiz MJ, Shariati S, Pakshir K, Rahimi MJ, Khashei R. Chemical composition and antimicrobial activities of essential oils from Nepeta cataria L. against common causes of food-borne infections. ISRN Pharm 2012; 2012: 1-6.
[http://dx.doi.org/10.5402/2012/591953] [PMID: 22779012]

[226] Pavela R. Insecticidal activity of some essential oils against larvae of *Spodoptera littoralis.* Fitoterapia 2005; 76(7-8): 691-6.
[http://dx.doi.org/10.1016/j.fitote.2005.06.001] [PMID: 16236461]

[227] Ghaninia M, Larsson M, Hansson BS, Ignell R. Natural odor ligands for olfactory receptor neurons of the female mosquito *Aedes aegypti* : use of gas chromatography-linked single sensillum recordings. J Exp Biol 2008; 211(18): 3020-7.
[http://dx.doi.org/10.1242/jeb.016360] [PMID: 18775939]

[228] Bibi T, Ahmad M, Edwards SE, Tareen NM, Jabeen R, Abdullah I. Ethnomedicinal uses of plants in the treatment of paediatric geohelminth infections in Kalat district of Northern Balochistan, Pakistan. J Ethnopharmacol 2016; 183: 176-86.

[http://dx.doi.org/10.1016/j.jep.2016.02.029] [PMID: 26927703]

[229] Mahnaz K, Alireza F, Hassan V, Mahdi S, Reza AM, Abbas H. Larvicidal activity of essential oil and methanol extract of *Nepeta menthoides* against malaria vector *Anopheles stephensi.* Asian Pac J Trop Med 2012; 5(12): 962-5.
[http://dx.doi.org/10.1016/S1995-7645(12)60182-5] [PMID: 23199714]

[230] Salehi B, Valussi M, Jugran AK, *et al.* Nepeta species: From farm to food applications and phytotherapy. Trends Food Sci Technol 2018; 80: 104-22.
[http://dx.doi.org/10.1016/j.tifs.2018.07.030]

[231] Seyoum A, Killeen GF, Kabiru EW, Knols BGJ, Hassanali A. Field efficacy of thermally expelled or live potted repellent plants against African malaria vectors in western Kenya. Trop Med Int Health 2003; 8(11): 1005-11.
[http://dx.doi.org/10.1046/j.1360-2276.2003.01125.x] [PMID: 14629767]

[232] Thyagarajan SP, Jayaram S, Gopalakrishnan V, Hari R, Jeyakumar P, Sripathi MS. Herbal medicines for liver diseases in India. J Gastroenterol Hepatol 2002; 17(s3): 293-304.
[http://dx.doi.org/10.1046/j.1440-1746.17.s3.30.x]

[233] Duthie GG. Parsley, polyphenols and nutritional antioxidants. Br J Nutr 1999; 81(6): 425-6.
[http://dx.doi.org/10.1017/S0007114599000768] [PMID: 10615216]

[234] Guesmi F, Beghalem H, Tyagi AK, *et al.* Prevention of H_2O_2 Induced Oxidative Damages of Rat Testis by *Thymus algeriensis.* Biomed Environ Sci 2016; 29(4): 275-85.
[PMID: 27241738]

[235] Guesmi F, Ben Ali M, Barkaoui T, *et al.* Effects of *Thymus hirtus sp. algeriensis* Boiss. et Reut. (Lamiaceae) essential oil on healing gastric ulcers according to sex. Lipids Health Dis 2014; 13(1): 138.
[http://dx.doi.org/10.1186/1476-511X-13-138] [PMID: 25159191]

[236] Guesmi F, Tyagi AK, Bellamine H, Landoulsi A. Antioxidant Machinery Related to Decreased MDA Generation by *Thymus Algeriensis* Essential Oil-induced Liver and Kidney Regeneration. Biomed Environ Sci 2016; 29(9): 639-49.
[PMID: 27806746]

[237] Cai L, Wu CD. Compounds from *Syzygium aromaticum* possessing growth inhibitory activity against oral pathogens. J Nat Prod 1996; 59(10): 987-90.
[http://dx.doi.org/10.1021/np960451q] [PMID: 8904847]

[238] Han X, Parker TL. Anti-inflammatory, tissue remodeling, immunomodulatory, and anticancer activities of oregano (*Origanum vulgare*) essential oil in a human skin disease model. Biochim Open 2017; 4: 73-7.
[http://dx.doi.org/10.1016/j.biopen.2017.02.005] [PMID: 29450144]

[239] Han X, Parker TL. Biological activity of vetiver (*Vetiveria zizanioides*) essential oil in human dermal fibroblasts. Cogent Med 2017; 4(1): 1298176.
[http://dx.doi.org/10.1080/2331205X.2017.1298176]

[240] Kafi S, Atashkar S, Alavi A, Rezvani S. Relationship of posttraumatic stress disorder with psychological defense styles in burn patients. Horiz Med Sci 2013; 19: 155-60.

[241] Nam Nabati M. The effect of distraction on the severity of the burns dressing pain in children in Isfahan Burns Hospital. Res Med Sci 2000; 7: 67-9.

[242] Seyyed-Rasooli A, Salehi F, Mohammadpoorasl A, Goljaryan S, Seyyedi Z, Thomson B. Comparing the effects of aromatherapy massage and inhalation aromatherapy on anxiety and pain in burn patients: A single-blind randomized clinical trial. Burns 2016; 42(8): 1774-80.
[http://dx.doi.org/10.1016/j.burns.2016.06.014] [PMID: 27575673]

[243] Filiptsova OV, Gazzavi-Rogozina LV, Timoshyna IA, Naboka OI, Dyomina YV, Ochkur AV. The essential oil of rosemary and its effect on the human image and numerical short-term memory.

Egyptian Journal of Basic and Applied Sciences 2017; 4(2): 107-11. [http://dx.doi.org/10.1016/j.ejbas.2017.04.002]

[244] Elmann A, Mordechay S, Rindner M, Ravid U. Anti-neuroinflammatory effects of geranium oil in microglial cells. J Funct Foods 2010; 2(1): 17-22. [http://dx.doi.org/10.1016/j.jff.2009.12.001]

[245] Inouye S, Yamaguchi H, Takizawa T. Screening of the antibacterial effects of a variety of essential oils on respiratory tract pathogens using a modified dilution assay method. J Infect Chemoher 2001; 7: 251-4.

[246] Inouye S, Takizawa T, Yamaguchi H. Antibacterial activity of essential oils and their major constituents against respiratory tract pathogens by gaseous contact. J Antimicrobial Chemoher 2001; 47: 565-73.

[247] Pattnaik S, Subramanyam VR, Bapaji M, Kole CR. Antibacterial and antifungal activity of aromatic constituents of essential oils. Microbios 1997; 89(358): 39-46. [PMID: 9218354]

[248] Santos FA, Rao VSN. 1,8-cineol, a food flavoring agent, prevents ethanol-induced gastric injury in rats. Dig Dis Sci 2001; 46(2): 331-7. [http://dx.doi.org/10.1023/A:1005604932760] [PMID: 11281182]

[249] Stein DJ, Hollander E, Rothbaum BO. Textbook of Anxiety Disorders. 2nd ed., Washington, DC: American Psychiatric Publishing, Inc. 2009.

[250] Kaplan HI, Sadoch BJ. Comprehensive Textbook of Psychiatry. 8th ed., Baltimore: Lippincott, Williams and Wilkins 2005.

[251] Grundmann O, Nakajima JI, Seo S, Butterweck V. Anti-anxiety effects of Apocynum venetum L. in the elevated plus maze test. J Ethnopharmacol 2007; 110(3): 406-11. [http://dx.doi.org/10.1016/j.jep.2006.09.035] [PMID: 17101250]

[252] Hossain MA, AL-Raqmi KAS, AL-Mijizy ZH, Weli AM, Al-Riyami Q. Study of total phenol, flavonoids contents and phytochemical screening of various leaves crude extracts of locally grown Thymus vulgaris. Asian Pac J Trop Biomed 2013; 3(9): 705-10. [http://dx.doi.org/10.1016/S2221-1691(13)60142-2] [PMID: 23998010]

[253] Komaki A, Hoseini F, Shahidi S, Baharlouei N. Study of the effect of extract of *Thymus vulgaris* on anxiety in male rats. J Tradit Complement Med 2016; 6(3): 257-61. [http://dx.doi.org/10.1016/j.jtcme.2015.01.001] [PMID: 27419090]

[254] Soto-Vásquez MR, Alvarado-García PAA. Aromatherapy with two essential oils from Satureja genre and mindfulness meditation to reduce anxiety in humans. J Tradit Complement Med 2017; 7(1): 121-5. [http://dx.doi.org/10.1016/j.jtcme.2016.06.003] [PMID: 28053898]

[255] Gadekar R, Singour PK, Chaurasiya PK, Pawar RS, Patil UK. A potential of some medicinal plants as an antiulcer agents. Pharmacogn Rev 2010; 4: 136-46.

[256] Malfertheiner P, Chan FKL, McColl KEL. Peptic ulcer disease. Lancet 2009; 374(9699): 1449-61. [http://dx.doi.org/10.1016/S0140-6736(09)60938-7] [PMID: 19683340]

[257] Awaad AS, El-Meligy RM, Soliman GA. Natural products in treatment of ulcerative colitis and peptic ulcer. J Saudi Chem Soc 2013; 17(1): 101-24. [http://dx.doi.org/10.1016/j.jscs.2012.03.002]

[258] Lakshmi V, Singh N, Shrivastva S, *et al.* Gedunin and Photogedunin of *Xylocarpus granatum* show significant anti-secretory effects and protect the gastric mucosa of peptic ulcer in rats. Phytomedicine 2010; 17(8-9): 569-74. [http://dx.doi.org/10.1016/j.phymed.2009.10.016] [PMID: 19962286]

[259] Klein LC Jr, Gandolfi RB, Santin JR, Lemos M, Filho VC, de Andrade SF. Antiulcerogenic activity of extract, fractions, and some compounds obtained from Polygala cyparissias St. Hillaire & Moquin

(Polygalaceae). Naunyn Schmiedebergs Arch Pharmacol 2010; 381(2): 121-6. [http://dx.doi.org/10.1007/s00210-009-0485-x] [PMID: 20054524]

[260] Sheen E, Triadafilopoulos G. Adverse effects of long-term proton pump inhibitor therapy. Dig Dis Sci 2011; 56(4): 931-50. [http://dx.doi.org/10.1007/s10620-010-1560-3] [PMID: 21365243]

[261] Zayachkivska OS, Konturek SJ, Drozdowicz D, Brzozowski T, Gzhegotsky MR. Influence of plant-originated gastroproteciive and antiulcer substances on gastric mucosal repair. Fiziol Zh 2004; 50(6): 118-27. [PMID: 15732769]

[262] Schmeda-Hirschmann G, Yesilada E. Traditional medicine and gastroprotective crude drugs. J Ethnopharmacol 2005; 100(1-2): 61-6. [http://dx.doi.org/10.1016/j.jep.2005.06.002] [PMID: 15993015]

[263] De Sousa DP. Medicinal Essential Oils: Chemical, Pharmacological and Therapeutic Aspects. 1st ed. New York, NY, USA: Nova Science Publishers 2012; pp. 1-236.

[264] Oliveira F, Andrade L, de Sousa É, de Sousa D. Anti-ulcer activity of essential oil constituents. Molecules 2014; 19(5): 5717-47. [http://dx.doi.org/10.3390/molecules19055717] [PMID: 24802985]

[265] Rozza AL, Hiruma-Lima CA, Takahira RK, Padovani CR, Pellizzon CH. Effect of menthol in experimentally induced ulcers: Pathways of gastroprotection. Chem Biol Interact 2013; 206(2): 272-8. [http://dx.doi.org/10.1016/j.cbi.2013.10.003] [PMID: 24121185]

[266] Vernin GA, Parkanyi C, Cozzolino F, Fellous R. GC/MS analysis of the volatile constituents of *Corymbia citriodora* Hook. from Réunion Island. J Essent Oil Res 2004; 16(6): 560-5. [http://dx.doi.org/10.1080/10412905.2004.9698798]

[267] Paik SY, Koh KH, Beak SM, Paek SH, Kim JA. The essential oils from *Zanthoxylum schinifolium* pericarp induce apoptosis of HepG2 human hepatoma cells through increased production of reactive oxygen species. Biol Pharm Bull 2005; 28(5): 802-7. [http://dx.doi.org/10.1248/bpb.28.802] [PMID: 15863882]

[268] Silva MIG, Moura BA, de Aquino Neto MR, *et al.* Gastroprotective activity of isopulegol on experimentally induced gastric lesions in mice: investigation of possible mechanisms of action. Naunyn Schmiedebergs Arch Pharmacol 2009; 380(3): 233-45. [http://dx.doi.org/10.1007/s00210-009-0429-5] [PMID: 19479241]

[269] Szabo S. Mechanisms of Mucosal Injury in the Stomach and Duodenum: Time-sequence Analysis of Morphologic, Functional, Biochemical and Histochemical Studies Scandina*vian*. J Gastroenterol 1987; 22: 21-8.

[270] Nguemfo EL, Dimo T, Dongmo AB, *et al.* Anti-oxidative and anti-inflammatory activities of some isolated constituents from the stem bark of Allanblackia monticola Staner L.C (Guttiferae). Inflammopharmacology 2009; 17(1): 37-41. [http://dx.doi.org/10.1007/s10787-008-8039-2] [PMID: 19127347]

[271] Rainsford KD. Structure-activity relationships of non-steroid anti-inflammatory drugs 1. Gastric ulcerogenic activity. Agents Actions 1978; 8(6): 587-605. [http://dx.doi.org/10.1007/BF01998888] [PMID: 742556]

[272] Wallace J. Nitric oxide, aspirin-triggered lipoxins and NO-aspirin in gastric protection. Inflamm Allergy Drug Targets 2006; 5(2): 133-7. [http://dx.doi.org/10.2174/187152806776383116] [PMID: 16613572]

[273] Moraes TM, Kushima H, Moleiro FC, *et al.* Effects of limonene and essential oil from *Citrus aurantium* on gastric mucosa: Role of prostaglandins and gastric mucus secretion. Chem Biol Interact 2009; 180(3): 499-505. [http://dx.doi.org/10.1016/j.cbi.2009.04.006] [PMID: 19410566]

[274] Al Moutaery AR. Protective effect of ketoconazole against experimentally induced gastric ulcers in rats. Res Commun Mol Pathol Pharmacol 2003; 113-114: 5-23.
[PMID: 15686104]

[275] Rozza AL, Moraes TM, Kushima H, *et al.* Gastroprotective mechanisms of Citrus lemon (Rutaceae) essential oil and its majority compounds limonene and β-pinene: Involvement of heat-shock protein-70, vasoactive intestinal peptide, glutathione, sulfhydryl compounds, nitric oxide and prostaglandin E_2. Chem Biol Interact 2011; 189(1-2): 82-9.
[http://dx.doi.org/10.1016/j.cbi.2010.09.031] [PMID: 20934418]

[276] Sanguinetti EE. Plantas Que Curam. 2nd ed. Porto Alegre, RS, Brazil: Editora Rígel 1989; p. 208.

[277] Sun J. D-Limonene: safety and clinical applications. Altern Med Rev 2007; 12(3): 259-64.
[PMID: 18072821]

[278] De Vincenzi M, Silano M, De Vincenzi A, Maialetti F, Scazzocchio B. Constituents of aromatic plants: eucalyptol. Fitoterapia 2002; 73(3): 269-75.
[http://dx.doi.org/10.1016/S0367-326X(02)00062-X] [PMID: 12048025]

[279] Mansour MA, Nagi MN, El-Khatib AS, Al-Bekairi AM. Effects of thymoquinone on antioxidant enzyme activities, lipid peroxidation and DT-diaphorase in different tissues of mice: A possible mechanism of action. Cell Biochem Funct 2002; 20(2): 143-51.
[http://dx.doi.org/10.1002/cbf.968] [PMID: 11979510]

[280] Al-Ali A, Alkhawajah AA, Randhawa MA, Shaikh NA. Oral and intraperitoneal LD_{50} of thymoquinone, an active principle of *Nigella sativa*, in mice and rats. J Ayub Med Coll Abbottabad 2008; 20(2): 25-7.
[PMID: 19385451]

[281] Souza R, Cardoso M, Menezes C, Silva J, De Sousa D, Batista J. Gastroprotective activity of α-terpineol in two experimental models of gastric ulcer in rats. Daru 2011; 19(4): 277-81.
[PMID: 22615669]

[282] Paisooksantivatana S, Bua-in Y. Essential oil and antioxidant activity of Cassumunar Ginger (Zingiberaceae: *Zingiber montanum* (Koenig) Link ex Dietr.) collected from various parts of Thailand. Witthayasan Kasetsat Witthayasat 2009; 43: 467-4705.

[283] Sukatta U, Rugthaworn P, Punjee P, Chidchenchey S, Keeratinijakal V. Chemical composition and physical properties of oil from Plai (*Zingiber cassumunar* Roxb.) obtained by hydro distillation and hexane extraction. Witthayasan Kasetsat Witthayasat 2009; 43: 212-7.

[284] Pazyar N, Yaghoobi R, Bagherani N, Kazerouni A. A review of applications of tea tree oil in dermatology. Int J Dermatol 2013; 52(7): 784-90.
[http://dx.doi.org/10.1111/j.1365-4632.2012.05654.x] [PMID: 22998411]

[285] Sellami IH, Maamouri E, Chahed T, Wannes WA, Kchouk ME, Marzouk B. Effect of growth stage on the content and composition of the essential oil and phenolic fraction of sweet marjoram (Origanum majorana L.). Ind Crops Prod 2009; 30(3): 395-402.
[http://dx.doi.org/10.1016/j.indcrop.2009.07.010]

[286] Jirovetz L, Buchbauer G, Shafi PM, Abraham GT. Analysis of the essential oil of the roots of the medicinal plant *Kaempferia galanga* L. (Zingiberaceae) from South India. Acta Pharm Turc 2001; 43: 107-10.

[287] Belsito D, Bickers D, Bruze M, *et al.* A toxicologic and dermatologic assessment of cyclic and non-cyclic terpene alcohols when used as fragrance ingredientes. Food Chem Toxicol 2008; 46: 1-71.

[288] Bhatia SP, Letizia CS, Api AM. Fragrance material review on elemol. Food Chem Toxicol 2008; 46(11): S147-8.
[http://dx.doi.org/10.1016/j.fct.2008.06.045] [PMID: 18640176]

[289] Matsunaga T, Hasegawa C, Kawasuji T, *et al.* Isolation of the antiulcer compound in essential oil from

the leaves of *Cryptomeria japonica.* Biol Pharm Bull 2000; 23(5): 595-8. [http://dx.doi.org/10.1248/bpb.23.595] [PMID: 10823671]

[290] Vila R, Mundina M, Muschietti L, *et al.* Volatile constituents of leaves, roots and stems from *Aristolochia elegans.* Phytochemistry 1997; 46(6): 1127-9. [http://dx.doi.org/10.1016/S0031-9422(97)00400-7]

[291] Péres VF, Moura DJ, Sperotto ARM, *et al.* Chemical composition and cytotoxic, mutagenic and genotoxic activities of the essential oil from *Piper gaudichaudianum* Kunth leaves. Food Chem Toxicol 2009; 47(9): 2389-95. [http://dx.doi.org/10.1016/j.fct.2009.06.035] [PMID: 19563855]

[292] Klopell FC, Lemos M, Sousa JPB, *et al.* Nerolidol, an antiulcer constituent from the essential oil of *Baccharis dracunculifolia* DC (Asteraceae). Z Naturforsch C J Biosci 2007; 62(7-8): 537-42. [http://dx.doi.org/10.1515/znc-2007-7-812] [PMID: 17913068]

[293] Freire RS, Morais SM, Catunda-Junior FEA, Pinheiro DCSN. Synthesis and antioxidant, anti-inflammatory and gastroprotector activities of anethole and related compounds. Bioorg Med Chem 2005; 13(13): 4353-8. [http://dx.doi.org/10.1016/j.bmc.2005.03.058] [PMID: 15890516]

[294] Capasso R, Pinto L, Vuotto ML, Di Carlo G. Preventive effect of eugenol on PAF and ethanol-induced gastric mucosal damage. Fitoterapia 2000; 71(Suppl. 1): S131-7. [http://dx.doi.org/10.1016/S0367-326X(00)00188-X] [PMID: 10930724]

[295] Maity P, Biswas K, Roy S, Banerjee RK, Bandyopadhyay U. Smoking and the pathogenesis of gastroduodenal ulcer--recent mechanistic update. Mol Cell Biochem 2003; 253(1/2): 329-38. [http://dx.doi.org/10.1023/A:1026040723669] [PMID: 14619984]

[296] Braquet P, Etienne A, Mencia-Huerta JM, Clostre F. Effects of the specific platelet-activating factor antagonists, BN 52021 and BN 52063, on various experimental gastrointestinal ulcerations. Eur J Pharmacol 1988; 150(3): 269-76. [http://dx.doi.org/10.1016/0014-2999(88)90007-6] [PMID: 3046952]

[297] Yang X, Eilerman RG. Pungent principal of Alpinia galangal (L.) swartz and its applications. J Agric Food Chem 1999; 47(4): 1657-62. [http://dx.doi.org/10.1021/jf9808224] [PMID: 10564034]

[298] Matsuda H, Pongpiriyadacha Y, Morikawa T, Ochi M, Yoshikawa M. Gastroprotective effects of phenylpropanoids from the rhizomes of *Alpinia galanga* in rats: structural requirements and mode of action. Eur J Pharmacol 2003; 471(1): 59-67. [http://dx.doi.org/10.1016/S0014-2999(03)01785-0] [PMID: 12809953]

[299] Tankam JM, Sawada Y, Ito M. Regular ingestion of cinnamomi cortex pulveratus offers gastroprotective activity in mice. J Nat Med 2013; 67(2): 289-95. [http://dx.doi.org/10.1007/s11418-012-0680-9] [PMID: 22760889]

[300] Furia TE, Bellanca N. Fenaroli's Handbook of Flavor Ingredients. Cleveland, OH, USA: Chemical Rubber Company Press 1975; p. 2.

[301] Ortiz MI, Ramírez-Montiel ML, González-García MP, Ponce-Monter HA, Castañeda-Hernández G, Cariño-Cortés R. The combination of naproxen and citral reduces nociception and gastric damage in rats. Arch Pharm Res 2010; 33(10): 1691-7. [http://dx.doi.org/10.1007/s12272-010-1020-9] [PMID: 21052946]

[302] Singh S, Khajuria A, Taneja SC, *et al.* The gastric ulcer protective effect of boswellic acids, a leukotriene inhibitor from *Boswellia serrata*, in rats. Phytomedicine 2008; 15(6-7): 408-15. [http://dx.doi.org/10.1016/j.phymed.2008.02.017] [PMID: 18424019]

[303] Al-Hader AA, Hasan ZA, Aqel MB. Hyperglycemic and insulin release inhibitory effects of *Rosmarinus officinalis.* J Ethnopharmacol 1994; 43(3): 217-21. [http://dx.doi.org/10.1016/0378-8741(94)90046-9] [PMID: 7990497]

[304] Talpur N, Echard B, Ingram C, Bagchi D, Preuss H. Effects of a novel formulation of essential oils on glucose– insulin metabolism in diabetic and hypertensive rats: A pilot study. Diabetes Obes Metab 2005; 7(2): 193-9.
[http://dx.doi.org/10.1111/j.1463-1326.2004.00386.x] [PMID: 15715893]

[305] Broadhurst CL, Polansky MM, Anderson RA. Insulin-like biological activity of culinary and medicinal plant aqueous extracts *in vitro*. J Agric Food Chem 2000; 48(3): 849-52.
[http://dx.doi.org/10.1021/jf9904517] [PMID: 10725162]

[306] Abdollahi M, Salehnia A, Mortazavi SH, *et al.* Antioxidant, antidiabetic, antihyperlipidemic, reproduction stimulatory properties and safety of essential oil of Satureja Khuzestanica in rat *in vivo*: A oxicopharmacological study. Med Sci Monit 2003; 9(9): BR331-5.
[PMID: 12960922]

[307] Barter P. The inflammation: Lipoprotein cycle. Atheroscler Suppl 2005; 6(2): 15-20.
[http://dx.doi.org/10.1016/j.atherosclerosissup.2005.02.004] [PMID: 15823492]

[308] Naderi GA, Asgary S, Ani M, Sarraf-Zadegan N, Safari MR. Effect of some volatile oils on the affinity of intact and oxidized low-density lipoproteins for adrenal cell surface receptors. Mol Cell Biochem 2004; 267(1/2): 59-66.
[http://dx.doi.org/10.1023/B:MCBI.0000049365.60694.81] [PMID: 15663186]

[309] Brophy JJ, Davies NW, Southwell IA, Stiff IA, Williams LR. Gas chromatographic quality control for oil of Melaleuca terpinen-4-ol type (Australian tea tree). J Agric Food Chem 1989; 37(5): 1330-5.
[http://dx.doi.org/10.1021/jf00089a027]

[310] Mondello L, Dugo P, Bartle KD, Dugo G, Cotroneo A. Automated HPLC-HRGC: A powerful method for essential oils analysis. Part V. identification of terpene hydrocarbons of bergamot, lemon, mandarin, sweet orange, bitter orange, grapefruit, clementine and mexican lime oils by coupled HPLC-HRGC-MS(ITD). Flavour Fragrance J 1995; 10(1): 33-42.
[http://dx.doi.org/10.1002/ffj.2730100106]

[311] Takahashi Y, Inaba N, Kuwahara S, Kuki W. Antioxidative effect of citrus essential oil components on human low-density lipoprotein *in vitro*. Biosci Biotechnol Biochem 2003; 67(1): 195-7.
[http://dx.doi.org/10.1271/bbb.67.195] [PMID: 12619696]

[312] Boateng JS, Matthews KH, Stevens HNE, Eccleston GM. Wound healing dressings and drug delivery systems: A review. J Pharm Sci 2008; 97(8): 2892-923.
[http://dx.doi.org/10.1002/jps.21210] [PMID: 17963217]

[313] Boateng J, Catanzano O. Advanced Therapeutic Dressings for Effective Wound Healing—A Review. J Pharm Sci 2015; 104(11): 3653-80.
[http://dx.doi.org/10.1002/jps.24610] [PMID: 26308473]

[314] Erel O. A novel automated direct measurement method for total antioxidant capacity using a new generation, more stable ABTS radical cation. Clin Biochem 2004; 37: 277-85.
[http://dx.doi.org/10.1016/j.clinbiochem.2003.11.015]

[315] Lehrner J, Marwinski G, Lehr S, Johren P, Deecke L. Ambient odors of orange and lavender reduce anxiety and improve mood in a dental office. Physiol Behav 2005; 86(1-2): 92-5.
[http://dx.doi.org/10.1016/j.physbeh.2005.06.031] [PMID: 16095639]

[316] Braden R, Reichow S, Halm MA. The use of the essential oil lavandin to reduce preoperative anxiety in surgical patients. J Perianesth Nurs 2009; 24(6): 348-55.
[http://dx.doi.org/10.1016/j.jopan.2009.10.002] [PMID: 19962101]

[317] Kim S, Kim HJ , Yeo JS, Hong S-J . The effect of lavender oil on stress, bispectral index values, and needle insertion pain in volunteers. J Alternatn Complemen Med 2011; 17(9): 823-6.

[318] Perry R, Terry R, Watson LK, Ernst E. Is lavender an anxiolytic drug? A systematic review of randomised clinical trials. Phytomedicine 2012; 19(8-9): 825-35.
[http://dx.doi.org/10.1016/j.phymed.2012.02.013] [PMID: 22464012]

[319] Goes TC, Antunes FD, Alves PB, Teixeira-Silva F. Effect of sweet orange aroma on experimental anxiety in humans. J Altern Complement Med 2012; 18(8): 798-804. [http://dx.doi.org/10.1089/acm.2011.0551] [PMID: 22849536]

[320] Pour FF, Jaafarzadeh M, Arman S. Effect of aromatherapy with orange essential oil on salivary cortisol and pulse rate in children during dental treatment: A randomized controlled clinical trial. Adv Biomed Res 2013; 2(1): 10. [http://dx.doi.org/10.4103/2277-9175.107968] [PMID: 23930255]

[321] Hongratanaworakit T. Relaxing effect of rose oil on humans. Nat Prod Commun 2009; 4(2): 1934578X0900400. [http://dx.doi.org/10.1177/1934578X0900400226] [PMID: 19370942]

[322] Hu PH, Peng YC, Lin YT, Chang CS, Ou MC. Aromatherapy for reducing colonoscopy related procedural anxiety and physiological parameters: A randomized controlled study. Hepatogastroenterology 2010; 57(102-103): 1082-6. [PMID: 21410035]

[323] Cho MY. Effects of aromatherapy on the anxiety, vital signs, and sleep quality of percutaneous coronary intervention patients in intensive care units. Evid-Based omplement Alterna Med 2013.

[324] de Jong M, Lucas C, Bredero H, van Adrichem L, Tibboel D, van Dijk M. Does postoperative 'M' technique ® massage with or without mandarin oil reduce infants' distress after major craniofacial surgery? J Adv Nurs 2012; 68(8): 1748-57. [http://dx.doi.org/10.1111/j.1365-2648.2011.05861.x] [PMID: 22050553]

[325] Kim JT, Ren CJ, Fielding GA, *et al.* Treatment with lavender aromatherapy in the post-anesthesia care unit reduces opioid requirements of morbidly obese patients undergoing laparoscopic adjustable gastric banding. Obes Surg 2007; 17(7): 920-5. [http://dx.doi.org/10.1007/s11695-007-9170-7] [PMID: 17894152]

[326] Soltani R, Soheilipour S, Hajhashemi V, Asghari G, Bagheri M, Molavi M. Evaluation of the effect of aromatherapy with lavender essential oil on post-tonsillectomy pain in pediatric patients: A randomized controlled trial. Int J Pediatr Otorhinolaryngol 2013; 77(9): 1579-81. [http://dx.doi.org/10.1016/j.ijporl.2013.07.014] [PMID: 23932834]

[327] Olapour A, Behaeen K, Akhondzadeh R, Soltani F, Razavi F, Bekhradi R. The Effect of Inhalation of Aromatherapy Blend containing Lavender Essential Oil on Cesarean Postoperative Pain. Anesth Pain Med 2013; 3(1): 203-7. [http://dx.doi.org/10.5812/aapm.9570]

[328] Tate S. Peppermint oil: A treatment for postoperative nausea. J Adv Nurs 1997; 26(3): 543-9. [http://dx.doi.org/10.1046/j.1365-2648.1997.t01-15-00999.x] [PMID: 9378876]

[329] Hines S, Steels E, Chang A, Gilshenan K. Aromatherapy for treatment of postoperative nausea and vomiting. Cochrane Database Syst Rev 2009; 4.

[330] Lane B, Cannella K, Bowen C, *et al.* Examination of the effectiveness of peppermint aromatherapy on nausea in women post C-section. J Holist Nurs 2012; 30(2): 90-104. [http://dx.doi.org/10.1177/0898010111423419] [PMID: 22034523]

[331] Lua PL, Zakaria NS. A brief review of current scientific evidence involving aromatherapy use for nausea and vomiting. J Altern Complement Med 2012; 18(6): 534-40. [http://dx.doi.org/10.1089/acm.2010.0862] [PMID: 22784340]

[332] Ferruggiari L, Ragione B, Rich ER, Lock K. The effect of aromatherapy on postoperative nausea in women undergoing surgical procedures. J Perianesth Nurs 2012; 27(4): 246-51. [http://dx.doi.org/10.1016/j.jopan.2012.01.013] [PMID: 22828020]

[333] Hunt R, Dienemann J, Norton HJ, *et al.* Aromatherapy as treatment for postoperative nausea: A randomized trial. Anesth Analg 2013; 117(3): 597-604. [http://dx.doi.org/10.1213/ANE.0b013e31824a0b1c] [PMID: 22392970]

[334] Hiki N, Kaminishi M, Yasuda K, *et al.* Multicenter phase II randomized study evaluating dose-response of antiperistaltic effect of L-menthol sprayed onto the gastric mucosa for upper gastrointestinal endoscopy. Dig Endosc 2012; 24(2): 79-86.
[http://dx.doi.org/10.1111/j.1443-1661.2011.01163.x] [PMID: 22348831]

[335] Shavakhi A, Ardestani SK, Taki M, Goli M, Keshteli AH. Premedication with peppermint oil capsules in colonoscopy: A double blind placebo-controlled randomized trial study. Acta Gastroenterol Belg 2012; 75(3): 349-53.
[PMID: 23082707]

[336] Halcón L, Milkus K. and wounds: A review of tea tree oil as a promising antimicrobial. Am J Infect Control 2004; 32(7): 402-8.
[http://dx.doi.org/10.1016/j.ajic.2003.12.008] [PMID: 15525915]

[337] Chin KB, Cordell B. The effect of tea tree oil (*Melaleuca alternifolia*) on wound healing using a dressing model. J Altern Complement Med 2013; 19(12): 942-5.
[http://dx.doi.org/10.1089/acm.2012.0787] [PMID: 23848210]

[338] Edmondson M, Newall N, Carville K, Smith J, Riley TV, Carson CF. Uncontrolled, open-label, pilot study of tea tree (Melaleuca alternifolia) oil solution in the decolonisation of methicillin-resistant Staphylococcus aureus positive wounds and its influence on wound healing. Int Wound J 2011; 8(4): 375-84.
[http://dx.doi.org/10.1111/j.1742-481X.2011.00801.x] [PMID: 21564552]

[339] Blackwood B, Thompson G, McMullan R, *et al.* Tea tree oil (5%) body wash versus standard care (Johnson's Baby Softwash) to prevent colonization with methicillin-resistant Staphylococcus aureus in critically ill adults: A randomized controlled trial. J Antimicrob Chemother 2013; 68(5): 1193-9.
[http://dx.doi.org/10.1093/jac/dks501] [PMID: 23297395]

[340] Cavalca Cortelli S, Cavallini F, Regueira Alves MF, *et al.* Clinical and microbiological effects of an essential-oil-containing mouth rinse applied in the "one-stage full-mouth disinfection" protocol—a randomized doubled-blinded preliminary study. Clin Oral Investig 2009; 13(2): 189-94.
[http://dx.doi.org/10.1007/s00784-008-0219-3] [PMID: 18716800]

[341] Osso D, Kanani N. Antiseptic mouth rinses: An update on comparative effectiveness, risks and recommendations. J Dent Hyg 2013; 87(1): 10-8.
[PMID: 23433693]

[342] Motealleh B, Zahedi P, Rezaeian I, Moghimi M, Abdolghaffari AH, Zarandi MA. Morphology, drug release, antibacterial, cell proliferation, and histology studies of chamomile-loaded wound dressing mats based on electrospun nanofibrous poly(ε-caprolactone)/polystyrene blends. J Biomed Mater Res B Appl Biomater 2014; 102(5): 977-87.
[http://dx.doi.org/10.1002/jbm.b.33078] [PMID: 24259351]

[343] Antonio F, Guillem R, Sonia T, *et al.* Cross-linked collagen sponges loaded with plant polyphenols with inhibitory activity towards chronic wound enzymes. Biotechnol J 2011; 6(10): 1208-18.
[http://dx.doi.org/10.1002/biot.201100194] [PMID: 21805643]

[344] Tan SP, McLoughlin P, O'Sullivan L, *et al.* Development of a novel antimicrobial seaweed extract-based hydrogel wound dressing. Int J Pharm 2013; 456(1): 10-20.
[http://dx.doi.org/10.1016/j.ijpharm.2013.08.018] [PMID: 23958753]

[345] Bhatnagar M, Parwani L, Sharma V, Ganguli J, Bhatnagar A. Hemostatic, antibacterial biopolymers from *Acacia arabica* (Lam.) Willd. and *Moringa oleifera* (Lam.) as potential wound dressing materials. Indian J Exp Biol 2013; 51(10): 804-10.
[PMID: 24266104]

[346] Muthukumar T, Prabu P, Ghosh K, Sastry TP. Fish scale collagen sponge incorporated with *Macrotyloma uniflorum* plant extract as a possible wound/burn dressing material. Colloids Surf B Biointerfaces 2014; 113: 207-12.
[http://dx.doi.org/10.1016/j.colsurfb.2013.09.019] [PMID: 24096157]

[347] Sharma A, Khanna S, Kaur G, Singh I. Medicinal plants and their components for wound healing applications. Future Journal of Pharmaceutical Sciences 2021; 7(1): 53. [http://dx.doi.org/10.1186/s43094-021-00202-w]

[348] Jain S, Shrivastave S, Nayak S. Recent trends in *Curcuma longa* Linn. Ph Cog Rev 2007; 1: 119.

[349] Ameri A, Rajive BB, Vaidya JG, Apte K, Deokule SS. Anti-staphylococcal and wound healing activities of Ganoderma praelongum and Glycyrrhiza glabra formulation in mice. Int J Appl Res Nat Prod 2013; 6(1): 27-31.

[350] Shukla A, Rasik AM, Jain GK, Shankar R, Kulshrestha DK, Dhawan BN. *in vitro* and *in vivo* wound healing activity of asiaticoside isolated from Centella asiatica. J Ethnopharmacol 1999; 65(1): 1-11. [http://dx.doi.org/10.1016/S0378-8741(98)00141-X] [PMID: 10350364]

[351] Chen YJ, Dai YS, Chen BF, *et al.* The effect of tetrandrine and extracts of *Centella asiatica* on acute radiation dermatitis in rats. Biol Pharm Bull 1999; 22(7): 703-6. [http://dx.doi.org/10.1248/bpb.22.703] [PMID: 10443466]

[352] Kumarasamyraja D, Jeganathan NS, Manavalan RA. Review on medicinal plants with potential wound healing activity. J Pharm Sci 2012; 2(4): 105-11.

[353] Georgescu M, Chifiriuc M, Marutescu L, *et al.* Bioactive wound dressings for the management of chronic wounds. Curr Org Chem 2016; 21(1): 53-63. [http://dx.doi.org/10.2174/1385272820666160510171040]

[354] Yang CS, Chen G, Wu Q. Recent scientific studies of a traditional chinese medicine, tea, on prevention of chronic diseases. J Tradit Complement Med 2014; 4(1): 17-23. [http://dx.doi.org/10.4103/2225-4110.124326] [PMID: 24872929]

[355] Rani S, Amanjot G, Surya P, Kanwar K, Kaur S. Wound healing potential of medicinal plants with their screening models: A comprehensive review. J Drug Deliv Ther 2016; 6(1): 56-6.

[356] Osunwokeemek O, Allison J, Theodore AO, Julius C. The wound healing effects of aqueous leave extracts of *Azadirachta indica* on Wistar rats. Int J Nat Res 2013; 3: 181-6.

[357] Kiran K, Asad M. Wound healing activity of *Sesamum indicum* L seed and oil in rats. Indian J Exp Biol 2008; 46(11): 777-82. [PMID: 19090349]

[358] Sapna S, Anju D, Sanju NS. Traditional Indian medicinal plants with potential wound healing activity: A review. Int J Pharm Sci Res 2016; 7(5): 1809-19.

[359] Himesh S, Singhai AK. A recent update of botanical for wound healing activity. Res J Pharm 2012; 3(7): 1-7.

[360] Muhammad AA, Karthivashan G, Arulselvan P, Fakurazi S. *in vitro* antioxidant properties of bioactive fraction of *Moringa oleifera.* J Natprod. Biomed Res 2015; 1(2): 51-6.

[361] Nayak BS, Isitor GN, Maxwell A, Bhogadi V, Ramdath DD. Wound-healing activity of Morinda citrifolia fruit juice on diabetes-induced rats. J Wound Care 2007; 16(2): 83-6. [http://dx.doi.org/10.12968/jowc.2007.16.2.27006] [PMID: 17319624]

[362] Manjunatha BK, Krishna V, Vidya SM, Mankani KL, Manohara YN. Wound healing activity of *Lycopodium serratum.* Indian J Pharm Sci 2007; 69(2): 283-7. [http://dx.doi.org/10.4103/0250-474X.33159]

[363] Nayak BS, Pinto Pereira LM. *Catharanthus roseus* flower extract has wound-healing activity in Sprague Dawley rats. BMC Complement Altern Med 2006; 6(1): 41. [http://dx.doi.org/10.1186/1472-6882-6-41] [PMID: 17184528]

[364] Mittal A, Sardana S, Pandey A. Herbal boon for wounds. Int J Pharma Sci 2013; 5(2): 1-12.

[365] Yogesh SG, Jeyabalan RSA. Potential wound healing agents from medicinal plants: A review. Pharmacol 2013; 4(5): 349-58.

[366] Chaudhary G, Goya S, Poonia P. *Lawsonia inermis* Linnaeus: A phytopharmacological review. Int J Pharm Sci Drug Res 2010; 2(2): 91-8.

[367] Asif A, Kakub G, Mehmood S, Khunum R, Gulfraz M. Wound healing activity of root extracts of *Berberis lyceum* royle in rats. Phytother Res 2007; 21(6): 589-91. [http://dx.doi.org/10.1002/ptr.2110] [PMID: 17295382]

[368] Galehdari H, Negahdari S, Kesmati M, Rezaie A, Shariati G. Effect of the herbal mixture composed of *Aloe Vera*, Henna, Adiantum capillus-veneris, and Myrrha on wound healing in streptozotocin-induced diabetic rats. BMC Complement Altern Med 2016; 16(1): 386. [http://dx.doi.org/10.1186/s12906-016-1359-7] [PMID: 27716154]

[369] Garcia-Orue I, Gainza G, Gutierrez FB, *et al.* Novel nanofibrous dressings containing rhEGF and Aloe vera for wound healing applications. Int J Pharm 2017; 523(2): 556-66. [http://dx.doi.org/10.1016/j.ijpharm.2016.11.006] [PMID: 27825864]

[370] Balekar N, Nakpheng T, Katkam NG, Srichana T. Wound healing activity of ent-kaura-9(11)16-d-en-19-oicacid isolated from *Wedelia trilobata* (L.) leaves. Phytomed 2012; 19(13): 1178-84. [http://dx.doi.org/10.1016/j.phymed.2012.07.014] [PMID: 22921749]

[371] Govindappa M. Antimicrobial, antioxidant and *in vivo* antiinflammatory activity of ethanol extract and active phytochemical screening of *Wedelia trilobata* (L.) Hitchc. J Med Plants Res 2011; 5(24): 5718-29.

[372] Vinothapooshan G, Sundar K. Wound healing effect of various extracts of *Adhatoda vasica.* Int J Pharma Bio Sci 2010; 1(4): 530-6.

[373] Mahmood A, Salmah I. Wound healing activity of *Carica papaya* L. aqueous leaf extract in rats. Int J Mol Med 2005; 1(4): 398-401.

[374] Selvaraj N, Lakshmanan B, Mazumder PM, Karuppasamy M, Jena SS, Pattnaik AK. Evaluation of wound healing and antimicrobial potentials of *Ixora coccinea* root extract. Asian Pac J Trop Med 2011; 4(12): 959-63. [http://dx.doi.org/10.1016/S1995-7645(11)60226-5] [PMID: 22118031]

[375] Fung TKH, Lau BWM, Ngai SPC, Tsang HWH. Therapeutic Effect and Mechanisms of Essential Oils in Mood Disorders: Interaction between the Nervous and Respiratory Systems. Int J Mol Sci 2021; 22(9): 4844. [http://dx.doi.org/10.3390/ijms22094844] [PMID: 34063646]

[376] Chaouki B. Essential oils and opportunities to mitigate enteric methane emissions from ruminants. Animal Feed Sci Technol 2011; 166-7.

[377] Ultee A, Kets EPW, Smid EJ. Mechanisms of action of carvacrol on the food-borne pathogen Bacillus cereus. Appl Environ Microbiol 1999; 65(10): 4606-10. [http://dx.doi.org/10.1128/AEM.65.10.4606-4610.1999] [PMID: 10508096]

[378] Ultee A, Kets EPW, Alberda M, Hoekstra FA, Smid EJ. Adaptation of the food-borne pathogen Bacillus cereus to carvacrol. Arch Microbiol 2000; 174(4): 233-8. [http://dx.doi.org/10.1007/s002030000199] [PMID: 11081791]

[379] Trombetta D, Castelli F, Sarpietro MG, *et al.* Mechanisms of antibacterial action of three monoterpenes. Antimicrob Agents Chemother 2005; 49(6): 2474-8. [http://dx.doi.org/10.1128/AAC.49.6.2474-2478.2005] [PMID: 15917549]

[380] Di Pasqua R, Betts G, Hoskins N, Edwards M, Ercolini D, Mauriello G. Membrane toxicity of antimicrobial compounds from essential oils. J Agric Food Chem 2007; 55(12): 4863-70. [http://dx.doi.org/10.1021/jf0636465] [PMID: 17497876]

[381] Paparella A, Taccogna L, Aguzzi I, *et al.* Flow cytometric assessment of the antimicrobial activity of essential oils against Listeria monocytogenes. Food Control 2008; 19(12): 1174-82. [http://dx.doi.org/10.1016/j.foodcont.2008.01.002]

[382] Xu J, Zhou F, Ji BP, Pei RS, Xu N. The antibacterial mechanism of carvacrol and thymol against *Escherichia coli*. Lett Appl Microbiol 2008; 47(3): 174-9. [http://dx.doi.org/10.1111/j.1472-765X.2008.02407.x] [PMID: 19552781]

[383] Di Pasqua R, Hoskins N, Betts G, Mauriello G. Changes in membrane fatty acids composition of microbial cells induced by addiction of thymol, carvacrol, limonene, cinnamaldehyde, and eugenol in the growing media. J Agric Food Chem 2006; 54(7): 2745-9. [http://dx.doi.org/10.1021/jf052722l] [PMID: 16569070]

[384] Bergen WG, Bates DB. Ionophores: their effect on production efficiency and mode of action. J Anim Sci 1984; 58(6): 1465-83. [http://dx.doi.org/10.2527/jas1984.5861465x] [PMID: 6378864]

[385] Waterman PG. Roles for secondary metabolites in plants. Ciba Found Symp 1992; 171: 255-69. [PMID: 1302182]

[386] Croteau R. Function of secondary metabolites in plants. 2000; 40: 115-7.

[387] Hamid A A, Aiyelaagbe OO, Usman LA. Medicinal and Pharmacological Uses. Int J Curr Res 2011; 33.

[388] Morales MT, Luna G, Aparicio R. Sensory and chemical evaluation of winey-vinegary defect in virgin olive oils. Eur Food Res Technol 2000; 211(3): 222-8. [http://dx.doi.org/10.1007/s002170050028]

[389] Stark AH, Madar Z. Olive oil as a functional food: epidemiology and nutritional approaches. Nutr Rev 2002; 60(6): 170-6. [http://dx.doi.org/10.1301/00296640260094574] [PMID: 12078915]

[390] Moldão-Martins M, Beirão-da-Costa S, Neves C, Cavaleiro C, Salgueiro L, Luísa Beirão-da-Costa M. Olive oil flavoured by the essential oils of *Mentha × piperita* and *Thymus mastichina* L. Food Qual Prefer 2004; 15(5): 447-52. [http://dx.doi.org/10.1016/j.foodqual.2003.08.001]

[391] Kalua CM, Bedgood DR Jr, Bishop AG, Prenzler PD. Changes in volatile and phenolic compounds with malaxation time and temperature during virgin olive oil production. J Agric Food Chem 2006; 54(20): 7641-51. [http://dx.doi.org/10.1021/jf061122z] [PMID: 17002434]

[392] Kalua CM, Allen MS, Bedgood DR Jr, Bishop AG, Prenzler PD, Robards K. Olive oil volatile compounds, flavour development and quality: A critical review. Food Chem 2007; 100(1): 273-86. [http://dx.doi.org/10.1016/j.foodchem.2005.09.059]

[393] Chipault JH, Mizuno GR, Hawkins JM, Lundberg WO. The antioxidant properties of natural spices. J Food Sci 1952; 17(1-6): 46-55. [http://dx.doi.org/10.1111/j.1365-2621.1952.tb16737.x]

[394] Yen HF, Hsieh CT, Hsieh TJ, Chang FR, Wang CK. *In vitro* anti-diabetic effect and chemical component analysis of 29 essential oils products. Yao Wu Shi Pin Fen Xi 2015; 23(1): 124-9. [PMID: 28911435]

[395] Jamshidi R, Afzali Z, Afzali D. Chemical composition of hydrodistillation essential oil of rosemary in different origins in Iran and comparison with other countries. Am-Eurasian J Agric Environ Sci 2009; 5: 78-81.

[396] Zaouali Y, Bouzaine T, Boussaid M. Essential oils composition in two Rosmarinus officinalis L. varieties and incidence for antimicrobial and antioxidant activities. Food Chem Toxicol 2010; 48(11): 3144-52. [http://dx.doi.org/10.1016/j.fct.2010.08.010] [PMID: 20728499]

[397] Yilmazer M, Karagoz S K, Ozkan G, Karacabey K. Aroma transition from rosemary leaves during aromatization of olive oil. J Food Drug Analy 2016; 24: 299-304.

[398] Reichling J. Plant-microbe interaction and secondary metabolites with antiviral, antibacterial and antifungal properties. In: Wink M, Ed. Functions of Plant Secondary Metabolites and Their Exploitation in Biotechnology. Sheffield: Sheffield Academic Press 1999; pp. 87-273.

[399] Reichling J, Schnitzler P, Suschke U, Saller R. Essential oils of aromatic plants with antibacterial, antifungal, antiviral, and cytotoxic properties--an overview. Forsch Komplement Med 2009; 16(2): 79-90.
[PMID: 19420953]

[400] Takaisi-Kikuni NB, Krüger D, Gnann W, Wecke J. Microcalorimetric and electron microscopic investigation on the effects of essential oil from *Cymbopogon densiflorus* on *Staphylococcus aureus.* Microbios 1996; 88(354): 55-62.
[PMID: 9121380]

[401] Hammer KA, Carson CF, Riley TV. Antifungal effects of *Melaleuca alternifolia* (tea tree) oil and its components on *Candida albicans, Candida glabrata* and *Saccharomyces cerevisiae.* J Antimicrob Chemother 2004; 53(6): 1081-5.
[http://dx.doi.org/10.1093/jac/dkh243] [PMID: 15140856]

CHAPTER 8

Future Perspective of Aromatherapy in Skin and Cancer Therapeutics

Deepti Chopra[1,*], **Saumya Shukla**[1,3], **Sakshi Yadav**[1,2], **Jyoti Singh**[1], **Divya Dubey**[1] and **Mohd. Danish Kamar**[1,4]

[1] *Photobiology Laboratory, Systems Toxicology and Health Risk Assessment Group, CSIR-Indian Institute of Toxicology Research, Vishvigyan Bhavan 31, P.O. Box No. 80, M.G. Marg, Lucknow-226001, India*

[2] *Department of Botany, University of Lucknow, Lucknow-226007, India*

[3] *Department of Biochemistry, School of Dental Sciences, Babu Banarasi Das University, BBD City, Faizabad Road, Lucknow-226028, Uttar Pradesh, India*

[4] *Academy of Scientific and Innovative Research, AcSIR Headquarters, CSIR-HRDC Campus, Sector 19, Kamla Nehru Nagar, Ghaziabad-201002, Uttar Pradesh, India*

Abstract: Essential oils have a direct influence on cancer cells along with an impact at a chemical level on the immune system. Essential oils work efficiently in getting rid of microorganisms and other foreign bodies from the human body by augmenting white blood cell activity. Many more small molecules change the way that the main components of many essential oils act. Furthermore, numerous components play an important part in various characteristics of essential oils like smell/fragrance, concentration, colour, texture, cell diffusion, lipophilicity/hydrophilicity, and fixation over cellular membranes and their distribution within the cell. Biologically, in the central nervous system disorders, volatile essential oils may affect synergistically along with the treatment drugs/chemicals. One of the important considerations is the specific time at which the plant possesses the highest quantity of volatile essential oils along with the chemical constituent mixture. Essential oils are a beneficial non-medicinal alternative and they could be included in routine conventional care for some particular health conditions when their protection and quality control issues have been calculated. Alternative medicine involving the usage of essential oils is hopeful to decrease the redundant effects of current medicine and if explored precisely, the therapy will benefit both the patients and the common man.

Keywords: Essential oil, Aromatherapy, Aromatherapeutic oils, Terpenoids, and Phenylpropanoids.

* **Corresponding author Deepti Chopra:** Photobiology Laboratory, Systems Toxicology and Health Risk Assessment Group, CSIR-Indian Institute of Toxicology Research, Vishvigyan Bhawan, 31, P.O. Box No. 80, M.G. Marg, Lucknow-226001, India; E-mails: deepti.ghar@gmail.com, choprad81@gmail.com

Pradeep Kumar Shukla, Ajeet Kumar Srivastav, Deepti Chopra, Shikha Agnihotry, Pragati Misra and Jyoti Singh (Eds.)

1. INTRODUCTION

Without a scientific basis, the practise of aromatherapy relies on the application of aromatic chemicals, such as essential oils (EOs) and aroma compounds, with the promise of improving psychological or physical well-being. This is offered in lieu of regular treatment, as an alternate solution, or as a substitute drug. Alternatively, precision-based treatment may be used in place of traditional medication. Those who specialise in practising aromatherapy, such as inhalation massage, the use of water immersion techniques, or the partial significance of healing essential oils, are known as aromachologists. Unfortunately, there is now no credible medical evidence that suggests aromatherapy can prevent, cure, or treat disease. Placebo-controlled experiments are difficult to correct because aromatherapy relies heavily on smell. The idea that it could prevent nausea and vomiting after surgery is quite alluring.

Essential oils (EOs) are a blend of low molecular weight plant-based molecules that are extracted using a variety of solvents and steam distillations. The primary components of EOs that give them their distinctive biological qualities and smell include terpenoids, phenylpropanoids, *etc.* Various physiological and pharmacological actions, including those that are anti-inflammatory, antiviral, antiprotozoal, anti-mycotic, anti-mutagenic, anti-tumourigenic, and anti-diabeticThe characteristics of nti-diabetes match EOs. The primary components of essential oils (EOs) of global relevance, particularly in the pharmaceutical and cosmetic industrics, have been identified and characterised by means of costly and precise phytochemical investigation. This chapter contains the current locations of the bioactive qualities and therapeutic potential of EOs (Fig. **1**). The volatile oils, also known as essential oils, are extracted using a variety of methods from the plant's flowers, leaves, stems, roots, fruits, and bark. The discovery of EOs' antimicrobial and antibacterial properties, as well as their skin absorptivity-based properties, led to their continued use.

The main methods used in aromatherapy that include the absorption of EOs on the skin's surface with perceptible feeling are fragrance inhalation, steam baths, baths, and local application. These lubricants change as they move through the system and exert a noticeable influence where the accentuated area is. This type of therapy makes use of a variety of adjustments and concoctions to provide relief from a range of issues, including insomnia, melancholy, gastrointestinal distress, headaches, back pain, respiratory issues, swollen joints, skin allergies, and urinary tract issues. When other aspects of diet and lifestyle are taken into account, EOs are proven to be more competent. Based on research on medicinal, therapeutic, improving, olfactory, massage, psychological, and safety issues, aromatherapy makes use of a range of plant parts. For cancer patients, there are benefits such as decreased anxiety and a decrease in the physical symptoms of stress, fatigue, and agitation [1].

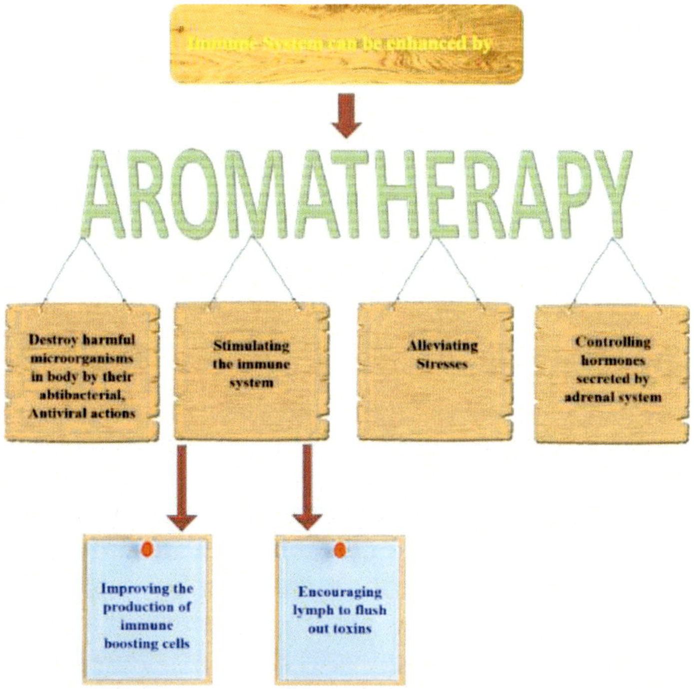

Fig. (1). Mechanism by which essential oil enhances the function of the immune system [24].

Any medicinal qualities that extra virgin olive oil (EO) may possess are derived from its biological components and structure. The advantages of essential oils and aromatherapy can be explained by a plethora of theories. The relationship between the brain's olfactory and paleomammalian cortical systems accounts for the majority of the mechanisms by which aromatherapy affects temperament and emotions, according to published research [2]. Biochemistry and psychology organisations, who may not be able to distinguish between the scent produced by EOs and fake perfumes and have a different take on the possible methods by which aroma influences the human brain, disproved these assertions [3]. The mechanism that EOs are supposed to have on different body parts is currently insufficient. These are mostly conjectural in nature due to the paucity of noteworthy research studies on the topic. Research delving deeply into the neurophysiology of smell and its connection to the limbic system is scarce [4]. The chapter covered the use of essential oils (EOs) in aromatherapy and how to increase well-being. The use of essential oils (EOs) in aromatherapy for personal care has improved in the United States throughout the previous few years [5].

Nevertheless, EOs have been in use for many eras, and EOs practices, along with aromatherapy, have been in use from generation to generation [6]. EOs from plants are natural pollinator attractants, repel insects, prevent microorganism growth, treat plant injury, and guard the plant against temperature variations [7]. Current EOs utilized in aromatherapy, which are vaporizable fluids, are generally extracted through a steam distillation procedure or by mechanical pressurizing from plants [8]. EOs have very specific pharmacological aspects that can very well relate to their physiological responses [9, 10]. For instance, the aroma of peppermint oil may alter the effects of the nervous system's endogenous opioids on anxiety and relaxation [11, 12]. EOs such as eucalyptus and thyme are remarkable anti-inflammatory and antioxidant [13, 14].

The latest meta-analysis along with orderly views assists the idea that aromatherapy may put onward clinical indication when analysed with standard or placebo treatment. The meta-analysis investigation in discomfort management has shown that aromatherapy is higher than placebo in treating postoperative obstetrical and antenatal aches [15]. An orderly assessment examining aromatherapy effects on menstrual cramps has shown that the menstrual ache was largely alleviated with aromatherapy interventions compared to placebo treatment [16]. In the meta-study, inhaling scent had favourable effects when compared to no treatment in controlled trials; this impact was mostly observed in subjective self-reports [17]. Sleep quality is influenced by aromatherapy as well. More beneficial than massage therapy was inhaling therapy [18]. Research on aromatherapy for depressive symptoms, however, discovered that massage aromatherapy performed noticeably better than inhaled aromatherapy [19]. The results of the literature review have demonstrated that the clinical effects of EO therapy may be relevant. Generally speaking, a variety of medical disorders can be treated using aromatherapy. It is chiefly efficient for emotional and attentional information processing along with autonomous nervous system function [12, 20].

A few benefits of aromatherapy for chronic pain, nervousness, and the value of life have been discovered in prior cancer diagnostics, but they also concluded that these benefits are not clinically relevant due to the paucity of studies [21]. Approximately 50% of the studies that were assessed had inadequate quality, outstanding results, the mode of administration, or suggested protocols for evaluation. The inaccuracy of the ingredients in aromatherapy is one important concern. Even the term "aromatherapy" has many ambiguities. Phytotherapy refers to the topical application or ingestion of these substances in the medical context. On the other hand, aromatherapy describes the inhalation of the volatile components of essential oils [22]. Any objective evaluation of EOs for clinical application becomes more difficult as a result of this conceptual uncertainty in high-level research articles. Different researchers seem unaware when testing any specific factors representing suspected aromatherapy. Moreover, this problem also relates to cellular metabolism studies of EOs. For instance, the authors of a study evaluating the mechanisms of action of limonene for treating various disorders mistook inhalation for ingestion and provided findings that were confused as to the functional pathways [23].

Similarly, a study that looked at the phytochemical mechanisms of aromatherapeutic oils in treating behavioural and psychological symptoms in dementia patients did not come to favourable conclusions regarding the practice [25]. According to a new review and meta-analysis, aromatherapy can help postmenopausal women with their psychological issues [26]. This study also was unable to conclude about aromatherapy massage improving psychological symptoms or about the clinical remunerations of aromatherapy. Thus, in terms of clinical pretext, the current knowledge based on the literature available about the effectiveness of EOs is inadequate.

EOs are utilised in cosmetic products for the face, body, and hair in cosmetic aromatherapy. These products include steps like toning, drying, cleaning, and moisturising. Understanding and using cosmetic aromatherapy with a foot or full body bath is simple and efficient. For example, a small bit of the right essential oil provides a thrilling and invigorating experience. The application of grape seed, almond, or jojoba oils in massage aromatherapy yields remarkable results. This is referred to as a massage treatment healing touch. In order to promote mental well-being, tranquility, relaxation, or bodily renewal, olfactory aromatherapy entails inhaling essential oils. EOs are no longer a strict substitute for clinical treatment; rather, they are used in conjunction with it. In psycho-aromatherapy, mood and feelings can be changed with the use of these oils, giving the delight of pastime invigoration or a pleasant reminiscence. Psycho-aromatherapy and aromachology are in agreement with each other whether the effects of aroma are natural or synthetic. Psycho-aromatherapy has a constrained or inadequate observation of natural EOs thus far.

2. NATIONAL STATUS OF AROMATHERAPY

Aromatherapy is a well-known alternative for cancer patients who use complementary therapies. According to quantitative studies using survey data, aromatherapy may help most cancer patients manage their symptoms better and lessen emotional distress. However, patients perceptions of the therapy are rarely considered. This investigation examined how patients experienced aromatherapy using a focus group interview. Concerning aromatherapy, eight themes were identified from the study, six of which have been discussed in some detail by previous authors. These topics include the ability of aromatherapy to reduce stress, the counselling function of the experts in this sector, the use of aromatherapy as compensation, patient empowerment, declarations made during contact, and unfavourable provider traits. The security of the scenario and preconceived beliefs about the expenditure of essential oils as a treatment option for cancer sufferers were the two main new difficulties that emerged. The results' implications are analysed in light of how counselling is believed to work in balancing other treatment approaches [4].

3. INTERNATIONAL STATUS OF AROMATHERAPY

Using essential oils (EOs) in aromatherapy can help treat, relieve, or even prevent the disease's telltale symptoms. The benefits of aromatherapy in treating chemotherapy-induced nausea and vomiting as well as cancer patients' discomfort was studied. In a study sixty chemotherapy patients from the Indian state of Kerala were chosen. Two patient groups were formed: the experimental design (n = 30) had aromatherapy-based massage sessions before and during chemotherapy, whereas the controlled study (n = 30) did not receive any of these services. Anxiety was first assessed at work and 24 hours following therapy. Within 24 hours of chemotherapy, the patients' levels of nausea and vomiting were recorded. The group receiving aromatherapy had a much higher reduction in anxiety as compared to the control group. It was also found that compared to controls, nausea was far less common in the experimental environment. Furthermore, there was a decrease in vomiting in the aromatherapy group compared to the control samples. This research demonstrates the noteworthy anxiolytic and antiemetic effects of aromatherapy rubdown, when used in addition to conventional antiemetics in patients undergoing chemotherapy. It was concluded that scientific specialists should consider aromatherapy as a possible treatment for typical side effects of anticancer chemotherapy, such as nausea, vomiting, and anxiety.

4. AROMATHERAPY IN SKIN TREATMENT

Overuse of chemotherapy and stem-mobile rescue have been used in the treatment of eighty breast cancer patients. Approximately 1% to 0.33 percent of the patients experienced various types of skin rashes. However, after the patients with skin allergies were divided into two groups, the aromatherapy group received treatment with an aqueous cream containing essential oils and plant extracts, while the prepared group received the preferred course of care. Regarding the metrics observed, there were no distinctions between organised corporations and aromatherapy [27, 28]. Since its founding in 1993, aromatherapy modifications at the Cancer Guide and Facts Centre (CSIC) of this local cancer centre have been continuously evaluated. Novel approaches to ascertaining supplementary therapy alternatives, exclusively grounded in the "remedy-as-practiced" approach, have been investigated. Following a preliminary pilot, the provider's following modifications were evaluated by the observation. Since formal questionnaires were insufficient for measuring the stress and despair associated with medical institutions, professional aromatherapists developed an estimation instrument known as the Hospital Anxiety and Depression Scale (HADS). With the assistance of medical professionals employed by the CSIC and the most cancers centres, standards have been set. The skin performs a wide range of tasks, including secretory, thermoregulatory, percutaneous amalgamation, and sensory activities. According to conventional data, skin-related illnesses account for 34% of all occupational ailments [29]. Although skin disorders rarely draw public condemnation, when they do—like in the case of onchocercal skin disorder (OSD), which is found in parts of Africa's rainforests—it's uncommon [30]. Skin disorders are difficult to manage in developing countries because most health care workers (HCWs) are not trained in treating skin, pores, and other skin concerns, which account for a large share of diseases in most Sub-Saharan African nations.

4.1. National Status

Asians possess a great array of skin types, ranging from pores and skin types II to VI, due to their diverse customs and civilizations. Asian patients with positive skin disorders present with unique symptoms and incidences. Similar to the West, where it is common for doctors to approach illnesses by assuming that they are caused by external factors, deterioration of the body element or organ, or a combination of both, Asians believe that the body is whole and that every aspect of it is connected to the overall health of the country. People in Asia typically remember that nutrition plays a major part in illness; certain cuisines are said to exacerbate certain conditions, while others may help them. After seeing their doctors, it is quite reasonable to ask Asian patients about any dietary restrictions they may be experiencing. The 20th-century version of symbol management and inflexible issues has greatly influenced the highly subjective market improvement of aromatherapy products. The effect is clear: aromatherapy explores and develops the customer's emotional reaction to the logo while concentrating mostly on the product's excellent attributes and the practical benefits of usage. Refocusing businesses and products on the emotional and environmental benefits that these items can offer is the main viewpoint. New tactics for enhancing fragrance execution will be discussed in the session, along with ways to provide customers with stronger, more emotionally engaging benefits. There is a growing push in developing countries to include conventional drugs—more especially, herbal remedies—into local health care systems.

4.2. International Status

Patients should consider the difficulties associated with choosing EOs aromatherapy as a complementary therapy option, as it is still gaining popularity in the US as a factor in self-care. It is equally necessary to improve understanding of potential drug interactions, potential negative effects, management options, and clinical implications related to EOs. Remember that using essential oils for aromatherapy can help to maintain and improve physical, mental, and emotional well-being. African nations have come to understand the need to develop improved conventional medicine treatments (ITMs) using readily available local plants that have long been used to treat a range of illnesses [31]. Research is being done to ascertain the significance of people interacting with soil-dwelling animals because of their potential benefits [32].

5. AROMATHERAPY IN CANCER TREATMENT

Aromatherapy treats cancer patients' mental stress, pain, muscle anxiety, and tiredness in addition to bridging the fear barrier. Methodical evaluation of the results of preclinical and clinical trials examining the safety and effectiveness of aromatherapy for cancer patients was done. The studied literature indicates that aromatherapy improves sadness, anxiety, and overall wellbeing right away. In particular, certain scientific research found that patients reported higher levels of inspiration, relaxation, mental ease, and better sleep. Additionally, some cause transitory improvements in pain management and raise anxiety and depressive levels (up to two weeks after treatment). While excessive consumption (*i.e.*, intentional misuse) of essential oils and community skin infections, especially those resulting from prolonged dermal contact, can raise the risk of allergic contact dermatitis and photoinduced toxicity (from certain oils), even though these side effects are rarely unpleasant [33]. Topical use of tea tree oil and lavender oil has been associated with reversible prepubescent gynecomastia over time [34].

5.1. National Status

A rapidly growing area of complementary and alternative medicine is aromatherapy. It involves using EOs to try to treat, reduce, or eliminate some of the symptoms associated with the disease. Sixty cancer patients from the Indian state of Kerala have been assigned to receive chemotherapy. Two patient groups were established: the treatment condition (n = 30) had a massage based on aromatherapy before to, during, and after chemotherapy, whereas the control group (n = 30) did not get any massage therapy. Tension levels in each group were assessed prior to and following the 24-hour post-chemotherapy period. The degree of gastrointestinal symptoms was evaluated in patients who had received treatment more than twenty-four hours prior. In contrast to the control group, individuals who had aromatherapy experienced a significant average decrease in stress. Significant anxiolytic and antiemetic effects have frequently been shown when aromatherapy rubdown is used in conjunction with conventional medicines in cancer patients undergoing chemotherapy. Results indicate that aromatherapy may be somewhat expensive for medical practitioners attempting to lessen the frequent side effects of anticancer treatment, such as nausea, vomiting, and stress [35].

5.2. International Status

Studies conducted in Australia indicate that about 1% of patients with most malignancies used aromatherapy [36]. The incidence rates in Turkey, Italy, and Spain vary from 1% to 2% [37]. Roughly 4% of Canadian surveys on its use by cancer patients were not recorded [38]. According to six UK polls, 46% of cancer patients said they used it [39]. A New Zealand survey found that 6% of cancer patients may utilise aromatherapy [40]. But it's unclear whether its use is meant as a therapeutic approach or just to enhance general health and, consequently, quality of life, rather than combating cancer directly.

6. EOS AS A THERAPEUTIC AGENT

The most popular ways to utilise essential oils for healing are topical application and indirect inhalation (or diffusion). Aromatherapy is the most common way to use essential oils for healing. Aromatherapy with essential oils has been incorporated into therapeutic rubdowns as an additional cure. The influence of essential oils on aromatherapy, however, is very tangible. For instance, the Olympic medalists' bouquets from the 2012 London Olympic had to have a "British smell," thus rosemary, mint, and lavender were used to create this fragrance [8].

Despite being widely accepted, U.S. fitness care specialists rarely acknowledge the use of EOs aromatherapy [41]. There is mounting evidence from research that using essential oils in aromatherapy can promote both physical and emotional well-being. The antifungal efficacy of extracts from 20 curry spices was tested against a variety of fungi, including *A. niger, C. albicans, C. blanki, C. cylindracea, C. glabrata, C. krusei, C. tropicalis,* and *S. cerevisiae*, using the disc diffusion method. By contrasting the susceptibility of several fungi to EOs with the preferred ketoconazole, an activity index (AI) was created. Different forms of inhibitory responses were observed in the studied species and the EOs that were used. Though ginger, turmeric, and pomegranate essential oils had little effect, thyme, clove, star, star anise, cumin, coriander, curry leaf,. basil, basil, and asafoetida essential oils inhibited the growth of the fungus. The fungus transformed a number of essential oils, including celery, black pepper, mace, cardamom, fennel, and nutmeg, into a particular inhibitory form. The anticandidal properties of EOs from thyme, cumin and cassia oil, which exhibit better antimycotic activity compared to alternative oils were examined using broth micro-dilution as well as broth macro-dilution techniques [42].

High-quality aromas can uplift us and help us deal with specific scientific symptoms and indicators. A few drops of lavender oil can help with insomnia9 or improve one's mood. There are studies on the calming and soothing effects of oils like sandalwood, chamomile, and bergamot as well as the mentally stimulating effects of jasmine, lemon, lemongrass, peppermint, and basil [43, 44]. Other aromas determined to be soothing were rose and lavender. Bright orange EOs were found to be effective in inducing anaesthesia in children as well as reducing their recovery time. When applied topically, EOs are diluted with provider oil, a cold-pressed vegetable oil. Cooking oils should not be used since they will be heated to high degrees, which will change their chemical composition and impede the absorption of their nutrients. Provider oils, which are available at fitness food stores, must be kept in the refrigerator and should be thrown out when they go rancid. EOs are colourless, usually first-class-smelling liquids that can create effective aromatherapy results that begin in the nose and mouth [45].

Inhaled EOs nearly straight away, act collectively on olfactory receptors, and affects the olfactory bulb in the brain. The olfactory bulb connects with the limbic device structures of the amygdala, hippocampus, hypothalamus, and cingulate gyrus; which play a vast position in emotional and physical responses in the human mind. The amygdala is concerned with feelings; the hippocampus performs a fantastic position in memory; the hypothalamus is chargeable for hormone regulation and autonomic frightening system reaction; and the cingulate gyrus regulates blood strain, pulse, awareness, and interest. Scents additionally have an impact on the mind by influencing the production of endorphins and noradrenaline, therefore inhibiting ache indicators, promoting relaxation and satisfaction, and increasing alertness and interest. In addition to the defined olfactory pathways tormented by EOs, inhaled EOs additionally go to the lungs which may be absorbed *via* the alveoli on the move and then ultimately affect the brain [46].

Moreover, essential oils have antibacterial properties that guarantee wound disinfection. One example is thymol made from the essential oil of Thymus vulgaris, the common thyme. Lister's discovery of thymol led to the creation of Listerine mouthwash. Thymol went on to become the primary antiseptic and is still used today. All essential oils (EOs) possess some antibacterial properties in addition to their antiseptic properties, despite varying in strength. As most bacteria are located inside the ulcer bed, it seems sense that excessive pressure should not be applied to wounds that are chronic in nature, as bacterial susceptibility varies. This implies that there will be direct contact between the diluted EOs and the impacted area. Applying essential oils (EOs) helps reduce inflammation, promote cell renewal, and get rid of infections. Only a few EOs, including peppermint *(Mentha piperita),* rosemary *(Rosmarinus occicinalis),* juniper *(Juniperus communis)*, and palmarosa *(Cymbopogon martini)*, are effective against *Pseudomonas aeruginosa*. Due to their mild chemical makeup, palmarosa and juniper would be the safest of those to employ in wound care. In addition to peppermint, lavender, juniper, tea tree, and methicillin- and vancomycin-resistant Enterococcus faecalis are efficient against these bacteria [47].

7. THE CURRENT USE OF AROMATHERAPY AS AN OCCUPATIONAL THERAPY

Aromatherapy, or the use of essential oils to promote health, is becoming more and more well-known among the general public. A growing number of specialists, including occupational therapists, are thinking about utilising it in a therapeutic setting. In the context of occupational therapy, this study investigates the therapeutic potential of aromatherapy and looks at a variety of unique applications for it [48]. It would be necessary to transfer the decision-making power from the occupational therapist to the client in order to implement a consumer-based paradigm for occupational therapy practise. To help guarantee that the version, if chosen, is understood and used, a radical debate of the version and its consequences on practise is an essential first step.

8. ANTIMUTAGENIC PROPERTIES AND DETOXIFICATION ENHANCEMENT

Some of the processes linked to the antimutagenic function of EOs include the direct scavenging of mutagens (antioxidant capture of radicals created by mutagens, stimulation of cellular antioxidative enzymes, prevention of metabolic transformation by P450 of pro-mutagens with active gene mutations, and stimulation of enzymatic cleanup of mutagens by employing EOs constituents). The effectiveness of antimutagenic drugs depends on whether they encourage error-free DNA repair or impede error-prone DNA restoration (Fig. **2**). There hasn't been any research on the antimutagenicity of using terpenic and phenolic chemicals from EOs to restore DNA [49].

Chemicals isolated from aromatic flora, such as α-terpinene, citral, α-terpineol, D-limonene, 1,8-cineole, camphor, and citronellal, altered hepatic mono-oxygenase action by associating with pro-mutagen xenobiotic bioconversion. Evidence has shown that EOs lessen Saccharomyces cerevisiae's apoptosis/necrosis and mitochondrial damage. Recent investigations revealed that positive EOs had antimutagenic properties against UV-induced mutations [50].

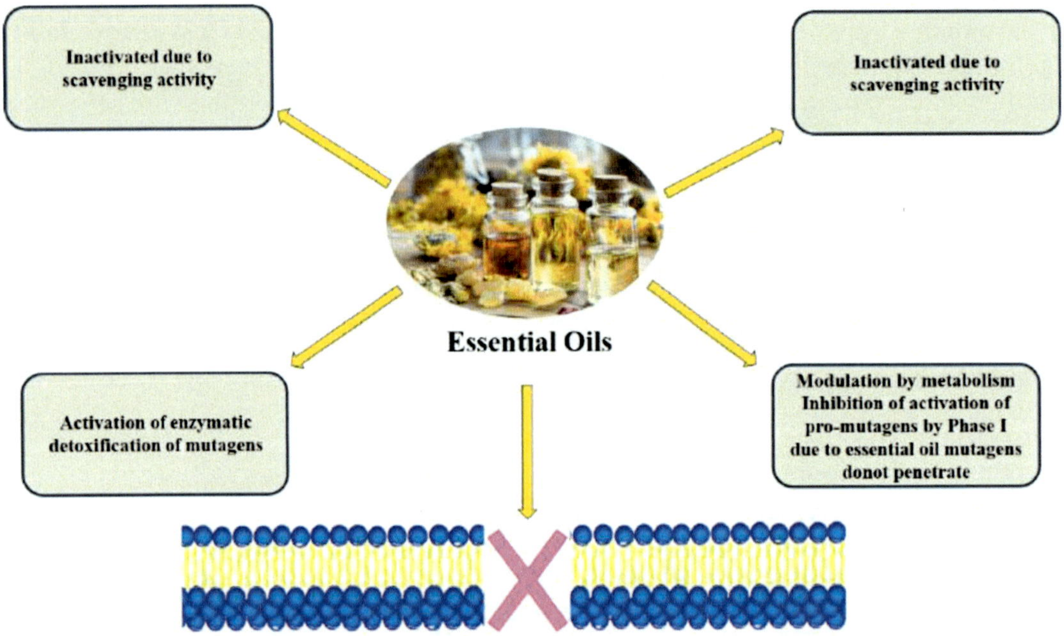

Fig. (2). Antimutagenic mechanism of EOs [24].

9. ANTIPROLIFERATIVE MECHANISM OF ACTION OF EOS

Natural EOs materials play an imperative function in most cancer prevention and remedies. EOs derived from dietary plants and aromatic herbs include, among other things, phenolics, oxygenated monoterpenes, oxygenated sesquiterpenes, sesquiterpenes and monoterpenes. Their chemopreventive properties are attributed to a variety of mechanisms, including antioxidant, antimutagenic, and antiproliferative properties, immune system development and monitoring, enzymes activating and improving cleaning, controlling multidrug susceptibility and synergistically using volatile ingredients. This analysis lists the structural groupings and mechanistic anticancer processes based on the most recent studies of ingredients found in dietary flora and aromatic plants [24]. Twenty-seven citrus flavonoids were tested for theirantiproliferative effects towards several tumours and ordinary human cellular strains. Seven flavonoids were therefore identified to have modest antiproliferative effects against mammalian cell lines that use eriodictyol normally while being active against tumour-mobile cells. Luteolin, quercetin, natsudaidain, nobiletin, tangeretin, and heptamethoxy flavones were the compounds with the highest levels of potency.

A C2-C3 double bond and the ortho-catechol group in ring B were important for the antiproliferative effect, as well as determined by the shape-hobby affiliation among those flavones and flavanones. C-3 hydroxyl and C-eight methoxyl moieties were required for significant interest in polymethoxylated flavones [51]. Ginger EOs (GEO) were tested for their ability to cause genetic modifications in S. typhimurium TA 98 and TA 100. The *in vitro* antiproliferative effects of *Satureja hortensis, Satureja montana, Salvia officinalis, Lavandula officinalis, Thymus vulgaris, Calamintha origanifolia, Foeniculum vulgare* and *Mentha arvensis* on human erythroleukemic K562 cells were investigated. The EOs produced from *S. montana* and *M. arvensis* demonstrated important pharmacological effects in reducing the growth of the K562 cell line, according to the researchers. α-pinene, β-terpene, α-terpineol, four-terpineol, and caryophyllene, which are the basic metabolic components of *Satureja hortensis* and *Satureja montana*, demonstrated antiproliferative interest. Other research has shown that the active ingredient eugenol found in nutmeg, clove, bay leaves, tulsi, and cinnamon has anti-proliferative effects against a variety of cancerous cell lines and mammalian models. Studies have revealed that *Citrus aurantifolia's* volatile components can prevent the multiplication of human colon carcinoma cells through apoptosis [52]. Human colon cancer cells (SW480) were 78% inhibited by oil at 100 g mL-1 concentration after 48 hours. After 24 and 48 hours, respectively, lime risky oil demonstrated DNA fragmentation and stimulation of caspase-3 could be connected to apoptosis. Analysis of the level of apoptosis-related proteins provided additional evidence in favour of lime volatile oil's ability to induce apoptosis and showed that it might be helpful in the prevention of colon cancer. *C. copticum, T. vulgaris*, and origanum volatile oils contain the phenolic monoterpene carvacrol. Carvacrol's antiproliferative effects on metastatic breast cancer cells (MDA-MB231) were mainly attributable to stimulation of the classical apoptosis reaction, which includes changes in the Bcl2/Bax ratio, mitochondrial cytochrome c release, caspase action, and the cleavage of poly (ADP-ribose) polymerase (PARP).

In HepG2 cells, it has been demonstrated that Curcuma wenyujin oil induces apoptosis *via* activating the caspase-3 and mitochondrial pathways. Additionally, they look at Curcuma wenyujin oil's antiapoptotic characteristics, which may aid in the identification of fresh compounds and ground-breaking drug targets for illnesses like liver cancer. The progression of the majority of malignancies and other chronic degenerative diseases is fundamentally influenced by mutations occurring in somatic cells as a result of intrinsic metabolic abnormalities [53]. One of the best strategies to prevent human cancer is to incorporate antimutagens and anticarcinogens into a daily diet. For the sake of human fitness, it is crucial to identify these food ingredients' antimutagenic and anticarcinogenic properties.

One of the often used spices from the Zingiberaceae family is ginger, *Zingiber officinale* Roscoe. It is frequently used to give food a unique flavour and scent. According to reports, ginger essential oils (GEO) obtained through steam distillation offer a variety of pharmacological properties, including characteristics that are antioxidant, antinociceptive, antimicrobial, and antimycotic [54]. The growing use of spices in the pharmaceutical, agricultural, and metallurgical industries, as food additives and preservatives, and as herbal medicines make it necessary to estimate their antimutagenic and anticarcinogenic potential [55]. The mutagenicity of EOs extracted from ginger (GEO), including and without microsomal activation, was examined using S. typhimurium TA 98, TA 100, TA 102, and TA 1535 strains. The effects of GEO on various microsomal-based cytochrome P450 enzyme isoforms were investigated, and its ability to correct the movement of section I carcinogen-metabolizing enzymes was examined. Significant inhibition of CYP1A1, CYP1A2, CYP2B1/2, aniline hydroxylase, and aminopyrine-N-demethylase were found *in vitro* and *in vivo* by GEO. The segment II carcinogen-metabolizing enzyme activities of glutathione S-transferase and uridine 5′-diphosphoglucuronyl transferase were also upregulated *in vivo* by GEO, demonstrating its use as both as an antimutagen and a chemopreventive drug [56].

10. CANCER CELL SPECIFICITY OF EOS

Essential oils (EOs) are derived from common aromatic molecules and possess a wide range of physiological and pharmacological qualities that make them useful for both preventive and curative medicine in almost every specialty. Women and men seem to react to essential oils (EOs) in the same ways, despite the fact that aromatherapy is beneficial to all ages. If the practitioner has the appropriate credentials and training, aromatherapy and aromatology can truly help with harmonization for a variety of patients, which is very different from the anti-stress rub-down rub-down method. Aromatic extracts have long been used with amazing results in medical therapies. Aromatherapy can be a useful supplementary clinical technique both inside and outside of healthcare settings. For instance, it can be used to treat cancer, depression, and dementia.

EOs are beneficial for a number of conditions, including reproductive wellness, backaches, urinary tract infections, stress, insomnia, and rectal abscesses. Patients with cancer or cells associated with cancer were also examined. The early benefits of aromatherapy massage were noted for anxiety, depression, and modern well-being up to eight weeks after treatment. A few clinical researches discovered that patients' sleep quality, psychological well-being, and consistent symptom alleviation were all enhanced. Many studies also reported improved pain management (up to two weeks after therapy) and short-term improvements in depression and anxiety levels.Taking an excessive amount, local skin irritation, especially with extended skin exposure, contact dermatitis, and UV-induced toxicity from exposure to sunlight are possible hazards even though EOs have generally shown few adverse effects (some oils). The regular use of tea tree oil and lavender topically has been associated with reversible prepubescent gynecomastia. By adding a tiny amount of the steaming water, EOs can be inhaled; a humidifier or atomizer then disperses the aroma throughout the space. Aromatic florals that have EOs in good amounts are frequently used in international cuisines as a seasoning for their tasty flavour and as food preservation due to their potent antibacterial properties.

Numerous EOs, including those have been found in this investigation to have powerful antimicrobial potential against several microbial species [57]. Examples of common food-borne pathogens that were resistant to *F. vulgare*, and *O. munitiflorum's* antibacterial action include *L. monocytogenes, E.coli, S. aureus,* and *S. typhimurium* [58]. The antimicrobial interest of the EOs of Ocimum basilicum and Origanum vulgare changed to found to have an outstanding antimicrobial hobby towards thirteen microorganisms [59]. The EOs of *Rosmarinus officinalis* were reportedly found to have potent antibacterial activity against a few oral pathogens [60]. As a result, *Satureja cuneifolia*, Ten., *Origanum onites, Mentha piperita, Mentha spicata, Ocimum basilicum,* and other terpenoid and aromatic ingredients found mainly in EOs were tested for their inhibitory effect against the distant traces of *Klebsiella pneumoniae.*

11. SYNERGISM OF EO EXTRACTS WITH CONVENTIONAL CHEMOTHERAPEUTIC AGENTS: THE POTENTIAL OF COMBINATION THERAPY USING EOS

The majority of the treatment advances for cancer over the past 10 years have been effectively attributed to the combination of radiation therapies and conventional chemotherapeutic drugs. In a similar vein, understanding the mechanisms by which chemotherapy boosts radiation's efficacy in patients and model structures will be necessary for future therapeutic advancements. In this assessment, the motion mechanisms of gemcitabine, platinum, and fluoropyrimidines are examined. When given both before and during radiation, five-fluorouracil and fluorodeoxyuridine, two fluoropyrimidines, boost the efficacy of radiation. Radiation sensitivity increases in cells that mistakenly develop into the S segment as a result of the medicine, suggesting a critical role for in the dysregulation of S-section checkpoints. Gemcitabine radiosensitizes by a related mechanism, however, it is yet unclear how much of a role apoptosis and particular DNA repair pathways (along with homologous halt rejoining) are related to one another. Sensitization most likely occurs for each of these medical categories when radiation-damaged DNA is incorrectly repaired by cells that are wrongly going through the S section. As a result, the lack of the S-phase checkpoint in cancer cells may also provide the biological basis for the selective death of tumours as opposed to normal problems. Cisplatin has several impact on cells, including the creation of adducts and the prevention of DNA damage repair, although the exact mechanism underlying its preference for cancer cells over normal cells has not yet been determined. With the potential to improve reaction prediction tests and therapeutic imaging tools, the discovery of enzymatic goals for these tablets opens up new research opportunities [61].

12. THE AIMS OF AROMATHERAPY

All blood types must be compared to the preliminary study (IgA), including red blood cells, white blood cells, granulocytes, CD4+, peripheral blood lymphocytes (PBLs), CD16+, and CD8+ leucocytes; additionally, the CD4+/CD8+ proportion, serum interferon-γ interleukin-6, and secretory immunoglobulin A counts must be compared. Eleven individuals (n = 11) who received an aromatherapy massage and oil rubdown utilising oils such as sweet marjoram, cypress, lavender, and almond were asked to complete the Self-rating Despair Scale (SDS) and the Nation-Trait Anxiety Inventory (STAI). There have been suggestions regarding Bacter pylori, methicillin-resistant Staphylococcus aureus (MRSA), and other infections. In Section I clinical investigations, it has been possible to inhibit the development of dental plaque, MRSA infection, and interdigital tineapedis [62].

CONCLUSIONS

Aromatherapy is healthful for the body, mind, and soul. I believe that any therapist who learns about aromatherapy will benefit from this dynamic and cutting-edge area of well-being and, in the long term, be able to instruct interested clients and their carers in a useful profession centred around well-being. Considering an EO as a whole, as opposed to just a few of its parts, is far more crucial because there is a higher chance of synergism. Thus, EOs, like many other plant-based therapies, are beneficial to variable degrees for a wide range of illnesses, including cancer. More evidence supporting the anticancer properties of unknown chemicals and distinctive EOs is considerably more desirable. Moreover, artificial modification of individual molecules is required to improve their attractiveness. The scientific community fervently supports additional research into the development of ecologically friendly medical protocols for this profoundly transformative subject, and the overall prognosis for the use of essential oils (EOs) in the treatment of cancer appears to be extremely great.

ACKNOWLEDGEMENTS

Deepti Chopra thanks Indian Council of Medical Research (ICMR), Delhi, India, for awarding Research Associateship (GAP-385) at CSIR-Indian Institute of Toxicology Research, Lucknow.

REFERENCES

[1] Fellowes D, Barnes K, Wilkinson SS. Aromatherapy and massage for symptom relief in patients with cancer. Coch Database Syst Rev 2004; 3. [http://dx.doi.org/10.1002/14651858.CD002287.pub2]

[2] Price L, Price S, Smith I. Carrier oils for aromatherapy & massage. Riverhead Publishing 1999.

[3] Perry N, Perry E. Aromatherapy in the management of psychiatric disorders: clinical and neuropharmacological perspectives. CNS Drugs 2006; 20(4): 257-80. [http://dx.doi.org/10.2165/00023210-200620040-00001] [PMID: 16599645]

[4] Boehm K, Büssing A, Ostermann T. Aromatherapy as an adjuvant treatment in cancer care--a descriptive systematic review. Afr J Tradit Complement Altern Med 2012; 9(4): 503-18. [http://dx.doi.org/10.4314/ajtcam.v9i4.7] [PMID: 23983386]

[5] Manion CR, Widder RM. Essentials of essential oils. Am J Health Syst Pharm 2017; 74(9): e153-62. [http://dx.doi.org/10.2146/ajhp151043] [PMID: 28438819]

[6] Boire NA, Riedel S, Parrish NM. Essential oils and future antibiotics: New weapons against emerging 'superbugs'. J Ancient Dis Prevent Remedies 2013; 1(2): 105. [http://dx.doi.org/10.4172/2329-8731.1000105]

[7] Price S, Price L, Eds. Aromatherapy for health professionals E-book. Elsevier 2011.

[8] Childers PM, Aleshire ME. What's that smell?: Essential oil aromatherapy. J Psychosoc Nurs Ment Health Serv 2020; 58(2): 4-5. [http://dx.doi.org/10.3928/02793695-20200117-01] [PMID: 32003858]

[9] Hongratanaworakit T. Physiological effects in aromatherapy. Songklanakarin J Sci Technol 2004; 26(1): 117-25.

[10] Edris AE. Pharmaceutical and therapeutic Potentials of essential oils and their individual volatile constituents: A review. Phytother Res 2007; 21(4): 308-23. [http://dx.doi.org/10.1002/ptr.2072] [PMID: 17199238]

[11] Bushnell MC, Čeko M, Low LA. Cognitive and emotional control of pain and its disruption in chronic pain. Nat Rev Neurosci 2013; 14(7): 502-11. [http://dx.doi.org/10.1038/nrn3516] [PMID: 23719569]

[12] Villemure C, Slotnick BM, Bushnell CM. Effects of odors on pain perception: deciphering the roles of emotion and attention. Pain 2003; 106(1): 101-8. [http://dx.doi.org/10.1016/S0304-3959(03)00297-5] [PMID: 14581116]

[13] Brochot A, Guilbot A, Haddioui L, Roques C. Antibacterial, antifungal, and antiviral effects of three essential oil blends. MicrobiologyOpen 2017; 6(4): e00459. [http://dx.doi.org/10.1002/mbo3.459] [PMID: 28296357]

[14] Divband K, Shokri H, Khosravi AR. Down-regulatory effect of Thymus vulgaris L. on growth and Tri4 gene expression in Fusarium oxysporum strains. Microb Pathog 2017; 104: 1-5. [http://dx.doi.org/10.1016/j.micpath.2017.01.011] [PMID: 28062283]

[15] Lakhan SE, Sheafer H, Tepper D. The effectiveness of aromatherapy in reducing pain: A systematic review and meta-analysis. Pain Res Treat 2016; 2016: 8158693. [http://dx.doi.org/10.1155/2016/8158693]

[16] Song JA, Lee M, Min E, Kim ME, Fike G, Hur MH. Effects of aromatherapy on dysmenorrhea: A systematic review and meta-analysis. Int J Nurs Stud 2018; 84: 1-11. [http://dx.doi.org/10.1016/j.ijnurstu.2018.01.016] [PMID: 29729556]

[17] Hur MH, Song JA, Lee J, Lee MS. Aromatherapy for stress reduction in healthy adults: A systematic review and meta-analysis of randomized clinical trials. Maturitas 2014; 79(4): 362-9. [http://dx.doi.org/10.1016/j.maturitas.2014.08.006] [PMID: 25234160]

[18] Hwang E, Shin S. The effects of aromatherapy on sleep improvement: A systematic literature review and meta-analysis. J Altern Complement Med 2015; 21(2): 61-8. [http://dx.doi.org/10.1089/acm.2014.0113] [PMID: 25584799]

[19] Sánchez-Vidaña DI, Ngai SPC, He W, Chow JKW, Lau BWM, Tsang HWH. The effectiveness of aromatherapy for depressive symptoms: A systematic review. Evid Based Complement Alternat Med 2017; 2017: 1-21. [http://dx.doi.org/10.1155/2017/5869315] [PMID: 28133489]

[20] Haze S, Sakai K, Gozu Y. Effects of fragrance inhalation on sympathetic activity in normal adults. Jpn J Pharmacol 2002; 90(3): 247-53. [http://dx.doi.org/10.1254/jjp.90.247] [PMID: 12499579]

[21] Shin ES, Seo KH, Lee SH, *et al.* Massage with or without aromatherapy for symptom relief in people with cancer. Coch Database Syst Rev 2016; 6. [http://dx.doi.org/10.1002/14651858.CD009873.pub3]

[22] Tisserand R, Young R, Williamson EM. Safety of Essential Oil, A Guide for Health Care Professionals, Churchill Livingstone. Elsevier 2013.

[23] Vieira AJ, Beserra FP, Souza MC, Totti BM, Rozza AL. Limonene: Aroma of innovation in health and disease. Chem Biol Interact 2018; 283: 97-106. [http://dx.doi.org/10.1016/j.cbi.2018.02.007] [PMID: 29427589]

[24] Bhalla Y, Gupta VK, Jaitak V. Anticancer activity of essential oils: A review. J Sci Food Agric 2013; 93(15): 3643-53. [http://dx.doi.org/10.1002/jsfa.6267] [PMID: 23765679]

[25] Scuteri D, Morrone LA, Rombolà L, *et al.* Aromatherapy and aromatic plants for the treatment of behavioural and psychological symptoms of dementia in patients with alzheimer's disease: Clinical evidence and possible mechanisms. Evid Based Complement Alternat Med 2017; 2017: 1-8. [http://dx.doi.org/10.1155/2017/9416305] [PMID: 28465709]

[26] Babakhanian M, Ghazanfarpour M, Kargarfard L, *et al.* Effect of aromatherapy on the treatment of psychological symptoms in postmenopausal and elderly women: A systematic review and meta-analysis. J Menopausal Med 2018; 24(2): 127-32. [http://dx.doi.org/10.6118/jmm.2018.24.2.127] [PMID: 30202763]

[27] Alexis AF, Barbosa VH, Eds. Skin of color: a practical guide to dermatologic diagnosis and treatment. Springer Science & Business Media 2012.

[28] Gravett P. Aromatherapy in the treatment of skin problems developing as a result of high dose chemotherapy. Int J Aromather 2001; 10(3-4): 132-4. [http://dx.doi.org/10.1016/S0962-4562(01)80008-4]

[29] Spiewak R. Occupational skin diseases among farmers. Lublin: Occupational and Para-Occupational Diseases in Agriculture Institute of Agricultural Medicine 2000; pp. 42-152.

[30] Vlassoff C, Weiss M, Ovuga EBL, *et al.* Gender and the stigma of onchocercal skin disease in Africa. Soc Sci Med 2000; 50(10): 1353-68. [http://dx.doi.org/10.1016/S0277-9536(99)00389-5] [PMID: 10741573]

[31] Inngjerdingen K, Nergård CS, Diallo D, Mounkoro PP, Paulsen BS. An ethnopharmacological survey of plants used for wound healing in Dogonland, Mali, West Africa. J Ethnopharmacol 2004; 92(2-3):

233-44.
[http://dx.doi.org/10.1016/j.jep.2004.02.021] [PMID: 15138006]

[32] Abrahams PW. Soils: their implications to human health. Sci Total Environ 2002; 291(1-3): 1-32. [http://dx.doi.org/10.1016/S0048-9697(01)01102-0] [PMID: 12150429]

[33] Kayne SB. Medical herbalism. Complementary and Alternative Medicine 2009; p. 269.

[34] Howard SR, de Roux N, Leger J, Carel JC, Dunkel L. Puberty and its disorders. Brook's clinical pediatric endocrinology. Wiley 2019. [http://dx.doi.org/10.1002/9781119152712.ch7]

[35] Santosh D, Joseph S, Jose A, *et al.* Anxiolytic and antiemetic effects of aromatherapy in cancer patients on anticancer chemotherapy. Pharmacologyonline 2011; 3: 736-44.

[36] Girgis A, Adams J, Sibbritt D. The use of complementary and alternative therapies by patients with cancer. Oncol Res 2005; 15(5): 281-9. [http://dx.doi.org/10.3727/096504005776404580] [PMID: 16261847]

[37] Johannessen H, Von Bornemann Hjelmborg J, Pasquarelli E, Fiorentini G, Di Costanzo F, Miccinesi G. Prevalence in the use of complementary medicine among cancer patients in Tuscany, Italy. Tumori 2008; 94(3): 406-10. [http://dx.doi.org/10.1177/030089160809400318] [PMID: 18705410]

[38] McKay DJ, Bendey JR, Grimshaw RN. Complementary and alternative medicine in gynecologic oncology. J Obstet Gynecol 2005; 27(6): 562-8.

[39] Shakeel M, Newton JR, Bruce J, Ah-See KW. Use of complementary and alternative medicine by patients attending a head and neck oncology clinic. J Laryngol Otol 2008; 122(12): 1360-4. [http://dx.doi.org/10.1017/S0022215108001904] [PMID: 18331656]

[40] Lawsin C, DuHamel K, Itzkowitz SH, *et al.* Demographic, medical, and psychosocial correlates to CAM use among survivors of colorectal cancer. Support Care Cancer 2007; 15(5): 557-64. [http://dx.doi.org/10.1007/s00520-006-0198-3] [PMID: 17205277]

[41] Boesl R, Saarinen H. Essential oil education for health care providers. Integr Med 2016; 15(6): 38-40. [PMID: 28223896]

[42] Kamble VA, Patil SD. Spice-derived essential oils: effective antifungal and possible therapeutic agents. J Herbs Spices Med Plants 2008; 14(3-4): 129-43. [http://dx.doi.org/10.1080/10496470802598677]

[43] Badia P, Wesensten N, Lammers W, Culpepper J, Harsh J. Responsiveness to olfactory stimuli presented in sleep. Physiol Behav 1990; 48(1): 87-90. [http://dx.doi.org/10.1016/0031-9384(90)90266-7] [PMID: 2236283]

[44] Manley CH. Psychophysiological effect of odor. Crit Rev Food Sci Nutr 1993; 33(1): 57-62. [http://dx.doi.org/10.1080/10408399309527612] [PMID: 8424855]

[45] Ali B, Al-Wabel NA, Shams S, Ahamad A, Khan SA, Anwar F. Essential oils used in aromatherapy: A systemic review. Asian Pac J Trop Biomed 2015; 5(8): 601-11. [http://dx.doi.org/10.1016/j.apjtb.2015.05.007]

[46] Buckle J. Clinical Aromatherapy. Essential oils in healthcare.

[47] Buckle J. Aromatherapy and Diabetes. Diabetes Spectr 2001; 14(3): 124-6. [http://dx.doi.org/10.2337/diaspect.14.3.124]

[48] Sanderson H, Ruddle J. Aromatherapy and occupational therapy. Br J Occup Ther 1992; 55(8): 310-4. [http://dx.doi.org/10.1177/030802269205500807]

[49] Bakkali F, Averbeck S, Averbeck D, Idaomar M. Biological effects of essential oils – A review. Food Chem Toxicol 2008; 46(2): 446-75. [http://dx.doi.org/10.1016/j.fct.2007.09.106] [PMID: 17996351]

[50] Manosroi J, Dhumtanom P, Manosroi A. Anti-proliferative activity of essential oil extracted from Thai medicinal plants on KB and P388 cell lines. Cancer Lett 2006; 235(1): 114-20. [http://dx.doi.org/10.1016/j.canlet.2005.04.021] [PMID: 15979235]

[51] Kawaii S, Tomono Y, Katase E, Ogawa K, Yano M. Effect of citrus flavonoids on HL-60 cell differentiation. Anticancer Res 1999; 19(2A): 1261-9. [PMID: 10368686]

[52] Patil JR, Jayaprakasha GK, Chidambara Murthy KN, Tichy SE, Chetti MB, Patil BS. Apoptosis-mediated proliferation inhibition of human colon cancer cells by volatile principles of Citrus aurantifolia. Food Chem 2009; 114(4): 1351-8. [http://dx.doi.org/10.1016/j.foodchem.2008.11.033]

[53] De Flora S, Izzotti A, Randerath K, *et al.* DNA adducts and chronic degenerative diseases. Pathogenetic relevance and implications in preventive medicine. Mutat Res Rev Genet Toxicol 1996; 366(3): 197-238. [http://dx.doi.org/10.1016/S0165-1110(96)00043-7] [PMID: 9033668]

[54] Singh G, Kapoor IPS, Singh P, de Heluani CS, de Lampasona MP, Catalan CAN. Chemistry, antioxidant and antimicrobial investigations on essential oil and oleoresins of Zingiber officinale. Food Chem Toxicol 2008; 46(10): 3295-302. [http://dx.doi.org/10.1016/j.fct.2008.07.017] [PMID: 18706468]

[55] Sacchetti G, Maietti S, Muzzoli M, *et al.* Comparative evaluation of 11 essential oils of different origin as functional antioxidants, antiradicals and antimicrobials in foods. Food Chem 2005; 91(4): 621-32. [http://dx.doi.org/10.1016/j.foodchem.2004.06.031]

[56] Jeena K, Liju VB, Kuttan R. Antioxidant, anti-inflammatory and antinociceptive activities of essential oil from ginger. Indian J Physiol Pharmacol 2013; 57(1): 51-62. [PMID: 24020099]

[57] Orhan IE, Ozcelik B, Kan Y, Kartal M. Inhibitory effects of various essential oils and individual components against extended-spectrum beta-lactamase (ESBL) produced by Klebsiella pneumoniae and their chemical compositions. J Food Sci 2011; 76(8): M538-46. [http://dx.doi.org/10.1111/j.1750-3841.2011.02363.x] [PMID: 22417594]

[58] Dadalioğlu I, Evrendilek GA. Chemical compositions and antibacterial effects of essential oils of Turkish oregano (Origanum minutiflorum), bay laurel (Laurus nobilis), Spanish lavender (Lavandula stoechas L.), and fennel (Foeniculum vulgare) on common foodborne pathogens. J Agric Food Chem 2004; 52(26): 8255-60. [http://dx.doi.org/10.1021/jf049033e] [PMID: 15612826]

[59] Bozin B, Mimica-Dukic N, Simin N, Anackov G. Characterization of the volatile composition of essential oils of some lamiaceae spices and the antimicrobial and antioxidant activities of the entire oils. J Agric Food Chem 2006; 54(5): 1822-8. [http://dx.doi.org/10.1021/jf051922u] [PMID: 16506839]

[60] Bernardes WA, Lucarini R, Tozatti MG, *et al.* Antibacterial activity of the essential oil from Rosmarinus officinalis and its major components against oral pathogens. Z Naturforsch C J Biosci 2010; 65(9-10): 588-93. [http://dx.doi.org/10.1515/znc-2010-9-1009] [PMID: 21138060]

[61] Lawrence TS, Blackstock AW, McGinn C. The mechanism of action of radiosensitization of conventional chemotherapeutic agents. Seminars in radiation oncology. WB Saunders 2003. [http://dx.doi.org/10.1053/srao.2003.50002]

[62] Kuriyama H, Watanabe S, Nakaya T, *et al.* Immunological and psychological benefits of aromatherapy massage. Evid Based Complement Alternat Med 2005; 2(2): 179-84. [http://dx.doi.org/10.1093/ecam/neh087] [PMID: 15937558]

SUBJECT INDEX

Pradeep Kumar Shukla, Ajeet Kumar Srivastav, Deepti Chopra, Shikha Agnihotry, Pragati Misra and Jyoti Singh (Eds.)

B

C

D

E

F

G

H

O

P

Q

R

S